Power and Sample Size in R

Power and Sample Size in R guides the reader through power and sample size calculations for a wide variety of study outcomes and designs and illustrates their implementation in R software. It is designed to be used as a learning tool for students as well as a resource for experienced statisticians and investigators.

The book begins by explaining the process of power calculation step by step at an introductory level and then builds to increasingly complex and varied topics. For each type of study design, the information needed to perform a calculation and the factors that affect power are explained. Concepts are explained with statistical rigor but made accessible through intuition and examples. Practical advice for performing sample size and power calculations for real studies is given throughout.

The book demonstrates calculations in R. It is integrated with the companion R package powertools and also draws on and summarizes the capabilities of other R packages. Only a basic proficiency in R is assumed.

Topics include comparison of group means and proportions; ANOVA, including multiple comparisons; power for confidence intervals; multistage designs; linear, logistic and Poisson regression; crossover studies; multicenter, cluster randomized and stepped wedge designs; and time to event outcomes. Chapters are also devoted to designing noninferiority, superiority by a margin and equivalence studies and handling multiple primary endpoints.

By emphasizing statistical thinking about the factors that influence power for different study designs and outcomes as well as providing R code, this book equips the reader with the knowledge and tools to perform their own calculations with confidence.

Key Features:
- Explains power and sample size calculation for a wide variety of study designs and outcomes
- Suitable for both students and experienced researchers
- Highlights key factors influencing power and provides practical tips for designing real studies
- Includes extensive examples with R code

Catherine M. Crespi is Professor in the Department of Biostatistics at the Jonathan and Karin Fielding School of Public Health, University of California Los Angeles. Her areas of specialization include trial design and analysis, multilevel modelling, longitudinal data and multivariate statistics. She is a Fellow of the American Statistical Association and an officer of the International Biometric Society.

Chapman & Hall/CRC Biostatistics Series
Series Editors: Mark Chang, *Boston University, USA*

ROC Analysis for Classification and Prediction in Practice
Christos Nakas, Leonidas Bantis and Constantine Gatsonis

Controlled Epidemiological Studies
Marie Reilly

Statistical Methods in Health Disparity Research
J. Sunil Rao

Case Studies in Innovative Clinical Trials
Edited by Binbing Yu and Kristine Broglio

Value of Information for Healthcare Decision Making
Edited by Anna Heath, Natalia Kunst, and Christopher Jackson

Probability Modeling and Statistical Inference in Cancer Screening
Dongfeng Wu

Development of Gene Therapies
Strategic, Scientific, Regulatory, and Access Considerations
Edited by Avery McIntosh and Oleksandr Sverdlov

Bayesian Precision Medicine
Peter F. Thall

Statistical Methods for Dynamic Disease Screening and Spatio-Temporal Disease Surveillance
Peihua Qiu

Causal Inference in Pharmaceutical Statistics
Yixin Fang

Applied Microbiome Statistics
Correlation, Association, Interaction and Composition
Yinglin Xia and Jun Sun

Association Models in Epidemiology
Study Design, Modeling Strategies, and Analytic Methods
Hongjie Liu

Likelihood Methods in Survival Analysis
with R Examples
Jun Ma, Malcolm Hudson, and Annabel Webb

Biostatistics for Bioassay
Ann Yellowlees and Matthew Stephenson

Power and Sample Size in R
Catherine M. Crespi

For more information about this series, please visit: www.routledge.com/Chapman--Hall-CRC-Biostatistics-Series/book-series/CHBIOSTATIS

Power and Sample Size in R

Catherine M. Crespi

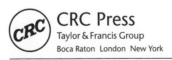

CRC Press
Taylor & Francis Group
Boca Raton London New York

CRC Press is an imprint of the
Taylor & Francis Group, an **informa** business

A CHAPMAN & HALL BOOK

Designed cover image: © Catherine M. Crespi

First edition published 2025
by CRC Press
2385 NW Executive Center Drive, Suite 320, Boca Raton FL 33431

and by CRC Press
4 Park Square, Milton Park, Abingdon, Oxon, OX14 4RN

CRC Press is an imprint of Taylor & Francis Group, LLC

© 2025 Taylor & Francis Group, LLC

Reasonable efforts have been made to publish reliable data and information, but the author and publisher cannot assume responsibility for the validity of all materials or the consequences of their use. The authors and publishers have attempted to trace the copyright holders of all material reproduced in this publication and apologize to copyright holders if permission to publish in this form has not been obtained. If any copyright material has not been acknowledged please write and let us know so we may rectify in any future reprint.

Except as permitted under U.S. Copyright Law, no part of this book may be reprinted, reproduced, transmitted, or utilized in any form by any electronic, mechanical, or other means, now known or hereafter invented, including photocopying, microfilming, and recording, or in any information storage or retrieval system, without written permission from the publishers.

For permission to photocopy or use material electronically from this work, access www.copyright.com or contact the Copyright Clearance Center, Inc. (CCC), 222 Rosewood Drive, Danvers, MA 01923, 978-750-8400. For works that are not available on CCC please contact mpkbookspermissions@tandf.co.uk

Trademark notice: Product or corporate names may be trademarks or registered trademarks and are used only for identification and explanation without intent to infringe.

ISBN: 978-1-138-59162-2 (hbk)
ISBN: 978-1-032-94244-5 (pbk)
ISBN: 978-0-429-48878-8 (ebk)

DOI: 10.1201/9780429488788

Typeset in CMR10 font
by KnowledgeWorks Global Ltd.

Publisher's note: This book has been prepared from camera-ready copy provided by the authors.

To my husband and children, and all of the students who have taught me how to teach over the years.

Contents

Preamble	xi
List of Figures	xiii
List of Tables	xv

1 Preliminaries   **1**
  1.1 R implementation 1
  1.2 Probability distributions 1
  1.3 Notation for common distributions 3
  1.4 R functions for common distributions 4
  1.5 Symmetric property of the normal distribution 5
  1.6 Standardizing a normal distribution 6

2 Getting started: a first calculation   **7**
  2.1 Steps in a sample size calculation 7
  2.2 Hypothesis testing 9
  2.3 A first calculation: one-sample z test 12
  2.4 Effect size 23
  2.5 Minimum detectable effect size 24
  2.6 A general formula when the test statistic is normally distributed   25
  2.7 R function for z tests 25
  2.8 Sample size adjustments 27
  2.9 Sensitivity analysis 28
  2.10 Estimating power using simulation 29
  2.11 Should I conduct a power analysis after my study is completed?   31

3 One or two means   **33**
  3.1 One-sample t test 33
  3.2 Two independent samples t test 46
  3.3 Relative efficiency 54
  3.4 Lognormal data 56
  3.5 Paired t test 59
  3.6 Remarks on R functions for t tests 61
  3.7 Nonparametric tests of location 62

4 Hypotheses for different study objectives   69
   4.1   Introduction 69
   4.2   Test for nonequality 71
   4.3   Test for superiority 71
   4.4   Test for noninferiority 73
   4.5   Test for superiority by a margin 77
   4.6   Test for equivalence 79
   4.7   Hypotheses when a lower mean corresponds to a better outcome   86
   4.8   Remarks 86

5 Analysis of variance for comparing means   88
   5.1   Introduction 88
   5.2   One-way analysis of variance 88
   5.3   Two-way analysis of variance 100
   5.4   Analysis of covariance 114
   5.5   Additional resources 117

6 Proportions: large sample methods   118
   6.1   Preliminaries 118
   6.2   One-sample proportion test 119
   6.3   Test of two independent proportions 124
   6.4   Test for two correlated proportions 132

7 Exact methods for proportions   137
   7.1   One proportion: exact binomial test 137
   7.2   Two-stage designs for single arm trials 141
   7.3   Two proportions: Fisher exact test 143
   7.4   Two correlated proportions: exact test 145

8 Categorical variables   148
   8.1   Chi-square goodness-of-fit test 148
   8.2   Chi-square test of independence 150
   8.3   Chi-square test for comparing two proportions 153
   8.4   Ordinal categorical responses 154
   8.5   Additional resources 156

9 Precision and confidence intervals   157
   9.1   Introduction 157
   9.2   Confidence intervals for means 158
   9.3   Confidence intervals for proportions 166
   9.4   Confidence intervals for relative risk 171
   9.5   Confidence intervals for odds ratio 172
   9.6   Additional resources 174

10 Correlation and linear regression — 175
- 10.1 Pearson correlation coefficient — 175
- 10.2 Simple linear regression — 179
- 10.3 Multiple linear regression — 182

11 Generalized linear regression — 193
- 11.1 Power for generalized linear models — 193
- 11.2 Logistic regression — 195
- 11.3 Poisson regression — 200
- 11.4 Additional resources — 202

12 Crossover studies — 203
- 12.1 Introduction — 203
- 12.2 2×2 crossover design — 205
- 12.3 $(2 \times 2)r$ crossover design — 209
- 12.4 Efficiency of crossover designs — 212
- 12.5 Additional resources — 214

13 Multisite trials — 216
- 13.1 Introduction — 216
- 13.2 Multilevel data structure — 216
- 13.3 Considerations for multisite trials — 217
- 13.4 Model for continuous outcomes — 218
- 13.5 Intraclass correlation coefficient — 221
- 13.6 Power for test of average treatment effect — 222
- 13.7 Power for test of heterogeneity of treatment effect — 230
- 13.8 Binary outcomes — 232
- 13.9 Additional resources — 236

14 Cluster randomized trials: parallel designs — 237
- 14.1 Introduction — 237
- 14.2 Continuous outcomes — 238
- 14.3 Binary outcomes — 253
- 14.4 Additional resources for parallel cluster randomized trials — 260
- 14.5 Individually randomized group treatment trials — 261
- 14.6 Other multilevel trial designs — 266

15 Cluster randomized trials: longitudinal designs — 269
- 15.1 Introduction — 269
- 15.2 Modeling framework for continuous outcomes — 271
- 15.3 Parallel cluster randomized trial with baseline measurement — 281
- 15.4 Cluster randomized crossover designs — 285
- 15.5 Stepped wedge designs — 291

16 Time to event outcomes — **302**
- 16.1 Introduction 302
- 16.2 Concepts for time to event studies 303
- 16.3 Logrank test 305
- 16.4 Tests based on the Kaplan-Meier estimator 310
- 16.5 Distributions for survival, accrual and loss to follow up . . . 312
- 16.6 Additional resources 315

17 Multiple primary endpoints — **316**
- 17.1 Introduction 316
- 17.2 Model 317
- 17.3 Co-primary endpoints 318
- 17.4 Alternative primary endpoints 324
- 17.5 Additional resources 327

Bibliography — **329**

Index — **349**

Preamble

This book was developed out of a course on the topic of power and sample size calculation that I teach at the UCLA Jonathan and Karin Fielding School of Public Health in Los Angeles, California. Through developing and teaching the course, I found that while there are some excellent reference-style textbooks on sample size calculation, such as Chow et al. [33], textbooks that were suitable for teaching a rigorous course or for self-learning and that were also integrated with software were in short supply. Hence this book was written.

I have attempted to make the material in the book accessible while not sacrificing rigor. The book assumes the reader understands basic probability concepts such as random variables, distributions of random variables and hypothesis testing, although there is a short refresher in Chapter 1. Most of the book should be accessible to graduate students who have had a one-year core sequence in statistics or biostatistics, who are the audience for the UCLA course, as well as scientists and investigators with some understanding of statistics. However, it is unavoidable that more statistical sophistication is needed to understand some of the more sophisticated modeling techniques and study designs. The material gets more challenging starting with Chapter 11 on generalized linear models.

The goal of the book is to emphasize statistical thinking about the factors that influence power for different study designs and outcomes. Therefore the book develops many of the mathematical formulas that lie behind sample size and power calculations rather than simply presenting formulas. This is not a cookbook of recipes. It is also not intended to be a complete inventory of sample size and power methods.

The book demonstrates calculations in R using examples. Only a basic proficiency in R is assumed. We use functions from the `powertools` package, which was developed as a companion R package to this book, as well as other packages. There are many packages for various types of power and sample size calculations available in R, and we try to summarize available resources in each chapter. The index includes not only concepts and topics but also the R functions and packages mentioned in the book.

This book focuses on applications to clinical and health-related research. However, the methods themselves can be applied in other areas. We focus on techniques for sample size and power analysis when planning a study in which the data will be analyzed using traditional "frequentist" methods of statistical inference rather than, for example, Bayesian methods. Data from most clinical studies are analyzed using traditional frequentist methods, e.g., t

tests, linear and logistic regression, and linear mixed models. Although there is a lively discussion in the scientific community about the merits and demerits of hypothesis testing (see, for example, Wasserstein and Lazar [225]), we sidestep these issues and assume that the study data will be analyzed using hypothesis testing or (less commonly) confidence intervals.

I am deeply indebted to the many individuals who have helped me produce this book and the companion R package. These include Analissa Avila, Zichen Liu, Kristen McGreevy, Phillip Sundin and Yixuan Zhou. You forever have my gratitude.

Catherine M. Crespi

List of Figures

1.1	Normal density function and cumulative distribution function	3
1.2	Illustration of symmetric property of the standard normal distribution.	5
2.1	Rejection and acceptance regions and critical values for one- and two-sided test.	11
2.2	Distribution of test statistic under null and alternative hypotheses for a lower-tailed z test.	16
2.3	Distribution of test statistic under null and alternative hypotheses for a upper-tailed z test.	18
2.4	Distribution of test statistic under null and alternative hypotheses for a two-tailed z test.	20
2.5	Power for two-sided, one-sample z test for range of μ_A values.	29
3.1	Density of noncentral t distributions for various degrees of freedom and noncentrality parameter values.	36
3.2	Power for lower-tailed one-sample t test.	37
3.3	Power for upper-tailed one-sample t test.	38
3.4	Factors affecting power for a one-sample t test.	40
3.5	Noncentral chi-square and F distribution.	43
3.6	Central and noncentral F distributions.	44
3.7	Power as a function of allocation ratio for a two-sample t test with equal variances.	53
3.8	Power as a function of allocation ratio for a two-sample t test with unequal variances.	54
3.9	Relationship between the lognormal and normal distributions. $X_1, \ldots, X_n$ are on the original scale and the log-transformed values are $Y_1 = \log(X_1), \ldots, Y_n = \log(X_n)$. The median on the original scale corresponds to the mean on the log-transformed scale.	56
4.1	Inference for test of nonequality based on confidence interval.	73
4.2	Inference for test of superiority based on confidence interval.	74
4.3	Relationships between μ_R, μ_T, and $m > 0$ when a lower or higher mean corresponds to a better outcome.	75
4.4	Inference for test of noninferiority based on confidence interval.	76

4.5	Inference for test of superiority by a margin based on confidence interval.	78
4.6	Inference for equivalence test based on confidence interval.	80
6.1	Variance of the sample proportion	119
10.1	Power versus number of predictors for an overall F test.	187
11.1	Variance inflation factor (VIF) as a function of $\rho^2_{X_1\|X_2X_3\ldots X_p}$, which is the population analogue of $R^2_{X_1\|X_2X_3\ldots X_p}$, the R^2 obtained when X_1 is regressed on $X_2,\ldots,X_p$.	199
12.1	Parallel versus crossover design	204
13.1	Data from multisite trials without and with a site-by-condition interaction.	220
14.1	Simulated data from two parallel cluster randomized trials showing the impact of variation of the cluster-level means.	239
15.1	Schematic representation of different cluster randomized trial designs.	270
15.2	Illustration of different correlation structures for a longitudinal cluster randomized trial	273
15.3	Schematic representation of a standard stepped wedge design trial with five clusters.	292
16.1	Depiction of accrual and loss to follow up processes for a survival study	303
16.2	Examples of survival curves in two groups	304
16.3	Kaplan-Meier survival curve estimator example	305
16.4	Survival curves from Example 16.3	312
16.5	Exponential distribution functions	313
17.1	Venn diagram representing co-primary versus alternative primary endpoints	317
17.2	Venn diagram showing impact of correlation for co-primary endpoints	323
17.3	Venn diagram showing impact of correlation for alternative primary endpoints	326

List of Tables

1.1	Notation for common distributions.	4
2.1	The four possible outcomes of a hypothesis test.	11
5.1	One-way ANOVA sources of variation table.	90
5.2	Multiple testing error rates	97
5.3	Sources of variation table for a two-way ANOVA with only main effects.	103
5.4	Sources of variation table for a two-way ANOVA with an interaction between the two factors.	108
6.1	Data set-up and notation for two correlated proportions.	133
7.1	Counts for a 2×2 table	144
8.1	Set-up and notation for chi-square goodness-of-fit test	149
8.2	Notation for chi-square test of independence for an $r \times c$ table.	150
8.3	Notation for ordinal categorical response model	154
9.1	Notation for cell counts in a 2×2 contingency table from a cohort or unmatched case-control study.	173
10.1	Linear regression model sources of variation table.	183
12.1	$(2 \times 2)r$ crossover design with $r = 2$ replicates.	210
14.1	Selected values of design effect	244
14.2	Design options for trials with multilevel structure.	267
15.1	Summary of models for longitudinal cluster randomized trials with a continuous outcome and their variance/correlation parameters. CAC, cluster autocorrelation; SAC, subject autocorrelation.	280
17.1	Samples sizes per group for two co-primary endpoints	323
17.2	Samples sizes per group for two alternative ("at least one") primary endpoints using Bonferroni adjustment	326

1
Preliminaries

1.1 R implementation

This book explains power and sample size calculations for many different study designs and outcomes and demonstrates their implementation in R. We assume that the reader has a basic proficiency in R. The book uses functions from the `powertools` package as well as other packages. To use the functions in an R package, it is necessary to first install the package and then load it in the current session using the `library` function, e.g.,

```
install.packages("powertools")
library(powertools)
```

The reader should be sure to consult the latest R documentation when using various functions and packages. To see the documentation for the function `ttest.2samp`, for example, enter at the R prompt

```
?ttest.2samp
```

1.2 Probability distributions

Calculating power entails calculating a probability, namely, the probability of rejecting the null hypothesis in favor of the alternative hypothesis when a specified alternative is true. A sample size calculation involves finding the number of subjects that are needed in order to achieve a desired level of power. These calculations involve working with random variables and their distributions. In particular, we will need to work with cumulative distribution functions (cdfs) and quantile functions of random variables.

The **probability density function** (pdf) of a random variable is a function such that the area under the curve between any two points a and b is equal to the probability that the random variable falls between a and b. The pdf of a normally distributed random variable Y with mean μ and variance σ^2 is the function $f(y) = \frac{1}{\sqrt{2\pi\sigma^2}} \exp[-\frac{1}{2}(\frac{y-\mu}{\sigma})^2]$. A standard normal random variable has mean 0 and variance 1. The pdf for a standard normal random variable is commonly denoted as $\phi(\cdot)$; thus $\phi(y) = \frac{1}{\sqrt{2\pi}} \exp[-\frac{1}{2}y^2]$.

DOI: 10.1201/9780429488788-1

In R, the dnorm function performs computations involving normal densities. This function takes as arguments the mean and standard deviation of the normal distribution and a quantile (which can be thought of as a value along the x-axis), and returns the height of the pdf at that quantile. For example,

```
dnorm(x = 12, mean = 10, sd = 5)
[1] 0.07365403
```

See Figure 1.1(A).

The **cumulative distribution function** (cdf) for a random variable Y evaluated at a quantile y gives the probability that Y is less than or equal to y, i.e., $P(Y \le y)$. The cdf for a standard normal random variable is commonly denoted $\Phi(\cdot)$; we have that $\Phi(y) = P(Y \le y) = \int_{-\infty}^{y} \frac{1}{\sqrt{2\pi}} \exp[-\frac{1}{2}u^2] du$. The cdf for a normally distributed random variable can be calculated using the pnorm function. For example, the probability that a normally distributed random variable with mean 10 and standard deviation 5 is less than or equal to 12 can be calculated as

```
pnorm(q = 12, mean = 10, sd = 5)
[1] 0.6554217
```

See Figure 1.1(B).

Another function that is important for power and sample size calculations is the **quantile function**, also called the **inverse cumulative distribution function**. While the cdf takes as an argument a quantile and returns a probability, the inverse cdf or quantile function takes as an argument a probability and returns the quantile corresponding to that probability (that is, the quantile such that the probability of the random variable being less than or equal to that quantile equals the given probability). The inverse cdf for the standard normal distribution is commonly denoted as $\Phi^{-1}(\cdot)$; if $\Phi(y) = P(Y \le y) = p$, then $\Phi^{-1}(p) = y$. The function qnorm computes the normal quantile function:

```
qnorm(p = 0.6554217, mean = 10, sd = 5)
[1] 12
```

The default values of the mean and standard deviation in these functions are 0 and 1, corresponding to the standard normal distribution. For example,

```
pnorm(q = 0)
[1] 0.5
qnorm(p = 0.5)
[1] 0

pnorm(q = -1.96)
[1] 0.0249979
qnorm(p = 0.0249979)
[1] -1.96
```

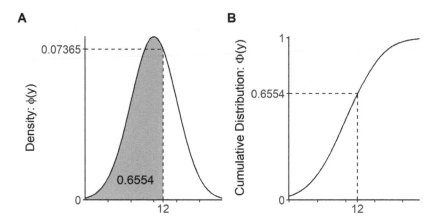

FIGURE 1.1: Normal distribution $Y \sim \mathcal{N}(10, 5)$. (A) Normal density function $\phi(y)$ showing $\phi(12) = 0.0737$ and (B) cumulative distribution function $\Phi(y)$ showing $\Phi(12) = 0.6554$.

1.3 Notation for common distributions

In this book, we will make extensive use of the normal, t, chi-square and F distributions, which are common distributions for test statistics. Chapter 3 introduces the noncentral t, chi-square and F distributions. Noncentral distributions generalize the more familiar "central" versions of these distributions. They include another parameter, called the **noncentrality parameter**, that creates a shift in location and sometimes other features. "Central" distributions are the special case of the noncentrality parameter equal to 0. Noncentral distributions play a key role in sample size and power calculations. We will usually use λ or Λ to denote the noncentrality parameter of a distribution and include it as the last parameter. If a distribution is not described as a noncentral distribution, this implies that it is a "central" distribution.

Our notation for these distributions is summarized in Table 1.1. The first three columns give notation for "central" versions of distributions and the last two columns give notation for noncentral versions. The t distribution with ν degrees of freedom will be denoted $t(\nu)$ and the noncentral t distribution with ν degrees of freedom and noncentrality parameter λ will be denoted $t(\nu, \lambda)$, for example. The corresponding cdfs are denoted $\mathcal{T}_\nu$ and $\mathcal{T}_{\nu,\lambda}$.

Let p denote a probability taking a value in the interval $(0, 1)$. The $100 \times p^{th}$ **quantile** of a random variable X is the value x_p such that $P(X \leq x_p) = p$. The notation for the $100 \times p^{th}$ quantile for various distributions is given in Table 1.1. For example, the $100 \times p^{th}$ quantile of a $\mathcal{N}(0, 1)$ distribution is z_p and that for a $t(\nu)$ distribution is $t_{p,\nu}$. We will not use the quantiles of noncentral distributions, so we will not introduce notation for them.

TABLE 1.1: Notation for common distributions.

Central distribution	Central cdf	$100 \times p^{th}$ quantile	Noncentral distribution	Noncentral cdf
$\mathcal{N}(0,1)$	Φ	z_p	–	–
$t(\nu)$	$\mathcal{T}_\nu$	$t_{p,\nu}$	$t(\nu, \lambda)$	$\mathcal{T}_{\nu,\lambda}$
$\chi^2(\nu)$	$\mathcal{X}^2_\nu$	$x^2_{p,\nu}$	$\chi^2(\nu, \Lambda)$	$\mathcal{X}^2_{\nu,\Lambda}$
$F(\nu_1, \nu_2)$	$\mathcal{F}_{\nu_1,\nu_2}$	f_{p,ν_1,ν_2}	$F(\nu_1, \nu_2, \Lambda)$	$\mathcal{F}_{\nu_1,\nu_2,\Lambda}$

When a random variable is approximately distributed as a particular distribution, we will use the symbol $\dot\sim$, for example, $X \dot\sim \mathcal{N}(0,1)$.

1.4 R functions for common distributions

It is a convention in R that pdfs begin with d, cdfs begin with p and quantile functions begin with q. The pdf, cdf and quantile functions for the normal distribution can be computed using

```
dnorm(x, mean, sd)
pnorm(q, mean, sd, lower.tail = TRUE)
qnorm(p, mean, sd, lower.tail = TRUE)
```

where x and q are vectors of quantiles and p is a vector of probabilities (the vectors can be of length one); mean = 0, sd = 1 and lower.tail = TRUE are default values. Similarly, the pdf, cdf and quantile functions for both central and noncentral t distributions can be computed using

```
dt(x, df, ncp)
pt(q, df, ncp, lower.tail = TRUE)
qt(p, df, ncp, lower.tail = TRUE)
```

and for the chi-square distribution, the functions are

```
dchisq(x, df, ncp)
pchisq(q, df, ncp, lower.tail = TRUE)
qchisq(p, df, ncp, lower.tail = TRUE)
```

and for the F distribution, the functions are

```
df(x, df1, df2, ncp)
pf(q, df1, df2, ncp, lower.tail = TRUE)
qf(p, df1, df2, ncp, lower.tail = TRUE)
```

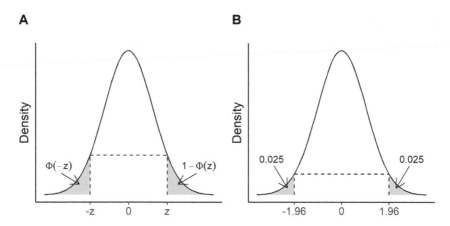

FIGURE 1.2: Illustration of symmetric property of the standard normal distribution.

For these functions, the default is ncp = 0. If the ncp argument is omitted, the central distribution is assumed. Another default is to compute the lower-tail probability of these distributions, $P(X \leq x)$. To compute the upper-tail probability, $P(X > x)$, set lower.tail = FALSE.

1.5 Symmetric property of the normal distribution

The normal distribution is symmetric about zero, with $\phi(z) = \phi(-z)$. Because it is symmetric and the probability under the pdf sums to 1,

$$\Phi(-z) = P(Z \leq -z) = P(Z \geq z) = 1 - P(Z \leq z) = 1 - \Phi(z).$$

For example, $\Phi(-1.96) = 1 - \Phi(1.96) = 0.0249979$, that is, the area in the lower tail beyond -1.96 or the upper tail beyond 1.96 is approximately 0.025. These relationships are illustrated in Figure 1.2. Furthermore, for a probability or percentile p, we have relationships among quantiles,

$$z_p = -z_{1-p}$$
$$z_{1-p} = -z_p$$

For example, $z_{0.975} = -z_{0.025} = 1.959964$ and $z_{0.025} = -z_{0.975} = -1.959964$.

1.6 Standardizing a normal distribution

Often we wish to perform probability calculations involving normally distributed variables with some specific mean and variance, $\mathcal{N}(\mu, \sigma^2)$. For example, if $X \sim \mathcal{N}(\mu, \sigma^2)$, what is $P(X < x_0)$? To solve such problems, we can convert the probability statement about X into an equivalent probability statement about a standard normal random variable using the relationship

$$\text{If } X \sim \mathcal{N}(\mu, \sigma^2) \text{ and } Z = \frac{X - \mu}{\sigma}, \text{ then } Z \sim \mathcal{N}(0, 1).$$

This is referred to as standardization of a normal random variable. For example, if $X \sim \mathcal{N}(\mu, \sigma^2)$

$$P(X < x_0) = P\left(\frac{X - \mu}{\sigma} < \frac{x_0 - \mu}{\sigma}\right) = P\left(Z < \frac{x_0 - \mu}{\sigma}\right) = \Phi\left(\frac{x_0 - \mu}{\sigma}\right)$$

where $Z \sim \mathcal{N}(0, 1)$.

2

Getting started: a first calculation

2.1 Steps in a sample size calculation

A fundamental part of planning a study is to determine the number of participants to include in it, that is, the **sample size**. Usually, we do not want the sample size for a study to be either too large or too small. If the sample size is too large, this means that we could have achieved our objectives with a smaller number of participants and thus we have wasted resources and possibly exposed participants to unnecessary risks. If the sample size is too small, the study may not provide clear answers to the research questions, and we have again used resources and exposed participants to risks without coming to a clear conclusion. The objective of sample size determination is to find the "just right" sample size – the sample size that will be adequate to achieve our objectives under realistic assumptions about how the study will unfold.

Performing a sample size calculation for a study is a process that is intertwined with the overall planning of the study itself. We can think of the process as involving the following steps. Often these steps are iterative; we may start the process but then go back, make refinements, and start again.

Step 1: Specify the essentials of the study plan: the research question, primary outcome and analysis method. Before we can conduct a sample size determination, we need the essential parts of the study plan to be in place. What is the research question? What outcome will be considered the primary outcome? What statistical method or model will we use to analyze the primary outcome? The answers to these questions provide the essential framework for calculating an appropriate sample size, which is usually based on providing adequate power for analyzing the primary outcome. For example, our research question may be whether Condition 1 results in lower mean depressive symptoms at a 3-month follow-up timepoint (primary outcome) than Condition 2, and the planned analysis may be an analysis of covariance (ANCOVA).

Step 2: Formulate the study hypotheses. The next step is to formally state the null and alternative hypotheses. Usually, the alternative hypothesis is what we seek to conclude and thus states our hypothesized "truth". The null hypothesis is then specified as the complement of the alternative, so that by rejecting the null hypothesis, we can conclude the alternative. For example, we may hypothesize (and seek to conclude) that the mean under Condition

1 will be less than the mean under Condition 2, which we can translate into $H_0: \mu_1 \geq \mu_2$ and $H_A: \mu_1 < \mu_2$.

Step 3: Determine the target effect size. An **effect size** is the magnitude of an effect, for example, the difference in means between two groups. Typically we seek to detect an effect size that is large enough to be clinically meaningful. For example, we may judge that a 4-point difference in mean depressive symptoms scores between conditions is clinically meaningful and reasonable to expect, and designate a 4-point mean difference as our target effect size. Expertise in the subject matter is needed to determine what magnitude of a difference is clinically meaningful.

Step 4: Specify the desired level of power and significance level. Power, as we discuss more formally later in this chapter, is the probability that we reject the null hypothesis and conclude that the alternative hypothesis is true. Typical desired levels of power are 0.8 or 0.9, that is, we typically seek to design a study such that, with our planned sample size, we will have a probability of 80% or 90% of reaching the desired conclusion. We also need to specify a significance level. As we discuss later in this chapter, the significance level is the probability that we mistakenly reject the null hypothesis when it is true. This is an undesirable outcome and so we typically want to keep this probability low. A common choice for the significance level (but not the only choice) is 0.05.

Step 5: Specify other parameters. A sample size calculation will usually require us to specify the values of various additional parameters. For example, to calculate sample size for an ANCOVA, we may need an estimate of the population variance of the outcome variable and the correlation between the baseline and follow-up scores. Other factors, such as participant dropout, may also need to be factored into the sample size calculation.

Step 6: Conduct the sample size calculation. The actual calculation of the required sample size comes after decisions have been made at the previous steps. These decisions will determine the appropriate method for calculating the sample size and reasonable values of parameters to use in the calculation. Thus there could be a lot of planning, research and discussion before actually performing the sample size calculation.

Step 7. Explore uncertainty. Because the calculation will involve making guesses about what the values of certain parameters will be in the future study, such as the effect size, population variance, correlation coefficient or dropout rate, the calculation should also include **sensitivity analyses** that explore how the sample size requirement varies when assumptions about these parameters are changed.

These steps assume that there is some flexibility in selecting a sample size for the study. In some situations, there is a fixed number of subjects available, and we would like to know the statistical power that we can achieve with the given sample size, or the smallest effect size that we could reasonably detect. In such situations, the steps are similar: we will need to specify the research question, primary outcome and analysis method; the study hypotheses; the values for various parameters; and then perform calculations.

This book is focused on methods for Step 6, the calculation step. But keep in mind that in real studies, the actual calculation is only one part of the larger overall process of planning a study.

2.2 Hypothesis testing

Hypothesis testing forms the basis for most sample size and power calculations. In this section, we review the basics of hypothesis testing.

When we conduct a study, we collect data from a sample of individuals and analyze it to draw inferences about the population from which the sample was selected. The term **population** refers to all members of a defined group; the term **sample** refers to the members of the population on which we collect data. For example, we may collect data on a sample of adults with diabetes drawn from the population consisting of all adults with diabetes.

Population **parameters** are quantities characterizing a population. An example is the mean value of some quantity in a population, which is commonly denoted μ. The values of population parameters are generally unknown because we do not have data on all population members. After we collect a sample, we compute sample statistics as estimates of population parameters. **Statistics** are quantities that we compute from data. The sample mean $\bar{Y} = \frac{1}{N}\Sigma_{i=1}^{N} Y_i$ is an example of a sample statistic. We commonly use the sample mean as an estimate of the population mean. We will use "hat" notation to denote the estimate of a population parameter. For example, the usual estimate of a population mean μ is the sample mean, $\hat{\mu} = \bar{Y}$.

Hypothesis testing uses sample statistics to test hypotheses about population parameters. The strategy of hypothesis testing is to set up a null hypothesis and see whether our data provide evidence against it. In a trial comparing a population mean μ to a reference value μ_0, a typical null hypothesis is

$$H_0: \mu = \mu_0$$

where μ_0 is some specified value, for example, 0. The complement of the null hypothesis is the alternative hypothesis. For the null hypothesis $H_0: \mu = \mu_0$, the alternative hypothesis is

$$H_A: \mu \neq \mu_0.$$

This alternative includes all values of μ other than μ_0.

The next step of hypothesis testing is to calculate a **test statistic** and determine its probability distribution when the null hypothesis is true, termed the **null distribution**. For a one-sample mean test, the typical test statistic

is
$$\frac{\bar{Y} - \mu_0}{SE(\bar{Y})}$$

where $SE(\bar{Y})$ denotes the standard error of $\bar{Y}$. When the observations $Y_1, ..., Y_N$ have mean μ_0 (that is, when the null hypothesis is true) and the sample size is large, this test statistic will have approximately a standard normal distribution. Other test statistics may have other null distributions, e.g., chi-square or F distributions.

We use the value of the test statistic to decide whether or not to reject H_0 and conclude that H_A is true. To do so, we find where the test statistic falls within the null distribution. Values of the test statistic that are unlikely to occur if H_0 is true provide evidence that H_0 may be false.

To formalize the decision-making process, we identify values of the test statistic for which we will reject H_0. These regions are called the **rejection regions**. If the test statistic is in the rejection region, we reject H_0; such an extreme value of the test statistic is not likely to be observed when the null hypothesis is true and so we reject H_0 and conclude that H_A is true. If the test statistic is not in the rejection region, we fail to reject H_0; our data do not provide sufficient evidence to contradict the null hypothesis. The do-not-reject region is also called the **acceptance region**. The values on the boundary between the rejection and acceptance regions are called the **critical values**.

The alternative hypothesis $H_A: \mu \neq \mu_0$ is a **two-sided alternative** and leads to a **two-sided test**. For two-sided alternatives, values of the test statistic that are either extremely low or extremely high will lead us to reject H_0 in favor of H_A. There will be two critical values defining the two thresholds. Figure 2.1(A) illustrates rejection regions for a two-sided test. We can also perform **one-sided tests** with **one-sided alternatives**. For example, we could test

$$H_0: \mu \leq \mu_0 \text{ versus } H_A: \mu > \mu_0,$$

which is called an **upper-tailed test**, or

$$H_0: \mu \geq \mu_0 \text{ versus } H_A: \mu < \mu_0$$

which is called a **lower-tailed test**. For one-sided tests, there will be one rejection region and one critical value. For upper-tailed tests, high values of the test statistic will lead us to reject the null; for lower-tailed tests, low values of the test statistic will lead us to reject the null. Figures 2.1(B) and 2.1(C) illustrate rejection regions for lower-tailed and upper-tailed tests.

One-sided hypotheses are sometimes written using equality in the null hypothesis, that is, $H_0: \mu = \mu_0$ versus $H_A: \mu > \mu_0$ or $H_0: \mu = \mu_0$ versus $H_A: \mu < \mu_0$. Such hypotheses should be treated as one-sided.

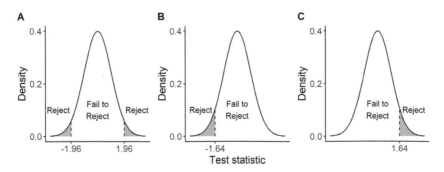

FIGURE 2.1: Rejection and acceptance regions for a (A) two-sided, (B) lower-tailed and (C) upper-tailed tests. In each panel, the null distribution is $\mathcal{N}(0,1)$ and the type I error rate or significance level α is 0.05. The critical values are -1.96 and 1.96 for the two-sided test and -1.64 and 1.64 for the lower- and upper-tailed tests, respectively. The shaded areas under the curves represent the type I error rate. In Panel (A), there is area of 0.025 in each tail and in Panels (B) and (C), the areas are each 0.05.

A hypothesis test entails deciding whether or not to reject H_0 and conclude that H_A is true. That decision may or may not agree with the truth. There are four possible scenarios for the outcome of a hypothesis test, as displayed in Table 2.1:

1. H_0 is true and we do not reject it. In this case, we have drawn a correct conclusion.

2. H_0 is true but we reject it. In this case, we have made a mistake that is called a **type I error**.

3. H_0 is false and we reject it. Here we have drawn a correct conclusion. Rejecting the null in favor of the alternative is the outcome that researchers usually hope for.

4. H_0 is false but we do not reject it. In this case, we have made a mistake called a **type II error**.

TABLE 2.1: The four possible outcomes of a hypothesis test.

	Do not reject H_0	Reject H_0
H_0 true	Correct conclusion	Type I error
H_0 false	Type II error	Correct conclusion

When conducting a hypothesis test, we are interested in the probabilities of these possible outcomes of the test. We use α to denote the probability that we reject H_0 when it is true, that is, the probability of a type I error:

$$\alpha = P(\text{Reject } H_0 \mid H_0 \text{ true}).$$

The value of α is specified by the researcher in advance of conducting the test. The most common value (but not the only choice) is 0.05. Specifying α of 0.05 means that we are willing to mistakenly reject the null hypothesis when it is true 5% of the time. The value of α is called the **significance level** of the test. In Figure 2.1, the shaded areas correspond to the type I error rates.

We use β to denote the probability that we do not reject H_0 when H_A is true, i.e., the probability of a type II error:

$$\beta = P(\text{Do not reject } H_0 \mid H_A \text{ true})$$

The **power** of a test is the probability that we reject H_0 when H_A is true. Power is equal to $1 - \beta$,

$$\text{Power} = 1 - \beta = P(\text{Reject } H_0 \mid H_A \text{ true}).$$

The power and type II error rate of a test depend not just on H_A being true but will vary depending on the particular true value of the population parameters under the alternative. For example, when testing the null hypothesis that two means are equal, $H_0: \mu_1 = \mu_2$, the power to reject the null hypothesis depends on the true difference between μ_1 and μ_2. Power will be higher for larger differences between μ_1 and μ_2 and lower for smaller differences.

While many studies focus on hypothesis testing for drawing inferences about population parameters, other studies are focused on estimating the values of parameters with a specified level of precision. Precision-based sample size calculations aim to determine the sample size that will lead to a confidence interval that is less than a specified width. Precision-based sample size calculation is discussed in Chapter 9.

2.3 A first calculation: one-sample z test

We now derive formulas for power and sample size for a one-sample mean test with normally distributed data. In these first calculations, we assume the value of the population variance σ^2 is known, to illustrate concepts without getting distracted by other issues. Tests for means for normally distributed data when the population variance is known are referred to as z tests. In Chapter 3, we cover the more realistic case that σ^2 will be estimated from the data; this leads to t tests.

A first calculation: one-sample z test

We will consider the following example, which involves a lower-tailed z test, then move on to upper-tailed and two-sided z tests:

Example 2.1. Suppose that hemoglobin A1c values in a population are normally distributed, with a standard deviation σ that is known to be 2. A hemoglobin A1c level above 5.7 percent is considered prediabetic or diabetic; values below 5.7 percent are considered non-diabetic. We plan to measure A1c values in a sample of 36 patients and test whether their population mean A1c is in the non-diabetic range. We formulate hypotheses with a one-sided alternative,

$$H_0: \mu \geq 5.7 \quad \text{versus} \quad H_A: \mu < 5.7$$

and plan to use significance level $\alpha = 0.05$. This is a lower-tailed test and low values of the test statistic will lead to rejection of H_0 and the conclusion that the population mean is less than 5.7 percent. If the true mean A1c level in this population is 4.9 percent, what is the power to reject H_0 and conclude $\mu < 5.7$?

Why did we specify this particular one-sided test? The following tip provides guidance on specifying null and alternative hypotheses:

▶ **The alternative hypothesis usually states the desired conclusion:** When designing and conducting a study, we typically hope to reject H_0 and conclude that H_A is true. A good rule of thumb is that the alternative hypothesis expresses the conclusion that we hope to reach. This rule of thumb can be especially helpful when designing noninferiority, superiority and equivalence studies, which are discussed in Chapter 4.

2.3.1 Power for a one-sided, lower-tailed z test

We now derive a formula for power for the scenario in Example 2.1. We assume that we have a random sample of N observations from a normal distribution. Specifically, we assume that $Y_1, ..., Y_N$ are independent and identically distributed (iid) normal random variables with unknown mean μ and known variance σ^2. The sample mean is $\bar{Y} = \frac{1}{N} \sum_{i=1}^{N} Y_i$. Suppose that we plan to conduct a one-sided, lower-tailed test

$$H_0: \mu \geq \mu_0 \quad \text{versus} \quad H_A: \mu < \mu_0$$

where μ_0 is some reference value. The significance level is set to α, e.g., 0.05. To conduct this test, the procedure is to calculate the test statistic

$$T = \frac{\bar{Y} - \mu_0}{\sigma/\sqrt{N}} \tag{2.1}$$

and determine its distribution under the condition that the null hypothesis is true. The null hypothesis states that $\mu \geq \mu_0$; we assume that the boundary value μ_0 is the true value under the null. Thus when H_0 is true, the Y_i's are iid $\mathcal{N}(\mu_0, \sigma^2)$, $\bar{Y} \sim \mathcal{N}(\mu_0, \sigma^2/N)$, and therefore the test statistic T has a standard normal distribution, $T \sim \mathcal{N}(0, 1)$. The use of the letter T here is not meant to imply that the test statistic has a t distribution, although when we use the estimate $\hat{\sigma}$ rather than the true value σ in the test statistic, as we do in Chapter 3, the test statistic will have a t distribution.

For a lower-tailed test, values below the critical value will lead to rejection of H_0. The next step is to determine the critical value. For significance level α, the critical value is the $100 \times \alpha^{th}$ percentile of the standard normal distribution, denoted z_α. The critical value can be computed in R using the qnorm function. For $\alpha = 0.05$, the critical value is $z_{0.05}$:

```
qnorm(p = 0.05)
[1] -1.644854
```

Thus for Example 2.1, we will reject H_0 if $T < -1.644854$.

The power of the test is the probability that the test statistic will fall in the rejection region given that a specific alternative is true. This is a conditional probability, i.e., a probability computed under a specific condition. We will denote the value of the mean when the alternative is true as μ_A. If the true population mean is μ_A, then $Y_i \sim \mathcal{N}(\mu_A, \sigma^2)$. Power is the conditional probability that the test statistic will fall in the rejection region given that $Y_i \sim \mathcal{N}(\mu_A, \sigma^2)$:

$$\text{Power} = P\left[T < z_\alpha \,\middle|\, Y_i \sim \mathcal{N}(\mu_A, \sigma^2)\right]. \tag{2.2}$$

How do we compute this probability? The first step is to find the distribution of T when the alternative is true. Now, if $Y_i \sim \mathcal{N}(\mu_A, \sigma^2)$, then

$$\bar{Y} \sim \mathcal{N}\left(\mu_A, \frac{\sigma^2}{N}\right)$$

$$\bar{Y} - \mu_0 \sim \mathcal{N}\left(\mu_A - \mu_0, \frac{\sigma^2}{N}\right)$$

$$T = \frac{\bar{Y} - \mu_0}{\sigma/\sqrt{N}} \sim \mathcal{N}\left(\frac{\mu_A - \mu_0}{\sigma/\sqrt{N}}, 1\right)$$

Thus when $\mu = \mu_A$, T has a normal distribution with mean $\frac{\mu_A - \mu_0}{\sigma/\sqrt{N}}$ and variance 1.

The next step is to convert T to a standard normal random variable in order to convert the probability calculation in (2.2) to a probability calculation involving the standard normal distribution (see Section 1.6). To standardize T, we subtract its mean then divide by its standard deviation, which is 1. We perform these operations on both sides of the inequality in (2.2), and also

A first calculation: one-sample z test

drop the conditioning notation for simplicity:

$$P\left[T - \frac{\mu_A - \mu_0}{\sigma/\sqrt{N}} < z_\alpha - \frac{\mu_A - \mu_0}{\sigma/\sqrt{N}}\right]$$
$$= P\left[Z < z_\alpha - \frac{\mu_A - \mu_0}{\sigma/\sqrt{N}}\right]$$
$$= \Phi\left(z_\alpha - \frac{\mu_A - \mu_0}{\sigma/\sqrt{N}}\right).$$

Thus power can be computed by evaluating the cdf of the standard normal distribution at the quantile $z_\alpha - \frac{(\mu_A - \mu_0)}{\sigma/\sqrt{N}}$. To summarize, the formula for power for a lower-tailed one-sample z test is

$$\text{Power (lower-tailed one-sample } z \text{ test)} = \Phi\left(z_\alpha - \frac{\mu_A - \mu_0}{\sigma/\sqrt{N}}\right). \quad (2.3)$$

Figure 2.2 shows the key relationships. When $H_0\colon \mu = \mu_0$ is true, $T \sim \mathcal{N}(0,1)$. When H_A is true and the mean is μ_A, $T \sim \mathcal{N}(\sqrt{N}(\mu_A - \mu_0)/\sigma, 1)$. Typically, when computing power for a lower-tailed test, we will assume that the true mean μ_A is less than μ_0; this is consistent with the alternative hypothesis being true. Power is the probability that a random variable that is distributed as $\mathcal{N}(\sqrt{N}(\mu_A - \mu_0)/\sigma, 1)$ falls below the critical value z_α. This is the area under the H_A curve from $-\infty$ to z_α, labeled as $1 - \beta$ (note that this includes the area labeled α).

We are now ready to calculate power for Example 2.1.

Example 2.2. Continuing Example 2.1, recall that we plan to measure hemoglobin A1c values in a sample of $N = 36$ patients from a population with known standard deviation $\sigma = 2$ and test, at $\alpha = 0.05$,

$$H_0\colon \mu \geq 5.7 \quad \text{versus} \quad H_A\colon \mu < 5.7.$$

If the true mean A1c level in this population is 4.9 percent, what is the power to reject H_0 and conclude $\mu < 5.7$?

Using formula (2.3), we can compute power as

```
pnorm(q = qnorm(p = 0.05) - (4.9 - 5.7) / (2 / sqrt(36)))
[1] 0.7749194
```

The power is about 0.775, or 77.5%. If the true mean A1c is 4.9 percent, there is probability of about 0.775 that we will reject the null hypothesis and conclude that the mean A1c in this population is less than 5.7 percent.

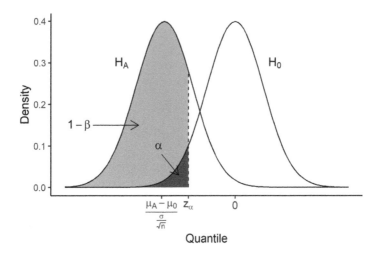

FIGURE 2.2: Distribution of test statistic under null and alternative hypotheses for a lower-tailed z test. Under H_0, $T \sim \mathcal{N}(0,1)$. Under H_A, $T \sim \mathcal{N}(\sqrt{N}(\mu_A - \mu_0)/\sigma, 1)$. Type I error rate α is indicated by the dark grey area under the H_0 curve. Power, $1-\beta$, is indicated by the light grey area under the H_A curve, which includes the α region. Type II error is the area under the H_A curve to the right of the dashed vertical line.

To summarize, these were the key steps in deriving a formula for power:

Keys steps in deriving a formula for power

After we have set up our hypotheses, specified the significance level α and determined the form of the test statistic, the key steps in deriving a formula for power are the following:

1. Determine the distribution of the test statistic when the null hypothesis is true, the critical values and the rejection region.

2. Determine the distribution of the test statistic when an alternative scenario about the values of population parameters is true.

3. Calculate power as the probability that the test statistic falls into the rejection region when the alternative is true.

2.3.2 Power for a one-sided, upper-tailed z test

Now we consider power for an upper-tailed test with hypotheses

$$H_0: \mu \leq \mu_0 \quad \text{versus} \quad H_A: \mu > \mu_0.$$

We conduct the test using the same test statistic, $T = \frac{\bar{Y} - \mu_0}{\sigma/\sqrt{N}}$, as for the lower-tailed test. However, for the upper-tailed test, the critical value is $z_{1-\alpha}$ and the rejection region consists of values above the critical value. Power can be calculated as the probability that the test statistic falls in the rejection region given that the true mean is μ_A:

$$\text{Power} = P\left[T > z_{1-\alpha} \,\middle|\, Y_i \sim \mathcal{N}(\mu_A, \sigma^2)\right]$$
$$= 1 - P\left[T < z_{1-\alpha} \,\middle|\, Y_i \sim \mathcal{N}(\mu_A, \sigma^2)\right].$$

When the alternative is true, $T \sim \mathcal{N}(\sqrt{N}(\mu_A - \mu_0)/\sigma, 1)$, which is the same as for the lower-tailed test (but we are likely to specify a different value for the true mean μ_A). Standardizing T by subtracting its mean from both sides of the inequality and dividing by its standard deviation, which is 1, we obtain (again we drop the conditioning notation for simplicity)

$$1 - P\left[T - \frac{\mu_A - \mu_0}{\sigma/\sqrt{N}} < z_{1-\alpha} - \frac{\mu_A - \mu_0}{\sigma/\sqrt{N}}\right]$$
$$= 1 - P\left[Z < z_{1-\alpha} - \frac{\mu_A - \mu_0}{\sigma/\sqrt{N}}\right]$$
$$= 1 - \Phi\left(z_{1-\alpha} - \frac{\mu_A - \mu_0}{\sigma/\sqrt{N}}\right)$$

Thus we have found that power for the upper-tailed one-sample z test can be calculated as

$$\text{Power (upper-tailed one-sample } z \text{ test)} = 1 - \Phi\left(z_{1-\alpha} - \frac{\mu_A - \mu_0}{\sigma/\sqrt{N}}\right). \quad (2.4)$$

Figure 2.3 illustrates the key relationships. For an upper-tailed test, we are usually interested in computing power for values of μ_A that are higher than μ_0 (which implies that the alternative hypothesis is in fact true), so the distribution of the test statistic under H_A will be to the right of its distribution under H_0. When $H_0: \mu = \mu_0$ is true, $T \sim \mathcal{N}(0,1)$ distribution. When the alternative is true and the mean is μ_A, $T \sim \mathcal{N}(\sqrt{N}(\mu_A - \mu_0)/\sigma, 1)$. Power is the probability that a random variable that is distributed as $\mathcal{N}(\sqrt{N}(\mu_A - \mu_0)/\sigma, 1)$ falls above the critical value $z_{1-\alpha}$. This is the area under the H_A curve from to $z_{1-\alpha}$ to ∞, labeled as $1 - \beta$ (which includes the area labeled α).

Calculating power for an upper-tailed one-sample z test is illustrated in the following example:

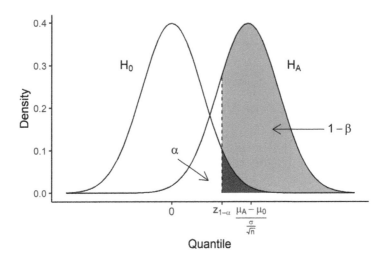

FIGURE 2.3: Distribution of test statistic under null and alternative hypotheses for a upper-tailed z test. Under H_0, $T \sim \mathcal{N}(0,1)$. Under H_A, $T \sim \mathcal{N}(\sqrt{N}(\mu_A - \mu_0)/\sigma, 1)$. Type I error rate α is indicated by the dark grey area under the H_0 curve. Power, $1-\beta$, is indicated by the light grey area under the H_A curve, which includes the α region. Type II error is the area under the H_A curve to the left of the dashed vertical line.

Example 2.3. For the hemoglobin A1c study, suppose we wish to test $H_0\colon \mu \leq 5.7$ versus $H_A\colon \mu > 5.7$ at $\alpha = 0.05$ when the true population mean is $\mu_A = 6.3$. For a sample of size $N = 36$ and known standard deviation $\sigma = 2$, what is the power to reject H_0 and conclude that H_A is true?

Using formula (2.4), we can compute power as

```
1 - pnorm(q = qnorm(p = 1 - 0.05) - sqrt(36) * (6.3 - 5.7) / 2)
[1]   0.561647
```

Power is about 0.562 or 56.2%.

It can be convenient to re-express power for an upper-tailed test as follows. Due to the symmetric property of the normal distribution (Section 1.5) equation (2.4) can also be written as

$$\text{Power (upper-tailed one-sample } z \text{ test)} = \Phi\left(z_\alpha + \frac{\sqrt{N}(\mu_A - \mu_0)}{\sigma}\right). \quad (2.5)$$

We can derive a unified expression for power for a one-sample, one-sided z test, either lower or upper, as follows. For a lower-tailed test, we are usually

A first calculation: one-sample z test   19

interested in power for $\mu_A < \mu_0$ so $\mu_A - \mu_0$ is negative; for an upper-tailed test, we are usually interested in power when $\mu_A > \mu_0$ so $\mu_A - \mu_0$ is positive. By using the absolute value $|\mu_A - \mu_0|$, equations (2.3) and (2.5) can both be expressed as

$$\text{Power (one-sided one-sample } z \text{ test)} = \Phi\left(z_\alpha + \frac{\sqrt{N}|\mu_A - \mu_0|}{\sigma}\right). \quad (2.6)$$

2.3.3 Power for a two-sided one-sample z test

For a two-sided test, the hypotheses are

$$H_0: \mu = \mu_0 \quad \text{versus} \quad H_A: \mu \neq \mu_0.$$

The test statistic is again $T = \frac{\bar{Y} - \mu_0}{\sigma/\sqrt{N}}$. We split α and allocate half to each tail, and we reject H_0 if the test statistic is beyond the lower or upper critical value. As for the one-tailed tests, when H_0 is true, $T \sim N(0,1)$ and when the alternative $\mu = \mu_A$ is true, $T \sim N(\sqrt{N}(\mu_A - \mu_0)/\sigma, 1)$. Figure 2.4 illustrates the relationships. To compute power, we sum the two probabilities corresponding to the two rejection regions:

$$\begin{aligned}
\text{Power} &= P\left[T < z_{\alpha/2} \text{ or } T > z_{1-\alpha/2} \mid Y_i \sim N(\mu_A, \sigma^2)\right] \\
&= \Phi\left(z_{\alpha/2} - \frac{\sqrt{N}(\mu_A - \mu_0)}{\sigma}\right) + 1 - \Phi\left(z_{1-\alpha/2} - \frac{\sqrt{N}(\mu_A - \mu_0)}{\sigma}\right) \\
&= \Phi\left(z_{\alpha/2} - \frac{\sqrt{N}(\mu_A - \mu_0)}{\sigma}\right) + \Phi\left(z_{\alpha/2} + \frac{\sqrt{N}(\mu_A - \mu_0)}{\sigma}\right) \quad (2.7)
\end{aligned}$$

Typically, one of the two probabilities will be very small and can be neglected. In Figure 2.4, the left tail of the H_A curve extends to the left with a very small area under it beyond $z_{\alpha/2}$. Thus we can approximate the power as the larger of the two probabilities, which can be calculated as

$$\text{Power (two-sided one-sample } z \text{ test)} \approx \Phi\left(z_{\alpha/2} + \frac{\sqrt{N}|\mu_A - \mu_0|}{\sigma}\right). \quad (2.8)$$

Example 2.4. Suppose we want to conduct a two-sided test $H_0: \mu = 5.7$ versus $H_A: \mu \neq 5.7$ at $\alpha = 0.05$. If the sample size is 36 and the true mean is 6.5, what is the power? We assume that σ is known to be 2.

Using power formula (2.7), we can find the probabilities of the test statistic falling into the lower and upper rejection regions and the power as follows:

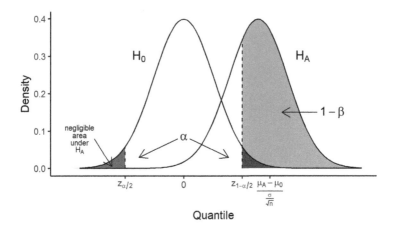

FIGURE 2.4: Distribution of test statistic under null and alternative hypotheses for a two-tailed z test. Under H_0, $T \sim \mathcal{N}(0,1)$. Under H_A, $T \sim \mathcal{N}(\sqrt{N}(\mu_A - \mu_0)/\sigma, 1)$. Type I error rate α is split between the two tails of the H_0 curve and indicated by dark grey. Power, $1 - \beta$, is indicated by the light grey area under the H_A curve. There is also a very small contribution to power due to area under the H_A curve to the left of $z_{\alpha/2}$. Type II error is the area under the H_A curve between the dashed vertical lines.

```
probL <- pnorm(q = qnorm(p = 0.05 / 2) - (6.5 - 5.7) * sqrt(36) / 2)
probL
[1] 6.504193e-06
probU <- pnorm(q = qnorm(p = 0.05 / 2) + sqrt(36) * (6.5 - 5.7) / 2)
probU
[1] 0.6700445
power <-   probL + probU   ;   power
[1] 0.670051
```

When the true population mean is high, the probability that the test statistic will be in the lower tail of the alternative distribution is very small (≈ 0.0000065). Thus the sum of the lower-tail and upper-tail probabilities is about equal to the upper-tail probability. The approximate power formula (2.8) gives the upper probability in this example.

2.3.4 What factors affect power?

Power for one- and two-sided one-sample z tests can be computed using equations (2.6) and (2.8). By examining these equations, we can see that power for these tests is a function of the sample size N, the magnitude of the difference

A first calculation: one-sample z test

between the null and alternative means $|\mu_A - \mu_0|$, the standard deviation of the outcome variable σ and the Type I error rate α. Each of these quantities helps to determine the argument (the quantile) of the standard normal cdf $\Phi(\cdot)$ used to compute power. How does each of these factors affect power?

Like all cdfs, $\Phi(x)$ is a monotone nondecreasing function (in fact it is strictly increasing); as x increases, $\Phi(x)$ increases. Using this fact, we can deduce how each of these factors affects power:

- As N increases, power increases.
- As the difference between the null and alternative means $|\mu_A - \mu_0|$ increases, power increases.
- As the standard deviation σ increases, power *decreases*.
- As the significance level α increases, z_α (or $z_{\alpha/2}$) increases and thus power increases.

Some of these factors may be under our control and some of them may not. For example, we may be able to increase the sample size, but we may not be able to change the variance of the observations. The significance level is usually prespecified and we generally will not vary it.

2.3.5 Finding required sample size

Rather than calculating the power for a given sample size, we often wish to find the sample size that will provide a desired level of power. To do so, the general approach is to solve a power formula for sample size. For a one-sided one-sample z test, we can use power formula (2.6) to set up an inequality

$$1 - \beta \leq \Phi\left(z_\alpha + \frac{|\mu_A - \mu_0|}{\sigma/\sqrt{N}}\right)$$

and solve it for N as follows. First, we apply the inverse cdf of the standard normal to each side:

$$\Phi^{-1}(1-\beta) \leq z_\alpha + \frac{|\mu_A - \mu_0|}{\sigma/\sqrt{N}}$$

Noting that $\Phi^{-1}(p) = z_p$, we obtain

$$z_{1-\beta} \leq z_\alpha + \frac{|\mu_A - \mu_0|}{\sigma/\sqrt{N}}$$

$$z_{1-\beta} - z_\alpha \leq \frac{|\mu_A - \mu_0|}{\sigma/\sqrt{N}}$$

Using the symmetric property $-z_p = z_{1-p}$ (see Section 1.5), we get

$$z_{1-\beta} + z_{1-\alpha} \leq \frac{|\mu_A - \mu_0|}{\sigma/\sqrt{N}}$$

$$\frac{(z_{1-\beta} + z_{1-\alpha})^2 \sigma^2}{(\mu_A - \mu_0)^2} \leq N.$$

Thus for a one-sided, one-sample z test, the sample size needed to achieve power of $1 - \beta$ with significance level α is

$$N \geq \frac{(z_{1-\beta} + z_{1-\alpha})^2 \sigma^2}{(\mu_A - \mu_0)^2}. \tag{2.9}$$

For a two-sided one-sample z test, using the same approach with equation (2.8) leads to the same formula but with $z_{1-\alpha/2}$ substituted for $z_{1-\alpha}$. The required sample size is

$$N \geq \frac{(z_{1-\beta} + z_{1-\alpha/2})^2 \sigma^2}{(\mu_A - \mu_0)^2}. \tag{2.10}$$

Example 2.5. Suppose that we wish to have 80% power for a two-sided one-sample z test at significance level 0.05 with $\mu_0 = 5.7$, $\mu_A = 6.5$ and known $\sigma = 2$. What is the required N?

We first find the normal distribution quantiles and then compute N:

```
zb <- qnorm(p = 0.8) ; zb
[1] 0.8416212
za <- qnorm(p = 1 - 0.05 / 2) ; za
[1] 1.959964
N <- ((zb + za)^2 * 2^2) / (6.5 - 5.7)^2 ; N
[1] 49.0555
```

We need a sample size of at least 49.0555 to achieve 80% power. The sample size should be rounded up to 50 to ensure power is not less than 80%.

Here, for the case of a one-sample z test, we were able to obtain a closed-form analytic expression for the sample size required to achieve a desired level of power. In other situations, we may not be able to find a closed-form expression for sample size; rather, we may need to use iterative numerical methods to find the smallest N that achieves the desired level of power (or have a computer do this for us).

> **Key steps to finding a formula for sample size**
>
> To find the sample size required to achieve a desired level of power, we solve the power formula for N. In some cases, we will be able to derive an explicit, closed-form formula for sample size. In other cases, we will not be able to get an explicit formula; we will need to use software to solve the power formula numerically and find N.

2.4 Effect size

In our example, the difference between the means under the null and under the alternative, $\mu_A - \mu_0$, is an effect size. An **effect size** is the magnitude of a difference. Effect sizes are important for characterizing the clinical or practical significance of a difference. For example, a difference in mean hemoglobin A1c of 0.2 percent may not be clinically meaningful, while a difference of 2 percent may be very meaningful for clinical outcomes. Effect sizes also arise in correlational analyses such as regression, where they pertain to the strength of association between two variables.

The effect size $\mu_A - \mu_0$ has the same units as μ; in our A1c example, $\mu_A - \mu_0$ has units of percent A1c. If we were comparing mean weights, $\mu_A - \mu_0$ could have units of kilograms, for example. It is sometimes convenient to work with standardized versions of such effect sizes. These are obtained by dividing the mean difference by the standard deviation. The quantity $d = (\mu_A - \mu_0)/\sigma$ is called a **standardized mean effect size**, **d effect size** or **Cohen's d effect size** after Cohen [36]. Cohen's 1988 book *Statistical Power Analysis for the Behavioral Sciences, 2nd edition* [36] is an influential text and we will refer to it again in this book. The standardized mean effect size expresses the difference between two means in units of standard deviation. Thus $d = 0.5$ indicates that μ_0 and μ_A are half of a standard deviation apart. Since statisticians are accustomed to thinking of differences in terms of standard deviation units, this can be a useful approach.

By substituting d into sample size equation (2.9), we get

$$N \geq \frac{(z_{1-\beta} + z_{1-\alpha})^2}{d^2}, \qquad (2.11)$$

which shows that for the one-sample z test, we can calculate sample size requirements based only on the significance level, desired power and standardized mean effect size.

Some rules of thumb for standardized mean effect sizes were given by Cohen [36], who suggested that d of 0.2, 0.5 and 0.8 represent small, medium and large effect sizes, respectively. Although we are discussing the standardized mean effect size here in the context of a one-sample test, d is also commonly used to characterize the difference between the means of two groups.

Example 2.6. The standardized mean effect size in the two-sided test in Example 2.5 is $d = (6.5 - 5.7)/2 = 0.4$. The two means are 0.4 standard deviations apart. This represents a small-to-medium effect size.

Standardized mean effect sizes are a convenient shorthand for the magnitude of the difference between two means. In later chapters, we will encounter other types of effect sizes.

2.5 Minimum detectable effect size

In some situations, we may be interested in the smallest effect size that can be detected with a given sample size and a specified level of power. This is called the **minimal** or **minimum detectable effect size**. When there is a closed-form, analytic expression for sample size such as equation (2.11), we can derive a formula for the minimum detectable effect size, which for the one-sided, one-sample z test, is

$$d \geq \frac{z_{1-\beta} + z_{1-\alpha}}{\sqrt{N}}. \qquad (2.12)$$

For a two-sided test, substitute $\alpha/2$ for α.

Example 2.7. Suppose that we have a sample size of 40 subjects available. We plan to conduct a one-sample z test. What is the smallest d effect size that can be detected with 90% power, when specifying two-sided α of 0.05?

```
(qnorm(p = 0.9) + qnorm(p = 1 - 0.05 / 2)) / sqrt(40)
[1] 0.5125286
```

The minimum detectable effect size is $d \approx 0.5$. With a sample of 40 subjects, we have 90% power to detect a difference between μ_0 and μ_A of about one half of a standard deviation.

2.6 A general formula when the test statistic is normally distributed

In the examples in this chapter, the test statistics have the form

$$\frac{\hat{\theta} - \theta_0}{\sqrt{Var(\hat{\theta})}}$$

and are normally distributed. In particular, in our examples, $\hat{\theta} = \bar{Y}$, $\theta_0 = \mu_0$ and $Var(\hat{\theta}) = Var(\bar{Y}) = \sigma^2/N$. This is a common form for a test statistic. When this is the case, we can set up the relationship

$$z_{1-\alpha} + z_{1-\beta} \approx \frac{|\theta_A - \theta_0|}{\sqrt{Var(\hat{\theta})}}$$

where θ_A is the assumed true value of θ. This is for a one-sided test; we use $z_{1-\alpha/2}$ for a two-sided test. A common approach to power and sample size calculation is to determine an expression for $Var(\hat{\theta})$, insert it in this relationship and then solve for a quantity of interest given values of the others. Expressions for $Var(\hat{\theta})$ will generally involve the sample sizes, with the variance decreasing as sample size increases. We will see this strategy to power and sample size calculation in many sections of this book.

2.7 R function for z tests

The preceding sections illustrate some general principles that will be widely applicable in many settings:

- Power is calculated as a function of inputs such as sample size, difference in means, population standard deviation and significance level.

- Once we have a formula for power, we can solve it for any of the inputs by specifying values for power and all of other inputs.

In some cases, we will be able to derive explicit closed-form formulas to solve for these inputs, for example, sample size or minimum detectable effect sizes. In other cases, we will need to use software to get the solution using numerical methods.

Many power and sample size functions in R use these principles. Their parameters include power and all of the inputs needed to calculate power (N, σ, α, etc.); we set the parameter for which we wish to solve to NULL, specify values for the other parameter, and the function solves for that parameter using the other values.

Example 2.8. The function ztest.1samp in the powertools package performs power and sample size calculations for a one-sample z test and has the syntax

```
library(powertools)
ztest.1samp(N, delta, sd, alpha, power, sides, v)
```

where delta is $\mu_A - \mu_0$ (true mean minus null mean). To use this function, we set one of the parameters N, delta, sd, alpha or power to NULL and specify values for the other parameters. For example, we can replicate Example 2.5 using the command

```
ztest.1samp(N = NULL, delta = 6.5 - 5.7, sd = 2, alpha = 0.05,
   power = 0.8, sides = 2)
[1] 49.05538
```

and we can replicate Example 2.7 using the command

```
ztest.1samp(N = 40, delta = NULL, sd = 1, alpha = 0.05, power = 0.9,
   sides = 2)
[1] 0.512518
```

Note how we set the standard deviation to 1. When we do this, delta becomes the standardized effect size d. In this function, sd = 1 is the default. Other defaults are alpha = 0.05 and sides = 2.

▶ **Specifying standardized effect sizes in R functions:** One can use d (standardized mean) effect sizes in functions that ask for a mean difference and standard deviation as inputs by specifying the mean difference as d and setting the standard deviation equal to 1.

Example 2.9. In functions in the powertools package, the parameter v stands for "verbose". Setting v = T gives verbose (long) output listing the values of key parameters and often other calculated output such as effect sizes and setting v = F gives short output; for most functions, this will be simply the value of the parameter that was solved for. The default is v = F. An example of output when specifying v = T is given below:

```
library(powertools)
```

```
ztest.1samp(N = 40, delta = NULL, sd = 1, alpha = 0.05, power = 0.9,
  sides = 2, v = T)

     One-sample z test power calculation

              N = 40
          delta = 0.512518
             sd = 1
          alpha = 0.05
          power = 0.9
          sides = 2
```

The powertools package also has functions for power and sample size for two-sample z tests (ztest.2samp) and paired z tests (ztest.paired). These functions assume that the variance is known and will not be estimated from the data. They are the known-variance analogues to two-sample and paired t tests, which are discussed in Chapter 3. In general, for real applications, you will want to use the t test functions. The z test functions are provided mostly for instructional purposes.

2.8 Sample size adjustments

In many studies, some participants drop out or otherwise do not provide useable outcome data, leaving a reduced number of **evaluable subjects** that can be included in the analysis. If we expect the outcomes of some participants to be lost due to attrition or other factors, the number of enrolled participants should be inflated so that the number of evaluable participants will provide adequate power.

If we expect that a proportion p of participants who enroll in the study will not provide evaluable outcome data, then the number of participants with evaluable outcome data is expected to be $N_{end} = N_{start}(1-p)$. Thus, if we need N_{end} participants to provide adequate power, the number enrolled should be

$$N_{start} \geq \frac{N_{end}}{1-p}.$$

Example 2.10. We found in Example 2.5 that we needed 50 evaluable participants to provide at least 80% power. If expect that about 10% of enrolled participants will drop out, then we need to enroll at least

```
50 / (1 - 0.1)
[1] 55.556
```

55.556 participants. This number should be rounded up to 56 to ensure adequate power.

A common mistake is to multiply N_{end} by $1 + p$; for example, if we expect 10% to drop out, we multiply N_{end} by 1.10. If we require 50 evaluable participants for adequate power, this would entail enrolling a sample size of $50 * 1.1 = 55$. But if 10% of those participants (5.5 participants) drop out, we will be left with 49.5 on average, which is less than 50 and therefore insufficient to achieve 80% power.

2.9 Sensitivity analysis

Calculating power or sample size involves making predictions about the true values that parameters will take in the future, such as the true value of the population mean. Of course our predictions could be wrong. Hence it is prudent to conduct a sensitivity analysis to see how power or sample size requirements change as assumed values of unknown parameters are changed.

Example 2.11. For the two-sided test in Example 2.4, we assumed $\mu_A = 6.5$. In reality, the true value of the mean in the population from which we will sample is unknown. Figure 2.5 displays power as μ_A ranges from 5.7 to 7.0. Power approaches 1 as μ_A (and the difference $|\mu_A - \mu_0|$) increases. As μ_A decreases toward μ_0, the power approaches the type I error rate α, which is 0.05 in this example. When $\mu_A = \mu_0$, the null hypothesis is true and thus the probability of rejecting H_0 is simply the type I error rate.

Code to produce a simplified version of Figure 2.5 is provided below:

```
library(powertools)
mu <- seq(from = 5.7, to = 7, by = 0.01)
power <- sapply(mu, function(x)
  ztest.1samp(N = 36, delta = x - 5.7, sd = 2, power = NULL,
    sides = 2, v = T)$power)
plot(mu, power, type = "l")
```

It is usually best to focus sensitivity analyses on parameters that are difficult to predict with accuracy in advance and/or have a large impact on the

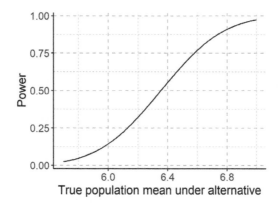

FIGURE 2.5: Power for a two-sided, one-sample z test when $\mu_0 = 5.7$, $\sigma = 2$, $N = 36$ and $\alpha = 0.05$ for values of μ_A ranging from 5.7 to 7.

power or sample size requirement. In the one-sample z test, such parameters include the true mean μ_A and the standard deviation σ. The type I error rate, α, is usually specified in advance and is not an unknown parameter.

2.10 Estimating power using simulation

In this chapter, we derived "closed-form" or "analytic" formulas for power and sample size for a one-sample z test. A closed-form or analytic formula is essentially a function: we can input specific values for various parameters and calculate an output. We provide many closed-form formulas for power in this book. When such formulas are available, power or sample size calculations can be performed quickly and are straightforward to reproduce.

However, in real world settings, we may encounter study design situations for which no suitable analytic formula for power exists. For example, the study may have data that do not conform to a normal or other distribution that is assumed by the statistical test, or the statistical model that we plan to fit to the data may not have a corresponding analytic formula for power, or we may plan to use a complex multiple comparison method to control the familywise error rate for multiple tests. In such situations, simulation can be a powerful and versatile tool for estimating power.

The basic steps in performing a power calculation using simulation are as follows:

1. Specify the data-generating model and write a function to generate a data set from the model. The data-generating model is the underlying "true" model for the population and describes how the data arise.

2. Write a function that performs the planned statistical test on a data set and outputs whether or not the null hypothesis was rejected.

3. Iterate steps (1) and (2) many times (at least 1000 for reliable results).

4. Estimate power as the proportion of the iterations in which the null hypothesis was rejected.

We do not need to use simulation to estimate power for a one-sample z test. However, for the sake of illustration, we show how to estimate power for a one-sample z test using simulation in the next example.

Example 2.12. We demonstrate how to use simulation to estimate power for a one-sample z test. We use the setting of Example 2.4: we have a sample of size 36 from a normal distribution with mean 6.5 and known standard deviation 2. We plan to conduct a two-sided test $H_0\colon \mu = 5.7$ versus $H_A\colon \mu \neq 5.7$ at $\alpha = 0.05$. What is the power to reject the null and conclude that $\mu \neq 5.7$?

The first step is to identify or create a function to generate a data set from the data-generating model. The data-generating model here is a normal distribution with $\mu = 6.5$ and $\sigma = 2$. A data set can be generated using:

```
ydata <- rnorm(n = 36, mean = 6.5, sd = 2)
```

Next, we apply the planned test to the simulated data. z tests can be conducted using the z.test function from the BSDA package. By default, the function performs a two-sided test at a significance level of 0.05, which is what we want. We set a random seed so the reader can reproduce the results:

```
library(BSDA)
set.seed(2345)
ydata <- rnorm(n = 36, mean = 6.5, sd = 2)
test <- z.test(x = ydata, mu = 5.7, sigma.x = 2) ; test

One-sample z-Test
data:  ydata
z = 2.1679, p-value = 0.03016
alternative hypothesis: true mean is not equal to 5.7
# some output omitted
```

Next, we capture whether the p-value is less than 0.05:

```
test$p.value < 0.05
[1] TRUE
```

Next, we replicate this code many times using the replicate function, which is in base R. Below, we run the code 10,000 times and save the results in an object called sim.pow. sim.pow is a vector of TRUE/FALSE values. TRUE/FALSE values are handled as 1/0 values in R. Taking the mean of sim.pow thus returns the proportion of TRUEs, which is an estimate of power, that is, the probability of rejecting H_0 when our specified data-generating model is true.

```
set.seed(2345)
sim.pow <- replicate(n = 10000, expr = {
  ydata <- rnorm(n = 36, mean = 6.5, sd = 2)
  test <- z.test(x = ydata, mu = 5.7, sigma.x = 2)
  test$p.value < 0.05
})
mean(sim.pow)
[1] 0.6676
```

Power is estimated to be 0.6676. For comparison, we use the analytic power formula, implemented by the ztest.1samp function:

```
library(powertools)
ztest.1samp(N = 36, delta = 6.5 - 5.7, sd = 2, alpha = 0.05,
   power = NULL, sides = 2)
[1] 0.670051
```

The analytic formula gives an exact calculation, assuming all assumptions are true. The power estimated using simulation is close to the exact power calculated from the formula.

There are specialized R packages that can be used for power simulation either generally or for specific types of models. For example, the Superpower package is designed for simulation-based power analysis for factorial designs and SimEngine is a general purpose package for statistical simulation. Helpful references concerning calculating power and sample size using simulation include Landau and Stahl [134].

2.11 Should I conduct a power analysis after my study is completed?

When investigators conduct a data analysis and fail to reject the null hypothesis, they are sometimes tempted to compute the "observed power", also called the "retrospective" or "post hoc power". A post hoc power analysis is an estimate of the power of a test given the observed effect size and sample size. The idea is to show that a non-significant result occurred because the power was insufficient.

The problem with this idea is that post hoc power is simply a one-to-one function of the p-value [96]. High p-values (i.e., non-significance) will always have low observed power. Low p-values will always have high observed power. Thus a post hoc power analysis does not provide any new or useful information.

To demonstrate, suppose we are conducting a lower-tailed, one-sample z test of $H_0\colon \mu \geq 0$ versus $H_A\colon \mu < 0$ with the values $\bar{Y} = -0.3$, $\sigma = 2$ and $N = 16$. We calculate the test statistic as $\bar{Y}/(\sigma/\sqrt{N})$, which equals a z-score, z_p;

```
-0.3 / (2 / sqrt(16))
[1] -0.6
```

$z_p = -0.6$. The p-value is calculated as $p = \Phi(z_p)$;

```
pnorm(-0.6)
1] 0.2742531
```

We obtain $p = 0.274$. The post hoc power analysis involves computing power using the formula $\Phi(z_\alpha - \mu_A/(\sigma/\sqrt{N}))$ (this is equation (2.3)) using $\bar{Y}$ for μ_A. Because $\bar{Y}/(\sigma/\sqrt{N}) = z_p$, this means post hoc power is computed as $\Phi(z_\alpha - z_p)$. This is a one-to-one function of the p-value.

A study may indeed be underpowered but a post hoc power calculation will do nothing to prove this. You will always get low post hoc power on a hypothesis test with a large p-value.

▶ Post hoc power calculations do not provide useful information and are not recommended.

3

One or two means

3.1 One-sample t test

In Chapter 2, we derived power and sample size for a one-sample test for a mean assuming the value of the population variance σ^2 was known. Now we assume σ^2 will be estimated from the data, which is usually the case. This leads to the one-sample t test.

The framework for power calculations that we develop for the one-sample t test in this section will be widely used in a variety of settings, including analysis of variance (Chapter 5), crossover trials (Chapter 12), multisite trials (Chapter 13) and cluster randomized trials (Chapters 14 and 15). The statistical procedures to compute power for t tests were developed by Neyman and colleagues in the 1930s [169, 170].

3.1.1 Test statistic and its distribution

The one-sample t test is used to test a hypothesis about the true value of the mean in a population based on a sample from the population. Let $Y_1, ..., Y_N$ be a random sample of size N from a normal distribution with mean μ and variance σ^2. The values of μ and σ^2 can be estimated using the sample mean $\bar{Y}$ and the sample variance $s^2 = \frac{1}{N-1}\sum_{i=1}^{N}(Y_i - \bar{Y})^2$, respectively. To test $H_0\colon \mu \leq \mu_0$, $H_0\colon \mu \geq \mu_0$ or $H_0\colon \mu = \mu_0$, the test statistic is

$$T = \frac{\bar{Y} - \mu_0}{s/\sqrt{N}}. \tag{3.1}$$

We set a significance level α, which specifies the probability of making a type I error by rejecting H_0 when it is true. For one-sided tests, we take "when H_0 is true" to mean the boundary case that the true mean μ is equal to μ_0.

To define the critical values and rejection regions, we need the distribution of T when H_0 is true and the mean is equal to μ_0. Dividing the numerator and denominator of T by σ and multiplying the denominator by $\sqrt{(N-1)/(N-1)}$, we can rewrite T as

$$T = \frac{\frac{\bar{Y}-\mu_0}{\sigma/\sqrt{N}}}{\sqrt{\frac{(N-1)s^2}{(N-1)\sigma^2}}}. \tag{3.2}$$

When H_0 is true, $\bar{Y} \sim \mathcal{N}(\mu_0, \sigma^2/N)$, and therefore the numerator is a standard normal random variable. The sample variance s^2 has a scaled chi-square distribution, specifically, $(N-1)s^2/\sigma^2 \sim \chi^2(N-1)$, and therefore the denominator takes the form of the square root of a $\chi^2(N-1)$ random variable divided by its degrees of freedom. One can also show that the numerator and denominator are independent. It follows that when H_0 is true, T has a t distribution with $N-1$ degrees of freedom, denoted $t(N-1)$ (see, e.g., [189]):

$$\frac{\mathcal{N}(0,1)}{\sqrt{\frac{\chi^2(N-1)}{N-1}}} \sim t(N-1).$$

Based on this null distribution, we identify the critical values as quantiles of the $t(N-1)$ distribution, and reject H_0 if $T < t_{\alpha, N-1}$ for a lower-tailed test, $T > t_{1-\alpha, N-1}$ for an upper-tailed test, and either $T < t_{\alpha/2, N-1}$ or $T > t_{1-\alpha/2, N-1}$ for a two-sided test.

As discussed in Section 2.3, power is computed as the conditional probability that H_0 will be rejected when a specific alternative about the values of the parameters is true. Here, the parameter of interest is the population mean. What is the distribution of T when the mean of the Y_i's is not μ_0 but rather some other value μ_A? In Section 2.3.1, we found that when the Y_i's are iid $\mathcal{N}(\mu_A, \sigma^2)$, then $\bar{Y} \sim \mathcal{N}(\mu_A, \sigma^2/N)$, $\bar{Y} - \mu_0 \sim \mathcal{N}(\mu_A - \mu_0, \sigma^2/N)$, and

$$\frac{\bar{Y} - \mu_0}{\sigma/\sqrt{N}} \sim \mathcal{N}\left(\frac{\mu_A - \mu_0}{\sigma/\sqrt{N}}, 1\right).$$

Thus when $\mu = \mu_A$, the T statistic in equation (3.2) has a distribution given by

$$\frac{\mathcal{N}\left(\frac{\mu_A - \mu_0}{\sigma/\sqrt{N}}, 1\right)}{\sqrt{\frac{\chi^2(N-1)}{N-1}}}. \tag{3.3}$$

This statistic takes the form of a **noncentral t distribution** with $N-1$ degrees of freedom and noncentrality parameter $\lambda = \frac{\mu_A - \mu_0}{\sigma/\sqrt{N}}$, which we denote as $t(N-1, \lambda)$.

Noncentral t distribution

A random variable of the form

$$\frac{\mathcal{N}(\lambda, 1)}{\sqrt{\frac{\chi^2(\nu)}{\nu}}}$$

where $\nu > 0$, $\lambda \in \mathbb{R}$ and the numerator and denominator are independent

---

has a noncentral t distribution with ν degrees of freedom and noncentrality parameter λ, denoted $t(\nu, \lambda)$. The "central" t distribution is the special case of $\lambda = 0$.

We denote the cdf of the $t(\nu, \lambda)$ distribution as $\mathcal{T}_{\nu,\lambda}$. When $\lambda = 0$, we will often omit it from the notation.

Examples of noncentral t densities are displayed in Figure 3.1. When $\lambda = 0$, the density is centered at zero and we have the usual "central" t distribution. As $|\lambda|$ increases, the location of the distribution shifts away from zero; hence the term "noncentrality parameter". When $\lambda = 0$, the density is symmetric; when $\lambda \neq 0$, the density is skewed. As the degrees of freedom increase, the density approaches that of a $\mathcal{N}(\lambda, 1)$ random variable.

Example 3.1. In R, the pdf, cdf and quantile function for both central and noncentral t distributions can be computed using the functions dt, pt and qt, respectively. The default value of the noncentrality parameter in these functions is zero.

The quantile of a $t(12, 10)$ distribution such that there is probability of 0.05 below that value can be computed as

```
qt(p = 0.05, df = 12, ncp = 10)
[1] 7.188817
```

This quantile is noted on the x-axis in Figure 3.1. Suppose $T \sim t(12, -10)$. The probability $P(T < -11) = \mathcal{T}_{12,-10}(-11)$ can be computed as

```
pt(q = -11, df = 12, ncp = -10)
[1] 0.3853194
```

This probability is indicated on the left-most density in Figure 3.1.

3.1.2 Power for one-sided tests

We have determined the distribution of the test statistic T for the one-sample t test when the mean of the Y_i's takes the null value μ_0 and when the mean takes an alternative value μ_A. These distributions are

$$\mu = \mu_0: T \sim t(N-1)$$

$$\mu = \mu_A: T \sim t(N-1, \lambda), \text{ where } \lambda = \frac{\mu_A - \mu_0}{\sigma/\sqrt{N}}$$

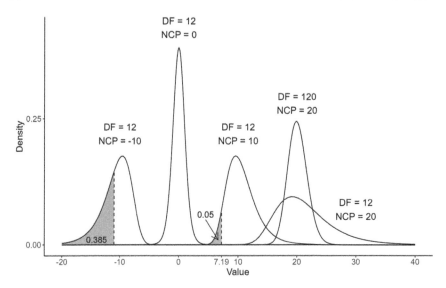

FIGURE 3.1: Density of noncentral t distributions for various degrees of freedom (DF) and noncentrality parameter (NCP) values.

We are ready to derive a formula for power. Suppose we plan to conduct a lower-tailed test with hypotheses

$$H_0: \mu \geq \mu_0 \quad \text{versus} \quad H_A: \mu < \mu_0$$

at level α. For a lower-tailed test, the critical value is $t_{\alpha, N-1}$, the $100 \times \alpha^{th}$ quantile of a $t(N-1)$ distribution. Power is the probability that the test statistic falls into the rejection region given that the alternative is true. This probability can be computed by evaluating the cdf of the $t(N-1, \lambda)$ distribution at the critical value:

$$\text{Power} = P\left[T < t_{\alpha, N-1} \mid T \sim t(N-1, \lambda)\right] \qquad (3.4)$$
$$= \mathcal{T}_{N-1, \lambda}(t_{\alpha, N-1}).$$

Figure 3.2 illustrates the relationships. In general, for a lower-tailed test, we will be interested in power for $\mu_A < \mu_0$ so $\mu_A - \mu_0$ and λ are negative. The critical value $t_{\alpha, N-1}$ will also be negative. Power is the area under the H_A density that is in the rejection region, which is the shaded area in Figure 3.2.

Power calculations for t tests can be conducted using several R functions (and other software), including functions in the **powertools** package. We use the **ttest.1samp** function to compute power in the next example and then perform the calculation step-by-step to facilitate understanding.

One-sample t test

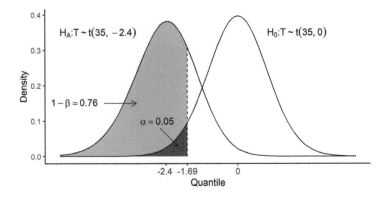

FIGURE 3.2: Power for lower-tailed one-sample t test.

Example 3.2. We repeat Example 2.2 assuming that σ will be estimated. We plan to measure hemoglobin A1c in a sample of 36 patients and conduct a lower-tailed test at $\alpha = 0.05$ of

$$H_0: \mu \geq 5.7 \quad \text{versus} \quad H_A: \mu < 5.7.$$

If the true value of σ is 2 (but will be estimated from the data) and the true population mean is 4.9, what is the power?

The ttest.1samp function in the powertools has the syntax

```
library(powertools)
ttest.1samp(N, delta, sd, alpha, power, sides)
```

The argument delta is $\mu_A - \mu_0$. To use this function, we set one of N, delta, sd, alpha or power to NULL and specify values for the other arguments. For this example,

```
ttest.1samp(N = 36, delta = 4.9 - 5.7, sd = 2, alpha = 0.05,
    power = NULL, sides = 1)
[1] 0.7606311
```

The power is about 0.76.

To facilitate understanding, we now perform the power calculation explicitly using formula (3.4). First, we create objects for the various parameters:

```
N <- 36
sigma <- 2
mu0 <- 5.7
muA <- 4.9
```

Next, we compute the critical value and value of the noncentrality parameter:

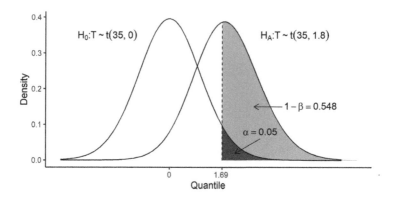

FIGURE 3.3: Power for upper-tailed one-sample t test.

```
crit <- qt(p = 0.05, df = N - 1)   ;   crit
[1] -1.689572
ncp <- (muA - mu0) * sqrt(N) / sigma   ;  ncp
[1] -2.4
```

Now we have the information needed to compute power, using the noncentral t distribution:

```
pt(q = crit, df = N - 1, ncp = ncp)
[1] 0.7606311
```

We obtain the same answer as we obtained using the function. Figure 3.2 shows the null and alternative distributions as well as the area under the alternative distribution from $-\infty$ to -1.6896, which corresponds to power.

For an upper-tailed test of

$$H_0: \mu \leq \mu_0 \quad \text{versus} \quad H_A: \mu > \mu_0,$$

the critical value is $t_{1-\alpha, N-1}$ and we reject H_0 for high values of T. Power can be calculated as

$$\begin{aligned} \text{Power} &= P\left[T > t_{1-\alpha, N-1} \mid T \sim t(N-1, \lambda)\right] \\ &= 1 - \mathcal{T}_{N-1, \lambda}(t_{1-\alpha, N-1}). \end{aligned} \quad (3.5)$$

Figure 3.3 illustrates the relationships. In general, for an upper-tailed test, we will be interested in power for $\mu_A > \mu_0$ so $\mu_A - \mu_0$ and λ are positive. The critical value $t_{1-\alpha, N-1}$ will also be positive.

One-sample t test 39

Example 3.3. Suppose we wish to test $H_0\colon \mu \leq 5.7$ versus $H_A\colon \mu > 5.7$ at $\alpha = 0.05$. If the true value of σ is 2 (and will be estimated from the data) and the true population mean is 6.3, what is the power with a sample of size 36?

First, we use the `ttest.1samp` function from the `powertools` package:

```
library(powertools)
ttest.1samp(N = 36, delta = 6.3 - 5.7, sd = 2, alpha = 0.05,
  power = NULL, sides = 1)
[1] 0.5478372
```

Power is about 0.55. To facilitate comprehension, we perform the calculation step-by-step using formula (3.5):

```
alpha <- 0.05
N <- 36
sigma <- 2
mu0 <- 5.7
muA <- 6.3
crit <- qt(p = 1 - alpha, df = N - 1)   ; crit
[1] 1.689572
ncp <- (muA - mu0) * sqrt(N) / sigma    ; ncp
[1] 1.8
# compute power:
1 - pt(q = crit, df = N - 1, ncp = ncp)
[1] 0.5478372
```

Figure 3.3 shows the null and alternative distributions as well as the area under the alternative distribution from 1.69 to $+\infty$, which corresponds to power.

In Section 2.3.1, we derived a unified expression for a one-sample one-sided z test, whether lower- or upper-tailed. Using similar logic, we can derive a **unified expression for power for a one-sided one-sample** t **test**, either lower or upper, as

$$\text{Power (one-sided one-sample } t \text{ test)} = 1 - \mathcal{T}_{N-1,|\lambda|}(t_{1-\alpha,N-1}). \qquad (3.6)$$

Example 3.4. For Example 3.2, we can also obtain power as

$$1 - \mathcal{T}_{35,|-2.4|}(1.6896) = 1 - \mathcal{T}_{35,2.4}(1.6896) = 0.7606$$

```
crit <- qt(p = 0.95, df = 35)
1 - pt(q = crit, df = 35, ncp = 2.4)
[1] 0.7606311
```

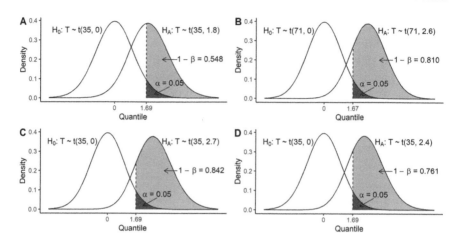

FIGURE 3.4: Factors affecting power for an upper-tailed, one-sample t test. (A) Power when $\mu_0 = 5.7$, $\mu_A = 6.3$, $\sigma = 2$ and $N = 36$. Compare to (B) $N = 72$, (C) $\mu_A = 6.6$ and (D) $\sigma = 1.5$.

3.1.3 What factors affect power?

Expression (3.6) shows that power for a one-sided, one-sample t test is a function of the significance level α, the sample size N and the noncentrality parameter $\lambda = \sqrt{N}(\mu_A - \mu_0)/\sigma$. How do each of these factors affect power?

The value of α determines the critical value, which is $t_{1-\alpha,N-1}$. If we specify a larger value for α, $t_{1-\alpha,N-1}$ decreases, the cdf value $\mathcal{T}_{N-1,|\lambda|}(t_{1-\alpha,N-1})$ decreases, and thus $1-\mathcal{T}_{N-1,|\lambda|}(t_{1-\alpha,N-1})$, which is power, increases. However, the increase in power comes at the expense of increasing the type I error rate, which may not be acceptable.

The sample size N impacts power in two ways: it affects the degrees of freedom of the test statistic (which are $N-1$) and it is a component of the noncentrality parameter, $\lambda = \sqrt{N}(\mu_A - \mu_0)/\sigma$. Figure 3.4 shows the impact on power of increasing N from 36 (Panel (A)) to 72 (Panel (B)), for Example 3.3. Due to the change in the degrees of freedom, the critical value has decreased slightly, from 1.69 to 1.67, which accounts for a small increase in power. Also due to the degrees of freedom change, the distribution of T under both the null and alternative becomes slightly less dispersed and closer to a normal distribution, which also has a small impact on power. However, by far the biggest impact on power comes from the change in the noncentrality parameter, which increases from 1.8 to 2.6, shifting the distribution of T under the alternative to the right. As a result, there is more area under the curve to the right of the critical value, increasing the power substantially.

Panel (C) of Figure 3.3 shows the effect of increasing μ_A from 6.3 to 6.6. Increasing the difference between μ_0 and μ_A increases the magnitude of the noncentrality parameter, which shifts the distribution of T under the alternative to the right, yielding a large increase in power. Panel (D) shows the effect of having a lower value of σ (1.5 rather than 2). This also increases the magnitude of the noncentrality parameter and results in increased power.

The main message is the following:

> ▶ When a power calculation involves a noncentrality parameter, parameters have their main impact on power through their effect on the noncentrality parameter. **Power increases as the magnitude of the noncentrality parameter increases.**

3.1.4 Power for two-sided tests

For a two-sided test of $H_0: \mu = \mu_0$ versus $H_A: \mu \neq \mu_0$ at level α, we reject H_0 if the test statistic $T = \frac{\bar{Y} - \mu_0}{\sqrt{s^2/N}}$ is in the lower or upper rejection region,

$$T < t_{\alpha/2, N-1} \text{ or } T > t_{1-\alpha/2, N-1}.$$

We can compute power as the sum of two tail probabilities,

$$\begin{aligned}\text{Power} &= P\left[T < t_{\alpha/2, N-1} \text{ or } T > t_{1-\alpha/2, N-1} \mid Y_i \sim \mathcal{N}(\mu_A, \sigma^2)\right] \\ &= 1 + \mathcal{T}_{N-1, \lambda}(t_{\alpha/2, N-1}) - \mathcal{T}_{N-1, \lambda}(t_{1-\alpha/2, N-1}).\end{aligned}$$

Another approach is to square the test statistic, which gives

$$T^2 = \frac{(\bar{Y} - \mu_0)^2}{s^2/N} = \frac{\left(\frac{\bar{Y} - \mu_0}{\sigma/\sqrt{N}}\right)^2}{\frac{(N-1)s^2}{(N-1)\sigma^2}} \quad (3.7)$$

where we multiplied the numerator and denominator by $(N-1)\sigma^2$ to obtain the second fraction. Under the null, the numerator and denominator have chi-square distributions with one and $N-1$ degrees of freedom, respectively, giving this statistic an $F(1, N-1)$ distribution:

$$T^2 = \frac{[\mathcal{N}(0,1)]^2}{\frac{\chi^2(N-1)}{N-1}} \sim F(1, N-1). \quad (3.8)$$

What is the distribution of T^2 when an alternative $\mu = \mu_A$ is true? Squaring (3.3), we have

$$\frac{\left[\mathcal{N}\left(\frac{\mu_A - \mu_0}{\sigma/\sqrt{N}}, 1\right)\right]^2}{\frac{\chi^2(N-1)}{N-1}} \quad (3.9)$$

The numerator is the square of a normal random variable with a nonzero mean and variance 1, which has a distribution called a **noncentral χ^2 distribution**.

When a noncentral chi-square is divided by a "central" chi-square and the two are independent, we obtain the **noncentral F distribution**.

Noncentral χ^2 and F distributions

Let $X_i, i = 1, \ldots, \nu$, be independent random variables distributed as $\mathcal{N}(\lambda_i, 1)$. A random variable of the form

$$\sum_{i=1}^{\nu} X_i^2$$

has a noncentral chi-square distribution with ν df and noncentrality parameter $\Lambda = \sum_{i=1}^{\nu} \lambda_i^2$. We denote this as $\chi^2(\nu, \Lambda)$. The standard "central" χ^2 distribution is the special case of $\Lambda = 0$, which occurs when all of the X_i are $\mathcal{N}(0, 1)$.

A random variable of the form

$$\frac{\chi^2(\nu_1, \Lambda)/\nu_1}{\chi^2(\nu_2)/\nu_2}$$

with a $\chi^2(\nu_1, \Lambda)$ in the numerator, $\chi^2(\nu_2)$ in the denominator, and the numerator and denominator independent, has a noncentral F distribution with ν_1 and ν_2 degrees of freedom and noncentrality parameter Λ, denoted $F(\nu_1, \nu_2, \Lambda)$. The noncentrality parameter for the F distribution corresponds to the noncentrality parameter for the χ^2 distribution in the numerator. We denote the cumulative noncentral F distribution as $\mathcal{F}_{\nu_1, \nu_2, \Lambda}$.

Figure 3.5 provides examples of noncentral χ^2 and F distributions. For the noncentral χ^2, increases in ν or Λ shift the distribution to the right. For the noncentral F, increases in ν_2 or Λ shift the distribution to the right. Increases in these parameter values also make the distributions more symmetric.

Now we know that the distribution of T^2 under $H_0: \mu = \mu_0$ is $F(1, N-1)$ and under an alternative specifying $\mu = \mu_A$ is $F(1, N-1, \Lambda)$, where $\Lambda = \frac{N(\mu_A - \mu_0)^2}{\sigma^2}$. To compute power, we also need the critical value. Noting that the square of a $t(\nu)$ random variable has an $F(1, \nu)$ distribution, the critical value is the F quantile $f_{1-\alpha, 1, N-1}$. Now we can calculate power for the two-sided one-sample t test as

$$\begin{aligned}
\text{Power (two-sided one-sample } t \text{ test)} \quad &(3.10)\\
= P[T^2 > f_{1-\alpha, 1, N-1} \mid T^2 \sim F(1, N-1, \Lambda)]&\\
= 1 - P[T^2 < f_{1-\alpha, 1, N-1} \mid T^2 \sim F(1, N-1, \Lambda)]&\\
= 1 - \mathcal{F}_{1, N-1, \Lambda}(f_{1-\alpha, 1, N-1}).&
\end{aligned}$$

One-sample t test

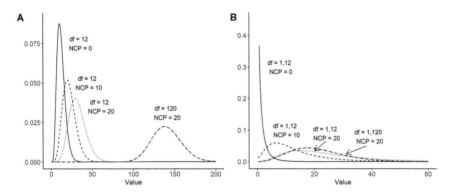

FIGURE 3.5: Examples of (A) noncentral χ^2 distributions and (B) F distributions.

The test is an upper-tailed test. Figure 3.6 depicts the relationships, which are further explained in the next example.

Example 3.5. Suppose we plan to conduct a two-sided test of H_0: $\mu = 5.7$ versus H_A: $\mu \neq 5.7$ at α of 0.05. The true mean is assumed to be $\mu_A = 4.9$ and the standard deviation is assumed to be $\sigma = 2$ and will be estimated. What is the power?

As depicted in Figure 3.6, under H_0, $T^2 \sim F(1, 35)$ and under H_A, $T^2 \sim F(1, 35, \Lambda)$ with $\Lambda = \frac{N(\mu_A - \mu_0)^2}{\sigma^2} = 5.76$. The critical value is $f_{0.95, 1, 35} = 4.1213$. Power is $P(T^2 > 4.1213) = 1 - \mathcal{F}_{1,35,5.76}(4.1213) \approx 0.646$. We can use the ttest.1samp function to conduct the calculation:

```
library(powertools)
ttest.1samp(N = 36, delta = 4.9 - 5.7, sd = 2, alpha = 0.05,
    power = NULL, sides = 2)
[1] 0.6457332
```

Power is about 0.65.

The following R code performs the calculation explicitly and is provided to facilitate understanding:

```
# The default for qf and pf is lower.tail = TRUE; specify
# lower.tail = FALSE to get upper-tail quantile and probability.

N <- 36
sigma <- 2
mu0 <- 5.7
muA <- 4.9
crit <- qf(p = 0.05, df1 = 1, df2 = N - 1, lower.tail = FALSE) ; crit
[1] 4.121338
```

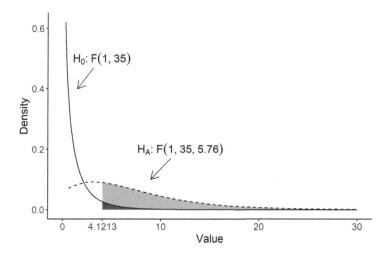

FIGURE 3.6: The $F(1, 35)$ density (solid line) and the $F(1, 35, 5.76)$ density (dashed line). For α of 0.05, the critical value is 4.1213. Shaded areas depict the type I error region (dark grey) and power (light plus dark grey).

```
ncp <- (muA - mu0) * sqrt(N) / sigma   ; ncp^2
[1] 5.76
pf(q = crit, df1 = 1, df2 = N - 1, ncp = ncp^2, lower.tail = FALSE)
[1] 0.6457332
```

What factors affect power? Power for a two-sided, one-sample t test is given in equation (3.10). Power is a function of α, N and Λ. As α increases, the critical value decreases and power is higher, but at the expense of increased type I error rate. Power increases as the degrees of freedom $N-1$ or $\Lambda = \frac{N(\mu_A - \mu_0)^2}{\sigma^2}$ increase.

3.1.5 Sample size for a one-sample t test

In Section 2.3.5, we found the sample size required to achieve a desired level of power for a lower-tailed, one-sample z test by setting $1-\beta \leq \Phi\left(z_\alpha + \frac{|\mu_A - \mu_0|}{\sigma/\sqrt{N}}\right)$ and solving for N. To find the sample size for a lower-tailed, one-sample t test, we might think to start with the equation

$$1 - \beta \leq \mathcal{T}_{N-1, \lambda}\left(t_{\alpha, N-1}\right)$$

where $\lambda = \sqrt{N}(\mu_A - \mu_0)/\sigma$ and solve for N. However, N is involved in the degrees of freedom and the noncentrality parameter of the noncentral t distribution as well as the quantile $t_{\alpha, N-1}$, and as a result there is no closed-form

One-sample t test

solution for N. There are two options for finding N. One option is to use software that uses numerical methods to solve for N. This will give us an "exact" solution. The other option is to use the one-sample z test formula to get an approximation of the required N. Using this normal approximation to the t distribution, the required sample size for a one-sided, one-sample t test at significance level α is

$$N \geq \frac{(z_{1-\beta} + z_{1-\alpha})^2 \sigma^2}{(\mu_0 - \mu_A)^2} = \frac{(z_{1-\beta} + z_{1-\alpha})^2}{d^2} \qquad (3.11)$$

For a two-sided test at level α, replace $z_{1-\alpha}$ with $z_{1-\alpha/2}$. This formula will tend to underestimate the required N. It has been suggested that adding a factor of $\frac{1}{2}z_{1-\alpha}^2$ ($\frac{1}{2}z_{1-\alpha/2}^2$ for a two-sided test) improves the approximation [80, 111]. However, when software that conducts the calculation using t distributions is readily available, it is prudent to use it to get a more accurate solution for N. We compare the required sample size computed using the normal approximation and the "exact" t distribution method in the following example.

Example 3.6. Suppose we want to find the number of participants needed for a study to have 80% power to detect an effect size of $d = 0.6$ when planning to conduct a lower-tailed, one-sample t test with $\alpha = 0.05$. Using the normal approximation sample size formula (3.11), which is equivalent to using a z test approach, we compute

```
library(powertools)
ztest.1samp(N = NULL, delta = 0.6, sd = 1, alpha = 0.05, power = 0.8,
    sides = 1)
[1] 17.17377
```

$N \approx 17.17$, which rounds up to 18 participants. We can compute the sample size requirement more precisely using software that uses t distributions:

```
library(powertools)
ttest.1samp(N = NULL, delta = 0.6, sd = 1, alpha = 0.05, power = 0.8,
    sides = 1)
[1] 18.60377
```

The required sample size is 18.60, which we should round up to 19 participants to ensure that the power is at least 80%. The normal approximation formula was reasonably close but underestimated the required N.

The example used a handy trick that was introduced in Section 2.7; the functions ask for both the mean difference and the standard deviation as inputs, but we were able to input a standardized mean effect size by specifying the mean difference as 0.6 (d) and the standard deviation as 1.

3.2 Two independent samples t test

The two-sample t test is used to test hypotheses about the difference between the means of two independent groups. The general framework for power calculation is the same as for a one-sample t test. However, when comparing two groups, there are additional factors to consider, including the relative sample sizes of the two groups and whether the two groups have equal or unequal variances, as well as the relative sizes of the variances if they are unequal. We begin with the case of equal variances.

3.2.1 Equal variances

For the two independent samples t test with equal variances, we assume we have normally distributed observations from two groups that have different means but the same variance, $Y_{i1} \sim \mathcal{N}(\mu_1, \sigma^2)$ and $Y_{i2} \sim \mathcal{N}(\mu_2, \sigma^2)$, with group sizes of n_1 and n_2 for a total sample size of $n_1 + n_2 = N$. Suppose we would like to conduct a lower-tailed test of the form

$$H_0: \mu_1 - \mu_2 \geq \Delta_0 \quad \text{versus} \quad H_A: \mu_1 - \mu_2 < \Delta_0.$$

Setting $\Delta_0 = 0$ corresponds to testing $H_0: \mu_1 \geq \mu_2$ versus $H_A: \mu_1 < \mu_2$. We estimate the common variance σ^2 using the pooled estimate

$$s_p^2 = \frac{(n_1 - 1)s_1^2 + (n_2 - 1)s_2^2}{n_1 + n_2 - 2}$$

that combines the sample variances s_1^2 and s_2^2. The test statistic is

$$T = \frac{\bar{Y}_1 - \bar{Y}_2 - \Delta_0}{s_p \sqrt{\frac{1}{n_1} + \frac{1}{n_2}}} = \sqrt{\frac{n_1 n_2}{n_1 + n_2}} \left(\frac{\bar{Y}_1 - \bar{Y}_2 - \Delta_0}{s_p} \right). \qquad (3.12)$$

To derive a formula for power, we need the distribution of the test statistic when H_0 is true and when an alternative about the mean difference is true. We can find that these distributions are (using an approach similar to that in Section 3.1):

$$\mu_1 - \mu_2 = \Delta_0: T \sim t(N - 2)$$
$$\mu_1 - \mu_2 = \Delta_A: T \sim t(N - 2, \lambda)$$

where

$$\lambda = \sqrt{\frac{n_1 n_2}{n_1 + n_2}} \left(\frac{\Delta_A - \Delta_0}{\sigma} \right). \qquad (3.13)$$

In a two-group randomized study, we often describe the allocation of participants to groups using the ratio of the sample sizes, $r = n_2/n_1$, called the **allocation ratio**. For example, when assigning participants to groups 2 and 1 with a 3:1 ratio, $r = 3$, $n_2 = 3n_1$ and $N = 4n_1$. We can express the noncentrality parameter using r and N as

$$\lambda = \sqrt{N\frac{r}{(1+r)^2}} \left(\frac{\Delta_A - \Delta_0}{\sigma}\right).$$

Another approach is to specify the proportion of observations that are assigned to each group. If we allocate a proportion $w \in (0,1)$ to group 1 and a proportion $1 - w$ to group 2, then $n_1 = Nw$ and $n_2 = N(1-w)$ and the noncentrality parameter becomes

$$\lambda = \sqrt{Nw(1-w)} \left(\frac{\Delta_A - \Delta_0}{\sigma}\right). \tag{3.14}$$

The box below provides formulas for converting between allocation ratio and proportion. Note that some authors or software may define the allocation ratio as n_1/n_2 so be sure to check definitions.

Converting between allocation ratio and proportion. When the allocation ratio is $r = n_2/n_1$, the proportions that are assigned to groups 1 and 2 are

$$w = \frac{1}{1+r} \quad \text{and} \quad 1 - w = \frac{r}{1+r}, \tag{3.15}$$

respectively, with $n_1 = \frac{N}{r+1}$ and $n_2 = \frac{Nr}{1+r}$. Note that

$$w(1-w) = \frac{r}{(1+r)^2}$$

and $r = (1-w)/w$.

When the group sizes are equal, $n_1 = n_2 = n$, $w = 0.5$, $r = 1$, and the noncentrality parameter simplifies to

$$\lambda = \sqrt{\frac{n}{2}}\left(\frac{\Delta_A - \Delta_0}{\sigma}\right) = \sqrt{\frac{N}{4}}\left(\frac{\Delta_A - \Delta_0}{\sigma}\right) \tag{3.16}$$

with total sample size $N = 2n$.

The **standardized effect size** $d = \frac{\mu_1 - \mu_2}{\sigma}$ is often used to quantify the difference between two means in a two-sample t test. This is the difference in means expressed in units of standard deviations. Standardized mean effect sizes were introduced in Section 2.4. When $\Delta_0 = 0$, the noncentrality parameter becomes $\lambda = d\sqrt{\frac{n_1 n_2}{n_1 + n_2}}$. For equal sized groups, $\lambda = d\sqrt{n/2} = d\sqrt{N/4}$.

Power can be found as the probability that the test statistic T falls into the rejection region given that $T \sim t(N - 2, \lambda)$. For lower-tailed, upper-tailed and two-sided tests, power can be calculated as

$$\text{Power (lower-tail test)} = P[T \leq t_{\alpha,N-2} \mid T \sim t(N-2,\lambda)] \quad (3.17)$$
$$= \mathcal{T}_{N-2,\lambda}(t_{\alpha,N-2})$$
$$\text{Power (upper-tail test)} = P[T \geq t_{1-\alpha,N-2} \mid T \sim t(N-2,\lambda)]$$
$$= 1 - \mathcal{T}_{N-2,\lambda}(t_{1-\alpha,N-2})$$
$$\text{Power (two-sided test)} = P[T^2 \geq f_{1-\alpha,1,N-2} \mid T^2 \sim F(1, N-2, \Lambda)]$$
$$= 1 - \mathcal{F}_{1,N-2,\Lambda}(f_{1-\alpha,1,N-2}).$$

where $\Lambda = \lambda^2$. A unified expression for power for a one-sided test, either lower- or upper-tailed, is

$$\text{Power (one-sided test)} = 1 - \mathcal{T}_{N-2,|\lambda|}(t_{1-\alpha,N-2}). \quad (3.18)$$

What factors affect power? By inspecting power formulas (3.17) and (3.18), we can see that power depends on the total sample size N, the magnitude of the noncentrality parameter λ, and the significance level α. As N increases, the degrees of freedom increase and the magnitude of λ also increases; both have the effect of increasing power. We can inspect λ to see how its other components affect its magnitude. Power increases as the magnitude of the difference $\Delta_A - \Delta_0$ increases or as σ decreases. The relative sizes of the two groups, n_1 and n_2, will also affect power; this is discussed in Section 3.2.4. As α increases, the critical value will shift to enlarge the rejection region and power will be higher; however, this will be at the expense of a higher type I error rate, which may not be acceptable.

Example 3.7. Suppose we wish to test $H_0: \mu_1 - \mu_2 \geq 0$ versus $H_A: \mu_1 - \mu_2 < 0$ at significance level 0.05 with sample sizes $n_1 = n_2 = 50$. We are interested in power when $\mu_1 - \mu_2 = 2$ and the true value of σ is thought to be 5.

In the ttest.2samp function, delta is $\Delta_A - \Delta_0$, which in this example is $2 - 0 = 2$. n1 is the sample size for group 1; by default, equal group sizes are assumed (nratio = 1). For a one-sided test, the power can be calculated as follows:

```
library(powertools)
ttest.2samp(n1 = 50, delta = 2, sd1 = 5, alpha = 0.05, power = NULL,
    sides = 1)
[1] 0.633565
```

For a two-sided test at the same significance level, power is substantially lower:

```
ttest.2samp(n1 = 50, delta = 2, sd1 = 5, alpha = 0.05, power = NULL,
    sides = 2)
[1] 0.5081857
```

Suppose that the hypotheses are instead H_0: $\mu_1 - \mu_2 \geq 1$ versus H_A: $\mu_1 - \mu_2 < 1$, that is, the mean difference under the null Δ_0 is 1. In this case, we specify delta as $\Delta_A - \Delta_0 = 2 - 1 = 1$:

```
ttest.2samp(n1 = 50, delta = 1, sd1 = 5, alpha = 0.05, power = NULL,
   sides = 1)
[1] 0.2572805
```

The power dropped from 0.63 to 0.26 because $\Delta_A - \Delta_0$ dropped from 2 to 1.

How does unequal allocation affect power? We discuss this topic in Section 3.2.4.

3.2.2 Unequal variances (Welch's t test)

The Welch's unequal variances t test [226] allows for the two groups to have unequal variances. The test statistic is

$$T = \frac{\bar{Y}_1 - \bar{Y}_2 - \Delta_0}{\sqrt{\frac{s_1^2}{n_1} + \frac{s_2^2}{n_2}}} \qquad (3.19)$$

where s_1^2 and s_2^2 are the sample variances for groups 1 and 2. One might ask, when designing a randomized trial, when might we design it assuming that the eventual analysis will use an unequal variances t test rather than an equal variances t test? If participants are randomized to groups, should we expect that the variances of the outcome in the two groups will be the same? Not necessarily. If the two groups experience different conditions, then the variance of the outcome in the two groups could be different. For example, in some studies, it might be sensible to assume that the variance will be higher in the intervention group than in the usual care control group because individuals may respond to the intervention condition in a variety of different ways.

When H_0 is true, the test statistic T in equation (3.19) has a t distribution with degrees of freedom given by the Welch-Satterthwaite formula [194, 226],

$$\frac{\left(\frac{\sigma_1^2}{n_1} + \frac{\sigma_2^2}{n_2}\right)^2}{\frac{\left(\frac{\sigma_1^2}{n_1}\right)^2}{n_1 - 1} + \frac{\left(\frac{\sigma_2^2}{n_2}\right)^2}{n_2 - 1}}. \qquad (3.20)$$

When the test is conducted, the variances are unknown and the degrees of freedom are approximated by substituting the sample variances for the unknown population variances.

Under a specific alternative $\mu_1 - \mu_2 = \Delta_A$, T has a noncentral t distribution with noncentrality parameter

$$\lambda = \frac{\Delta_A - \Delta_0}{\sqrt{\frac{\sigma_1^2}{n_1} + \frac{\sigma_2^2}{n_2}}} = \sqrt{N \frac{r}{(1+r)(r\sigma_1^2 + \sigma_2^2)}} (\Delta_A - \Delta_0) \tag{3.21}$$

and degrees of freedom given by (3.20). When the group sizes are equal ($n_1 = n_2 = n$), λ simplifies to

$$\lambda = \sqrt{\frac{n}{\sigma_1^2 + \sigma_2^2}} (\Delta_A - \Delta_0) \tag{3.22}$$

and when the variances are also equal, we get $\lambda = \sqrt{\frac{n}{2}} \left(\frac{\Delta_A - \Delta_0}{\sigma}\right)$, as in (3.16).

Rather than specify the variances for each group, we could specify the variance for one group and the ratio of the two variances, or the standard deviation for one group and the ratio of the standard deviations. Define the ratio of the standard deviations as $f = \sigma_2/\sigma_1$. Then

$$\lambda = \sqrt{N \frac{r}{(r+1)(r+f^2)}} \left(\frac{\Delta_A - \Delta_0}{\sigma_1}\right). \tag{3.23}$$

Power can be approximated using this formula for λ in power formulas (3.17), with the Welch-Satterthwaite degrees of freedom (3.20) substituted for $N - 2$.

Example 3.8. Suppose we wish to compute power for a two-sample t test with hypotheses $H_0\colon \mu_1 - \mu_2 \geq 0$ versus $H_A\colon \mu_1 - \mu_2 < 0$ at level 0.025. We specify a true mean difference of $\Delta_A = \mu_1 - \mu_2 = 3$. The variance in group 1, the usual care group, is expected to be $\sigma_1 = 4$. The variance in the intervention group, group 2, is expected to be higher, with $\sigma_2 = 6$. If the group sizes are $n_1 = 25$ and $n_2 = 75$, what is the power?

In the function ttest.2samp, n1 is the sample size for group 1, n.ratio is n_2/n_1 and sd.ratio is σ_2/σ_1. The function computes power and sample size for a Welch's (unequal variances) t test by default.

```
library(powertools)
ttest.2samp(n1 = 25, n.ratio = 3, delta = 3, sd1 = 4, sd.ratio = 1.5,
    alpha = 0.025, power = NULL, sides = 1)
[1] 0.7969349
```

3.2.3 Sample size using normal approximation

Echoing our discussion in Section 3.1 for the one-sample t test, we cannot get closed-form solutions for sample size for a two-sample t test by solving the power formulas for sample size because the group sizes determine the degrees of freedom and the noncentrality parameter in these formulas. Thus we do not know what degrees of freedom to use unless we know the group sizes, but that is what we want to solve for.

For relatively large N, the normal approximation to the t distribution can provide an estimate of the required sample size. The normal approximation is equivalent to using a two-sample z test, which assumes the variances are known. The z test formulas are helpful for understanding how various factors affect the sample size requirement, and so we provide them here. However, we recommend using the more accurate t-based formulas, implemented in software, for calculations.

The normal approximation-based sample size formula for total sample size N for a two-sided, two-sample t test to provide power of $1 - \beta$ with type 1 error rate α is

$$N \geq \frac{(z_{1-\alpha/2} + z_{1-\beta})^2}{(\Delta_A - \Delta_0)^2} \left(\frac{r+1}{r}\right)(r\sigma_1^2 + \sigma_2^2). \qquad (3.24)$$

When specifying a standard deviation ratio, the last term becomes $(r+f^2)\sigma_1^2$. When we have equal variances, the formula is

$$N \geq \frac{(z_{1-\alpha/2} + z_{1-\beta})^2}{(\Delta_A - \Delta_0)^2} \frac{(r+1)^2 \sigma^2}{r}. \qquad (3.25)$$

For a one-sided test, use $z_{1-\alpha}$ rather than $z_{1-\alpha/2}$.

Example 3.9. Suppose that we wish to determine the sample size needed to detect a medium effect size of $d = 0.5$ for a two-sample t test with equal allocation, with 80% power in a two-sided test with $\alpha = 0.05$. Using the normal approximation approach, which is implemented by the ztest.2samp function, the total N needed is approximately:

```
library(powertools)
ztest.2samp(n1 = NULL, n.ratio = 1, delta = 0.5, sd1 = 1, alpha = 0.05,
    power = 0.8, sides = 2)
[1] 62.79088
```

We round this up to 63 in each group, suggesting that we need a total of 126 subjects. We can calculate a more accurate sample size requirement using a t-based calculation:

```
library(powertools)
ttest.2samp(n1 = NULL, n.ratio = 1, delta = 0.5, sd1 = 1, alpha = 0.05,
    power = 0.8, sides = 2)
[1] 63.76561
```

Rounding up, we need 64 in each group, for a total of 128 subjects. The normal approximation slightly underestimates the required sample size.

3.2.4 How does allocation affect power?

While many randomized trials allocate equal numbers of participants to each group, there are several reasons why unequal allocation might be chosen. Reasons include patient preference (patients may be more likely to participate if the chance of being assigned in the experimental arm is higher), cost (one condition may be less costly than the other), a desire for increased data on safety or other outcomes in the experimental condition, or an expectation of higher dropout rates in one condition compared to the other [60, 81]. In most trials with unequal allocation, more patients are assigned to the experimental condition, but sometimes more are assigned to the control condition.

How does allocation ratio affect power? First, we consider the case of equal group variances. Recall that power increases as the magnitude of λ increases. When the group variances are equal, λ is

$$\lambda = \sqrt{N\frac{r}{(1+r)^2}}\left(\frac{\Delta_A - \Delta_0}{\sigma}\right) = \sqrt{Nw(1-w)}\left(\frac{\Delta_A - \Delta_0}{\sigma}\right).$$

For N and other parameters fixed, the magnitude of λ is maximized when the function $f(r) = r/(1+r)^2$ is maximized, which occurs when $r = 1$, that is, equal allocation. Equivalently, power will be highest when $f(w) = w(1-w)$ is maximized, which occurs when $w = 0.5$, which is equal allocation. This can be proven by using derivatives to find the maximum of the function.

How do imbalances in group sample sizes affect power? We explore this in the following example.

Example 3.10. Suppose we have a fixed total sample size of 120 for a two-arm trial comparing means. If $d = 0.5$ and $\alpha = 0.05$ two-sided, what is the power associated with different allocation ratios? Equal variances is assumed.

We can produce a plot of power versus r for a range of different allocation ratios using this code:

```
library(powertools)
r <- seq(from = 1/3, to = 3, by = 0.1)
power <- sapply(r, function(x)
    ttest.2samp(n1 = 120 / (1 + x), n.ratio = x, delta = 0.5, sd1 = 1,
        sd.ratio = 1, alpha = 0.05, sides = 2, v = T)$power)
plot(r, power, type = "l")
```

A version of this figure is presented in Figure 3.7. The curve is asymmetric; this is because power for r of 2, i.e., $(n_1, n_2) = (40, 80)$ is equal to power for r of $1/2$, i.e., $(n_1, n_2) = (80, 40)$. Highest power is obtained with $r = 1$, equal allocation. However, small imbalances in group sizes have minimal impacts on power. Larger imbalances have a more appreciable impact on power, but this might be a reasonable tradeoff if unequal allocation enhances other study objectives, e.g., enticing more participants to enroll in the study by offering a

Two independent samples t test

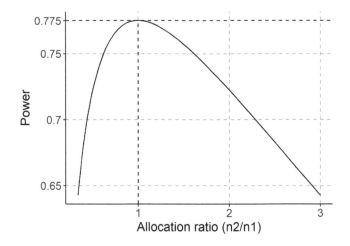

FIGURE 3.7: Power as a function of allocation ratio for Example 3.10, an equal variances scenario.

higher probability of receiving the experimental treatment or accruing a larger sample of intervention participants to support secondary analyses or analysis of safety endpoints.

When the group variances are unequal, the noncentrality parameter is

$$\lambda = \sqrt{N\frac{r}{(r+1)(r+f^2)}}\left(\frac{\Delta_A - \Delta_0}{\sigma_1}\right)$$

where $f = \sigma_2/\sigma_1$ is the standard deviation ratio. In this case, the allocation that maximizes power is $n_2/n_1 = \sigma_2/\sigma_1$; that is, power is maximized when the ratio of the sample sizes equals the ratio of the population standard deviations ($r = f$), with more participants in the group with higher variance (again, this can be shown using calculus). If we are specifying the fraction w in group 1, power is maximized when $w = 1/(1+f)$.

Example 3.11. In Example 3.8, the standard deviation ratio was $f = 1.5$. Figure 3.8 displays power as a function of the allocation ratio for this example. Highest power is achieved when the allocation ratio equals the standard deviation ratio. However, power is not sensitive to small deviations from the optimal allocation ratio.

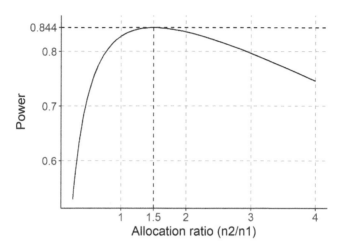

FIGURE 3.8: Power as a function of allocation ratio for Example 3.11, an unequal variances scenario.

3.3 Relative efficiency

Suppose that our parameter of interest is θ (for example, θ might be the difference in means between two conditions) and we are comparing two different study designs, A and B, to estimate the parameter. Let $\hat{\theta}_A$ and $\hat{\theta}_B$ denote the estimators of θ under the two designs and let $Var(\hat{\theta}_A)$ and $Var(\hat{\theta}_B)$ denote the variances of these estimators. The **relative efficiency** of Design A compared to Design B is defined as

$$\text{RE(A, B)} = \frac{1/Var(\hat{\theta}_A)}{1/Var(\hat{\theta}_B)} = \frac{Var(\hat{\theta}_B)}{Var(\hat{\theta}_A)}. \qquad (3.26)$$

If $Var(\hat{\theta}_A) < Var(\hat{\theta}_B)$, then $\text{RE}(\hat{\theta}_A, \hat{\theta}_B) > 1$ and A is a more efficient design than B.

In many cases, the relative efficiency of two designs is equal to the ratio of the sample sizes required to achieve the same power under the two designs, that is, $\text{RE}(\hat{\theta}_A, \hat{\theta}_B) = N_B/N_A$. This will be true when $Var(\hat{\theta}) \propto 1/N$ for A and B. This is the case for many normal approximation-based sample size formulas, such as those for a two-sample t test in Section 3.2.3. We illustrate in the following example.

Example 3.12. Suppose our estimator of interest is the difference of means, $\theta = \mu_1 - \mu_2$. We plan to estimate θ using a two independent group design with a total sample size of N, and we want to compare designs that use different allocations to the two groups. Assuming equal variances, $Var(\hat{\theta}) = \sigma^2 \left(\frac{1}{n_1} + \frac{1}{n_2} \right) = \frac{\sigma^2}{N} \frac{(1+r)^2}{r}$, where $N = n_1 + n_2$ and $r = n_2/n_1$. The relative efficiency of two designs using different allocations, r_A and r_B, with the same total N is

$$\text{RE}(\hat{\theta}_A, \hat{\theta}_B) = \frac{Var(\hat{\theta}_B)}{Var(\hat{\theta}_A)} = \left(\frac{1+r_B}{1+r_A} \right)^2 \frac{r_A}{r_B}.$$

Using normal approximation-based sample size formula (3.24), the ratio of the sample sizes required to achieve the same power is

$$\frac{N_B}{N_A} = \left(\frac{1+r_B}{1+r_A} \right)^2 \frac{r_A}{r_B} = \text{RE}(\hat{\theta}_A, \hat{\theta}_B).$$

For example, comparing 1:1 to 2:1 allocation ($r_A = 1$ and $r_B = 2$), RE is 1.125; Design A is 12.5% more efficient than Design B. Further, $N_B = 1.125 N_A$, so we need 12.5% more subjects for Design B compared to Design A in order to achieve the same power.

Higher efficiency is usually a desirable property of a study design. However, in some studies, the increase in overall sample size due to using a less efficient design might be acceptable if the less efficient design helps to achieve other objectives, e.g., lower cost or faster accrual of participants due to a higher probability of receiving the experimental rather than the standard treatment.

3.3.1 Remarks on estimating the d effect size from prior data

Often, to perform power or sample size calculations, we use effect size estimates calculated from data from prior studies to inform our calculations. For example, to estimate the Cohen d effect size from a two-group study, we may use the formula

$$\hat{d} = \frac{\bar{Y}_1 - \bar{Y}_2}{\sqrt{\frac{(n_1-1)s_1^2 + (n_2-1)s_2^2}{n_1+n_2-2}}}.$$

However, this formula gives an upwardly biased estimate of the population effect size [84], meaning that it overestimates the true effect size, especially for small samples. A corrected effect size estimate called Hedges's g [84] has been shown to be unbiased for the true d effect size [46]:

$$g = \hat{d} \left(1 - \frac{3}{4(n_1 + n_2) - 9} \right).$$

See [132] for more discussion.

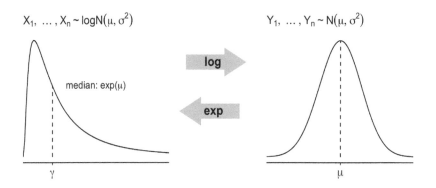

FIGURE 3.9: Relationship between the lognormal and normal distributions. $X_1, \ldots, X_n$ are on the original scale and the log-transformed values are $Y_1 = \log(X_1), \ldots, Y_n = \log(X_n)$. The median on the original scale corresponds to the mean on the log-transformed scale.

3.4 Lognormal data

In many studies, the outcome variables are right-skewed and become approximately normal when log-transformed. In these cases, the log-transformed observations better satisfy the normality assumption of the t test, and a t test may be used to compare the means of the log-transformed data. Log transformations are commonly used on pharmacokinetic data, for example [32]. Unless noted otherwise, log in this text refers to the natural logarithm, which has base e.

Consider a sample of observations $X_1, \ldots, X_n$. If the log-transformed observations, $Y_1 = \log(X_1), \ldots, Y_n = \log(X_n)$, are distributed $\mathcal{N}(\mu, \sigma^2)$, then the observations on the original scale, $X_1, \ldots, X_n$, have a **lognormal distribution** with parameters μ and σ^2, which we denote $log\mathcal{N}(\mu, \sigma^2)$. Figure 3.9 shows the relationship between the lognormal and normal distributions. For the normal distribution, the mean is also the median, and exponentiating μ yields the median of the corresponding lognormal distribution, which we denote as γ; $\gamma = \exp(\mu)$. γ is also the geometric mean of the lognormal distribution. We will generally refer to γ as the median. A lognormal distribution is often characterized by its median, $\gamma = \exp(\mu)$, and its coefficient of variation (CV), which is equal to $\sqrt{\exp(\sigma^2) - 1}$. The **coefficient of variation** of a random variable X is the ratio of its standard deviation to its arithmetic mean, $SD(X)/E(X)$. It is a measure of the variability of X expressed in relation to its mean and is often expressed as a percent, $\%CV = 100\% \, SD(X)/E(X)$.

Lognormal data

For lognormal data, if we have a null hypothesis comparing the means of the log-transformed observations for two groups,

$$H_0: \mu_1 - \mu_2 = \Delta_0$$

we can get back to the original scale by exponentiating,

$$\exp(\mu_1 - \mu_2) = \exp(\Delta_0)$$
$$\frac{\exp(\mu_1)}{\exp(\mu_2)} = k_0$$
$$\frac{\gamma_1}{\gamma_2} = k_0$$

where γ_1 and γ_2 are the medians of the two groups on the original scale and $k_0 = \exp(\Delta_0)$ is the null value of the ratio of the medians. Thus a test of the difference in means on the log-transformed scale is a test of the ratio of the medians on the original scale. A typical null hypothesis might specify $\Delta_0 = 0$, in which case $k_0 = \exp(0) = 1$. This corresponds to a null hypothesis that $\gamma_1 = \gamma_2$. A value $k_0 = 1.5$ represents a null hypothesis that γ_1 is 50% higher than γ_2, that is, the median in group 1 is 50% higher than the median in group 2.

> ▶ **Hypothesis tests on log-transformed data:** For lognormal data, a test of the difference in means $\mu_1 - \mu_2$ on the log-transformed scale corresponds to a test of the ratio of the medians γ_1/γ_2 on the original scale.

Power and sample size calculations for comparing means of log-transformed data can be conducted using standard formulas for comparing means. However, sometimes, rather than having the expected values of μ_1, μ_2, σ_1^2 and σ_2^2 for the log-transformed data, we may have information on the expected medians and CVs of the outcome variable on the original scale. In this case, we need to convert:

$$\mu_1 = \log(\gamma_1), \, \mu_2 = \log(\gamma_2), \, \Delta_A = \mu_1 - \mu_2$$
$$\sigma_1^2 = \log(CV_1^2 + 1), \, \sigma_2^2 = \log(CV_2^2 + 1)$$
$$\Delta_0 = \log(k_0)$$

Then we can use these values in a power function designed for t tests.

Example 3.13. The elimination half-life of a compound is the time for its plasma concentration to fall by one-half. Suppose that elimination half-life is right-skewed, such that when we log-transform the values, the data are approximately normal. We plan a study that hopes to conclude that the median elimination half-life of Compound 1 is longer than that of Compound 2. This corresponds to the hypotheses

$$H_0: \gamma_1/\gamma_2 \leq 1 \quad \text{versus} \quad H_A: \gamma_1/\gamma_2 > 1.$$

Based on prior studies, Compound 2 has a median half-life of 20 hours and CV of 0.8. Assuming that the true half-life of Compound 1 is 25% longer than that of Compound 2, what is the sample size required to achieve 80% power for a study with equal allocation and one-sided α of 0.025?

To conduct the sample size calculation, we need to get the parameters for the normally distributed, log-transformed data. We assume equal CVs.

```
gamma2 <- 20
gamma1 <- 1.25 * gamma2   ;  gamma1
[1] 25
mu1 <- log(gamma1) ; mu1
[1] 3.218876
mu2 <- log(gamma2) ; mu2
[1] 2.995732
Delta_A <- mu1 - mu2 ; Delta_A
[1] 0.2231436
```

The difference in means on the log-transformed scale is about 0.223. Now we get the standard deviation on the log-transformed scale:

```
cv <- 0.8
sd <- sqrt(log(0.8^2 + 1)) ; sd
[1] 0.7033465
```

The standard deviation on the log-transformed scale is about 0.703. We use these values in the function:

```
library(powertools)
ttest.2samp(n1 = NULL, delta = 0.223, sd1 = 0.703, power = 0.8,
   alpha = 0.025, sides = 1)
[1] 156.9712
```

We need 157 subjects in each group. Note that the standardized effect size is $0.2232/0.7033 \approx 0.32$, which is relatively small.

3.5 Paired t test

In a paired-sample design, measurements are taken from each individual under two different conditions. For example, one measurement may be taken under a control condition and the other under an intervention condition. Paired samples may also arise from measurements on pairs of individuals who were matched on some criteria, such as age and sex, but experience different conditions. The paired t test is used to test hypotheses about the difference between two means when the observations are paired.

Let N denote the number of pairs and let Y_{i1} and Y_{i2} represent the observations taken under different conditions for pair i. For each pair, we calculate the difference, $d_i = Y_{i1} - Y_{i2}$. Hypotheses in a paired t test involve the difference in means between conditions, $\mu_d = \mu_1 - \mu_2$. Hypotheses for a two-sided test take the form

$$H_0: \mu_d = \Delta_0 \quad \text{versus} \quad H_A: \mu_d \neq \Delta_0$$

where Δ_0 is often equal to zero. The test procedure is the same as for a one-sample t test (Section 3.1) but we consider the observations to be the d_i's. The test statistic is

$$T = \frac{\bar{d} - \Delta_0}{s_d/\sqrt{N}} \tag{3.27}$$

where $\bar{d} = \frac{1}{N}\sum_{i=1}^{N} d_i$ and $s_d^2 = \frac{1}{N-1}\sum_{i=1}^{N}(d_i - \bar{d})^2$. When H_0 is true, $T \sim t(N-1)$. When the difference in means equals an alternative value Δ_A, the test statistic has a noncentral t distribution, $T \sim t(N-1, \lambda)$, where the noncentrality parameter is

$$\lambda = \frac{\Delta_A - \Delta_0}{\sigma_d/\sqrt{N}} \tag{3.28}$$

and σ_d^2 is the population variance of the differences. This variance is $\sigma_d^2 = Var(d_i) = Var(Y_{i1} - Y_{i2}) = Var(Y_{i1}) + Var(Y_{i2}) - 2Cov(Y_{i1}, Y_{i2}) = \sigma_1^2 + \sigma_2^2 - 2\rho\sigma_1\sigma_2$, where σ_1^2 and σ_2^2 are the variances of observations Y_{i1} and Y_{i2} and $\rho = Corr(Y_{i1}, Y_{i2})$ is the correlation between the two observations taken on the same pair. If the variances under the two conditions are the same, $\sigma_1^2 = \sigma_2^2 = \sigma^2$, then $\sigma_d^2 = 2\sigma^2(1-\rho)$. Power can be calculated as the probability that T is in the rejection region given $T \sim t(N-1, \lambda)$:

$$\text{Power (one-sided test)} = 1 - \mathcal{T}_{N-1,|\lambda|}(t_{1-\alpha, N-1}) \tag{3.29}$$
$$\text{Power (two-sided test)} = 1 - \mathcal{F}_{1, N-1, \Lambda}(f_{1-\alpha, 1, N-1}).$$

where $\Lambda = \lambda^2$ and λ is given in equation (3.28).

3.5.1 Sample size using normal approximation

As discussed in Section 3.1.5, when a power formula involves a noncentral t or F distribution, the parameters of the distribution depend on the sample size, and as a result, we cannot directly solve the power formula for N and get a closed-form expression for the sample size. Sample size calculations can be performed using software that numerically inverts power formulas to solve for N. This approach will give "exact" solutions. We can get an approximation of the required sample size by using the normal rather than the t distribution. Using a normal approximation, the required sample size for a two-sided paired t test is

$$N \geq \frac{(\sigma_1^2 + \sigma_2^2 - 2\rho\sigma_1\sigma_2)(z_{1-\alpha/2} + z_{1-\beta})^2}{(\Delta_A - \Delta_0)^2}. \quad (3.30)$$

When the variances under the two conditions are equal, this simplifies to

$$N \geq \frac{2\sigma^2(1-\rho)(z_{1-\alpha/2} + z_{1-\beta})^2}{(\Delta_A - \Delta_0)^2}. \quad (3.31)$$

In these formulas, N is the number of pairs, each of which contributes two observations. The total number of observations is $2N$. For a one-sided test, substitute $z_{1-\alpha}$ for $z_{1-\alpha/2}$.

Normal approximation-based sample size formulas are helpful for understanding how various factors affect the sample size requirement, but will generally underestimate the required N. It is prudent to use software to conduct a precise calculation rather than rely on a normal approximation formula.

What factors affect power and sample size? The factors affecting power and sample size can be gleaned by inspecting the formulas. As expected, higher variance decreases power (and increases N) and greater null and alternative mean difference $|\Delta_A - \Delta_0|$ increases power (and decreases N). Higher correlation between two measurements on the same individual, ρ, leads to increased power (and smaller N). This occurs because higher values of ρ lead to lower values of σ_d.

Example 3.14. A single-arm study will measure participants on a continuous outcome before and after an intervention is applied. The true difference in means from pre- to post-intervention is expected to be 4. Previous studies suggest that the measurements will have a standard deviation of $\sigma_1 = \sigma_2 = 10$ and that the correlation between the pre and post measurements is likely to be between 0.4 and 0.6. How many participants are needed for 80% power to test $H_0: \mu_d = 0$, with two-sided α of 0.05?

We find sample size for a range of values of ρ as follows:

```
library(powertools)
rho <- seq(from = 0.4, to = 0.6, by = 0.05)
N <- sapply(rho, function(x)
  ttest.paired(N = NULL, delta = 4, sd1 = 10, sd2 = 10, rho = x,
               alpha = 0.05, power = 0.8, sides = 2, v = T)$N
)
```

```
cbind(rho, N)
     rho     N
[1,] 0.40 60.81515
[2,] 0.45 55.91206
[3,] 0.50 51.00945
[4,] 0.55 46.10745
[5,] 0.60 41.20630
```

The required N goes down as ρ increases. N is quite sensitive to the value of ρ, which should be kept in mind when selecting a sample size.

If we expect that some individuals will only provide the pre measurement and drop out of the study before the post, the number enrolled in the study should be inflated accordingly; see Section 2.8.

The function `ttest.paired` takes as input the standard deviations of the two measurements and the correlation between them. Some functions for power and sample size for paired t tests take as input the standard deviation of the differences, σ_d. If we do not have a direct guesstimate of σ_d but rather have information about the standard deviations of the observations and the correlation, we can calculate the standard deviation of the differences as $\sigma_d = \sqrt{\sigma_1^2 + \sigma_2^2 - 2\rho\sigma_1\sigma_2}$ if the two variances are expected to be different or $\sigma_d = \sqrt{2\sigma^2(1-\rho)}$ if the variances are expected to be equal, $\sigma_1^2 = \sigma_2^2 = \sigma^2$.

3.6 Remarks on R functions for t tests

In addition to the functions in the `powertools` package, there are R functions in other packages that compute power and sample size for t tests. One is the `power_t_test` function in the `MESS` package. For this function, `delta` must be positive in order to get the correct calculation. In the t test functions in `powertools`, `delta` is to be set equal to $\mu_A - \mu_0$ for a one-sample test or $\Delta_A - \Delta_0$ for a two-sample test, and the value can be positive or negative. The function `AB_t2n` in the `pwrAB` package also computes power and sample size for two-sample t tests. This function takes as input the proportion of the sample in one group rather than the allocation ratio. The `TrialSize` package also offers functions. In general, different functions often use different arguments and conventions and it is important to read the documentation carefully when using them.

3.7 Nonparametric tests of location

t tests are tests for location, meaning that they test hypotheses about location parameters, which describe the central tendency of distributions. For t tests, the location parameters are means. t tests are also **parametric tests**, meaning that they rely on assumptions about the parametric form of the distribution from which the data are sampled. In particular, t tests assume that the underlying populations are normally distributed.

In practice, the underlying data may be non-normal, which violates the normal distribution assumption of a t test. Nevertheless, t tests are generally still valid for non-normal data as long as the sample sizes are not very small [145]. When sample sizes are small and the data are non-normal, one may use **nonparametric tests**, which make few or no assumptions about the underlying distributions of the populations. There are various resources on the choice between parametric and nonparametric tests, for example, [11, 65, 205].

In this section, we discuss power and sample size calculation for three nonparametric tests that are often used in the place of t tests when data are non-normal: the sign test, signed-rank test, and rank-sum test. The sign test and signed-rank test are used in place of a one-sample t test or a paired t test; these are one-sample tests of location. The rank-sum test, also called the Mann–Whitney–Wilcoxon test, is used to compare two independent samples and is a nonparametric alternative to the two independent sample t test; it is a two-sample test of location.

3.7.1 Sign test

The sign test is often used in place of a one-sample or paired t test as a one-sample test of location. We discuss the sign test in the context of paired observations. Suppose that each participant i provides two measurements, Y_{i1} and Y_{i2}, taken under different conditions. It is assumed that the measurements are on a continuous scale and that it is possible to rank them. For each participant, we calculate the difference, $d_i = Y_{i1} - Y_{i2}$. The sign of d_i provides information on whether an individual's outcome under condition 1 was better or worse than under condition 2.

The null hypothesis of the sign test is that the median difference, denoted M, is zero, meaning that differences are equally likely to be less than or greater than zero. H_A can be one- or two-sided. $H_A: M > 0$ implies that outcomes tend to be higher under condition 1 and $H_A: M < 0$ implies that outcomes tend to be higher under condition 2.

The test statistic is the number of participants with positive d_i, denoted as S. Under H_0, $P(d_i > 0) = 0.5$ and S has a binomial distribution, $S \sim \text{Bin}(N, 0.5)$, where N is the number of participants with nonzero d_i values. Ties with $d_i = 0$ are not used to calculate the test statistic.

Nonparametric tests of location　　　　　　　　　　　　　　　　　　　　63

Performing a sign test as well as calculating power or sample size for it can be handled using a normal approximation or an exact approach. Using the normal approximation to the binomial distribution (see Section 6.1), if the true probability of a positive d_i is p, the sample size needed for power of $1 - \beta$ for a two-sided sign test at level α is approximately (see Noether [172])

$$N \approx \frac{(z_{1-\alpha/2} + z_{1-\beta})^2}{4(p - 0.5)^2}$$

and power is approximately

$$1 - \beta \approx \Phi\left(z_{\alpha/2} + 2\sqrt{N}|p - 0.5|\right).$$

The calculations require specification of a value for $p = P(d_i > 0)$ under the alternative. We illustrate a calculation in the following example.

Example 3.15. A study will ask participants to rate two conditions on a visual analog scale from 0 to 10. The investigators expect that 75% of participants will rate condition 1 higher than condition 2. If the study will yield 20 participants with non-zero difference scores, what is the power to reject the null hypothesis of the sign test and conclude that ratings under condition 1 tend to be higher than those under condition 2? We specify a significance level of 0.05 for a one-sided test.

```
library(powertools)
signtest(N = 20, p = 0.75, power = NULL, alpha = 0.05, sides = 1)
[1] 0.7228116
```

Power is approximately 72%.

More accurate calculations can be performed by viewing the sign test as a special case of the one-sample binomial test, discussed in Section 7.1, with $H_0\colon p = 0.5$. One can plan to conduct an exact binomial test and perform the corresponding power calculation for the exact test.

Example 3.16. We revisit Example 3.15 and conduct a power calculation for an exact sign test using the exact binomial test. We use the `power_binom_test` function from the `MESS` package:

```
library(MESS)
power_binom_test(n = 20, p0 = 0.5, pa = 0.75, sig.level = 0.05,
    power = NULL, alternative = "greater")
```

One-sample exact binomial power calculation

```
            n = 20
           p0 = 0.5
           pa = 0.75
    sig.level = 0.05
        power = 0.6171727
  alternative = greater
```

Power for the exact test is about 62%. We expect this calculation to be more accurate than the normal approximation.

3.7.2 Signed-rank test

Like the sign test, the signed-rank test is a nonparametric alternative to a one-sample or paired t test. While the sign test only considers whether the differences $d_i = Y_{i1} - Y_{i2}$ are positive or negative, i.e., their sign, the signed-rank test [230] also considers their magnitude and is a more powerful test. We focus on using the signed-rank test for paired observations.

Like the sign test, the signed-rank test uses the differences d_i to test the null hypothesis that the median difference is zero, $H_0\colon M = 0$, versus a one- or two-sided alternative. The test assumes that the differences arise from a continuous and symmetric distribution and can be ranked. The test statistic is obtained by ordering the absolute values of the differences, $|d_i|$, and assigning each value a rank, R_i. The test statistic is the sum of the ranks for subjects with positive d_i's, denoted R^+. A large R^+ is evidence against the null. Under H_0, for a sample of size N, R^+ has expected value $E(R^+) = N(N+1)/4$ and variance $Var(R^+) = N(N+1)(2N+1)/24$ [230] and $[R^+ - E(R^+)]/\sqrt{Var(R^+)}$ has an asymptotic standard normal distribution. Under an alternative with $p = P(d_i > 0)$ and $p' = P(d_i + d_j > 0)$ for $i \neq j$, $E(R^+) = Np + N(N-1)p'/2$. Sample size using a normal approximation as presented by Noether [171] is

$$N \approx \frac{(z_{1-\alpha/2} + z_{1-\beta})^2}{3(p' - 0.5)^2}.$$

This formula assumes the variance under the alternative is equal to that under the null. The parameter p' can be difficult to specify. It might be based on a pilot sample, if available. Another formula, provided by Chow et al [33], requires specification of three probabilities. Another approach is to directly specify the distribution of d_i under the alternative and perform a Monte Carlo simulation of power. This approach is offered by the `sim.ssize.wilcox.test` function from the `MKpower` package. Power by simulation is discussed in Section 2.10.

Nonparametric tests of location

Example 3.17. The `sim.ssize.wilcox.test` function from the MKpower package can be used to find sample size for the signed-rank test (as well as the rank-sum test, discussed in Section 3.7.3.). In this function, the input `rx` is a function that specifies the distribution under the alternative. To meet the assumptions of the test, this should be specified as a continuous and symmetric distribution. We specify a shifted t distribution, in particular, a t with $\nu = 4$ degrees of freedom shifted to the right by 0.6 units. This distribution has mean 0.6 and variance $\nu/(\nu - 2) = 2$, with heavy tails compared to a normal distribution. Note that a shifted t distribution is not the same as a noncentral t distribution, which is not symmetric. The function performs a search for the required sample size using simulation to compute power for various values of N:

```
library(MKpower)
rxy <- function(n) rt(n, df = 4) + 0.6
sim.ssize.wilcox.test(rx = rxy, mu = 0, type = "paired", power = 0.9,
   n.max = 100, iter = 10000)

    Wilcoxon signed rank test

              n = 10, 20, 30, 40, 50
             rx = rt(n, df = 4) + 0.6
      sig.level = 0.05
      emp.power = 0.2934, 0.5470, 0.7352, 0.8567, 0.9196
    alternative = two.sided

NOTE: n is number in *each* group
# For paired data, n is the number of pairs.
```

This indicates that a sample size of about 50 pairs will provide 90% power. Because the function uses Monte Carlo simulation, there will be random variation in the output. A higher number of iterations leads to more accuracy.

Although it is not necessary to specify $p = P(d_i > 0)$ or $p' = P(d_i + d_j > 0)$ when using this approach, it is instructive to estimate them, which we can do using simulation. We then use p' in Noether's approximate sample size formula for the signed-rank test for comparison:

```
x1 <- rt(n = 100000, df = 4) + 0.6
p <- sum(x1>0)/length(x1)   ;  p
[1] 0.71049
x2 <- c(rt(n = 100000, df = 4) + 0.6 + rt(n = 100000, df = 4) + 0.6)
ps <- sum(x2>0)/length(x2)   ;  ps
1] 0.7617

library(powertools)
signedrank(N = NULL, ps = ps, power = 0.9, sides = 2)
[1] 51.1408
```

We estimate $p \approx 0.71$ and $p' \approx 0.76$. Noether's formula suggests a sample size of about 52. In general, these calculations should be taken as a rough guide to required sample size, given the need to make various assumptions and approximations.

Given that the underlying distribution in the above example is not terribly different from a normal distribution, the effect size can be roughly characterized as the difference in locations under the null and alternative divided by the standard deviation under the alternative, which gives $0.6/\sqrt{2} = 0.42$, a "medium" effect size. Effect size for the signed-rank test can also be characterized by the rank correlation [122].

We have seen in this section that even though the signed-rank test itself involves few assumptions, power calculations for the test require assumptions such as the expected distribution of the sample or the value of p', which can be difficult to specify. A reasonable approach to determining a sample size for a signed-rank test might be to perform a sample size calculation for a sign test due to its simplicity.

3.7.3 Rank-sum test

The Wilcoxon-Mann-Whitney rank-sum test [149], also called the Mann-Whitney U test, is the nonparametric analog of the two independent sample t test. Suppose that $X_1, \ldots, X_{n_1}$ and $Y_1, \ldots, Y_{n_2}$ are two independent samples from populations with continuous cdfs F and G, respectively. The rank-sum test is used to test the null hypothesis that the distributions are the same, $F = G$, against the alternative that one distribution is stochastically larger than the other distribution, i.e., the Y observations tend to be larger than X observations or vice versa. The test is performed by ordering the $N = n_1 + n_2$ observations from smallest to largest and assigning a rank to each observation. The test statistic U is the sum of the ranks assigned to the Y_j's. Letting R_j denote the rank of Y_j,

$$U = \sum_{j=1}^{n_2} R_j = \frac{n_2(n_2+1)}{2} + \sum_{i=1}^{n_1}\sum_{j=1}^{n_2} I(Y_j - X_i > 0) \qquad (3.32)$$

where $I(Y_j - X_i > 0) = 1$ if $Y_j - X_i > 0$ and 0 otherwise. Under H_0, the double summation in (3.32) has expected value $n_1 n_2/2$, and U is asymptotically normal with mean $n_2(N+1)/2$ and variance $n_1 n_2 (N+1)/12$ [93]. To compute power, we need the distribution of U under some alternative, which is complicated to derive. Several authors have presented approximations. Noether [172] presented the sample size formula

$$N \approx \frac{(1+r)^2}{r} \frac{(z_{1-\alpha} + z_{1-\beta})^2}{12(p-0.5)^2}$$

Nonparametric tests of location

where $r = n_2/n_1$ and $p = P(Y_j > X_i)$, the probability that an observation from G is greater than an observation from F under the alternative. We can think of p as the effect size for a rank-sum test. Power is approximately

$$1 - \beta \approx \Phi\left(z_\alpha + \sqrt{12N\frac{r}{(1+r)^2}}(p - 0.5)\right).$$

Example 3.18. Suppose we want to calculate the power to compare the distance between two mutations on a DNA strand in two groups of people. Each group has 10 individuals. We do not want to assume that the distances are normally distributed and choose a rank-sum test for analysis. If the probability that the distance in the second group is greater than the distance in the first group, $P(Y > X)$, is 0.8, what is the power to reject H_0 and conclude that the groups tend to have different distances between mutations? The desired type I error is 0.05 for a two-sided test.

```
library(powertools)
ranksum(n1 = 10, n.ratio = 1, p = 0.8, alpha = 0.05, power = NULL,
    sides = 2)
[1] 0.642006
```

Power is computed to be about 64%.

Noether's formula is based on approximating the asymptotic variance of U under the alternative using the variance under the null. The approximation is reasonable when the location shift is small but problematic for larger location shifts [202]. A more accurate approximation was presented by Lehmann [136], who derived an expression for the variance under the alternative as

$$n_1 n_2 p_1 (1 - p_1) + n_1 n_2 (n_1 - 1)(p_2 - p_1^2) + n_1 n_2 (n_2 - 1)(p_3 - p_1^2)$$

where $p_1 = P(Y_j > X_i)$, $p_2 = P(Y_j > X_i \text{ and } Y_j > X_h)$ and $p_3 = P(Y_j > X_i \text{ and } Y_k > X_i)$. The values of p_1, p_2 and p_3 could be estimated based on pilot data, if available. Shieh et al. [202] provide analytical forms for some distributions. Another option is to compute power using Monte Carlo simulation. This is illustrated using the `wmwpowd` function from the `wmwpow` package in the next example.

Example 3.19. The `wmwpow` package has functions that facilitate Monte Carlo power calculations for the rank-sum test. The function `wmwpowd` performs Monte Carlo power calculations based on user-specified distributions for F and G. For example, suppose we specify $F \sim \text{Unif}(0,1)$ and $G \sim \text{Unif}(0.5, 1.5)$. With 10 subjects in each group, what is the power?

```
library(wmwpow)
wmwpowd(n = 10, m = 10, distn = "unif(0, 1)", distm = "unif(0.5, 1.5)",
   sides = "two.sided", alpha = 0.05, nsims = 10000)

Supplied distribution 1: unif(0, 1); n = 10
Supplied distribution 2: unif(0.5, 1.5); m = 10

p: 0.875
WMW odds: 7
Number of simulated datasets: 10000
Two-sided WMW test (alpha = 0.05)

Empirical power: 0.908
```

The power is about 91%. The output also indicates that $P(Y > X) = 0.875$, the effect size in this context, and that this corresponds to an odds, $P(Y > X)/P(Y < X)$, of 7.

The function wmwpowp from this package performs Monte Carlo power calculations based on specifying one distribution and $P(Y > X)$. Other resources in R for power for the rank-sum test include the functions sim.ssize.wilcox.test and sim.power.wilcox.test in the MKpower package and the n.wilcox.ord function in the samplesize package.

4
Hypotheses for different study objectives

4.1 Introduction

The objective of many studies is to reach a conclusion about outcomes under one condition compared to outcomes under another condition. In this chapter, we label the two conditions as Treatment R for reference — this could be the usual care, standard care or the control group — and Treatment T for the test or experimental treatment. What exactly do we hope to conclude regarding the relationship of outcomes under Treatment R and Treatment T? Several different objectives can be distinguished. We may want to conclude that outcomes under Treatment T are

1. different from,
2. better than,
3. not substantially worse than,
4. substantially better than or
5. essentially the same as

outcomes under Treatment R. These different study objectives can be translated into different study hypotheses, namely, hypotheses that test for

1. nonequality,
2. superiority,
3. noninferiority,
4. superiority by a margin and
5. equivalence.

This chapter discusses these five types of hypothesis tests and how they affect the calculation of power and sample size requirements. When reading this chapter, it is helpful to keep in mind the following tip:

> ▶ To understand the different trial objectives and hypotheses, **focus on the alternative hypothesis**. The alternative hypothesis is typically the conclusion that the investigators would like to reach, and thus states the hoped-for result.

The reader should be aware that the terms **"equality"**, **"noninferiority"**, **"superiority" and "equivalence" are not used in a consistent manner in the literature**. Different authors use different terms. It is important to understand the actual study design that the author is referring to. One person's "noninferiority" study may be another person's "equivalence" study.

Throughout the chapter, we will assume that we are comparing two conditions by comparing their means, μ_T and μ_R. The same concepts apply to outcomes other than means, e.g., proportions.

To set up the appropriate hypotheses for the study objective and conduct power calculations correctly, it is vitally important to pay attention to whether a higher mean corresponds to a better or a worse outcome and the direction of inequalities. For consistency, throughout most of this chapter, we will assume that a higher mean indicates a better outcome. Section 4.7 addresses the situation in which a lower mean corresponds to a better outcome.

To illustrate power and sample size calculations for the various study objectives and hypotheses, we will use the situation of a two-sample t test with equal variances and equal allocation. In Chapter 3, we learned that to test the hypotheses

$$H_0: \mu_T - \mu_R = \Delta_0 \text{ versus } H_A: \mu_T - \mu_R \neq \Delta_0$$

at significance level α for a two-sample t test with equal variances and equal allocation, we use the test statistic

$$T = \frac{\bar{Y}_T - \bar{Y}_R - \Delta_0}{s_p\sqrt{4/N}}$$

where s_p^2 is the pooled variance estimate. When H_0 is true, $T \sim t(N-2)$. When an alternative $\Delta_A = \mu_T - \mu_R$ is true, T has a noncentral t distribution, $T \sim t(N-2, \lambda)$, where

$$\lambda = \frac{\Delta_A - \Delta_0}{\sigma\sqrt{4/N}}.$$

Using the normal approximation to the t distribution, the total sample size N needed to achieve power of $1 - \beta$ is (this is usually a slight underestimate)

$$N \geq \frac{4(z_{1-\alpha/2} + z_{1-\beta})^2 \sigma^2}{(\Delta_A - \Delta_0)^2}.$$

For a one-sided test at level α, we substitute $z_{1-\alpha}$ for $z_{1-\alpha/2}$.

In the following sections, we will find that the hypotheses and therefore the appropriate power and sample size calculations will follow from answering the following questions:

> ➤ To formulate the hypotheses and conduct an appropriate power or sample size calculation for a particular trial objective, we need to answer the questions:
>
> 1. What do we specify for Δ_0?
>
> 2. Do we use a one-sided or two-sided test?
>
> 3. For a one-sided test, what is the direction of the inequality?

4.2 Test for nonequality

If the study objective is to conclude that two means are not equal, and there is no *a priori* expectation that one mean will be higher than the other, the logical hypothesis test is a two-sided **test for nonequality**:

$$H_0\colon \mu_T - \mu_R = 0 \text{ versus } H_A\colon \mu_T - \mu_R \neq 0.$$

If we reject H_0, we conclude that $\mu_T \neq \mu_R$. This test is sometimes called a "test for equality", but to better reflect the conclusion under the alternative, we prefer to call it a test for <u>non</u>equality. Such a test may also be called a "test for inequality".

Power and sample size for tests of nonequality. Two-sided tests with $\Delta_0 = 0$ are tests for nonequality.

4.3 Test for superiority

Often we want to conclude that one mean is higher than the other, rather than that the means are merely not equal. In this case, it may be sensible to use a one-sided test. For example, if a higher mean corresponds to a better outcome, and we hope to conclude that outcomes under Treatment T are better than outcomes under Treatment R, we could set up the hypotheses as

$$H_0\colon \mu_T - \mu_R \leq 0 \text{ versus } H_A\colon \mu_T - \mu_R > 0.$$

Note that H_A states the desired conclusion, that $\mu_T > \mu_R$. We refer to such a test as a **test for superiority**. As previously noted, terminology differs from author to author. Such a test may sometimes be called a "test for inequality". Further, some authors may use the term "superiority test" to mean a test for superiority by a margin, which we discuss in Section 4.5.

Often the significance level α for a one-sided test is specified to be half of the α level that would be conventional for a two-sided test. For example, we often set $\alpha = 0.025$ for a one-sided test when $\alpha = 0.05$ is conventional for a two-sided test. This retains the type I error rate associated with a two-sided test but by using a one-sided test, we clearly state the expected ordering of the means.

Power and sample size for tests of superiority. One-sided tests with $\Delta_0 = 0$ are tests for superiority. In general, the power or required sample size for a two-sided test at level α is the same as for a one-sided test at level $\alpha/2$. For practical purposes, either one can be used.

4.3.1 Hypotheses and confidence intervals

We have focused thus far on inference using hypotheses tests, but some studies use confidence intervals for inference. Hypotheses and confidence intervals have the relationship that if H_0 is rejected at significance level α using a two-sided test, then a $100(1 - \alpha)\%$ confidence interval does not contain the null value, and vice versa. For example, if H_0 is rejected at the 0.05 level in a two-sided test, then a 95% confidence interval will exclude the null value and vice versa.

Example 4.1. For a two-sided, two-sample t test with equal variances and equal allocation, we reject the null hypothesis for a test of nonequality $H_0 \colon \mu_T - \mu_R = 0$ in favor of $H_A \colon \mu_T - \mu_R \neq 0$ at the 0.05 level if

$$\frac{|\bar{Y}_T - \bar{Y}_R|}{s_p\sqrt{4/N}} > t_{N-2, 0.975}$$

This is equivalent to rejecting H_0 if the 95% confidence interval

$$(\bar{Y}_T - \bar{Y}_R) \pm t_{N-2, 0.975}\, s_p\sqrt{4/N}$$

does not include the null value of zero.

Figure 4.1 illustrates situations in which we would conclude or not conclude nonequality of two means using confidence intervals.

Test for noninferiority

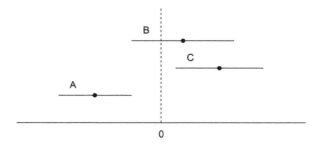

FIGURE 4.1: Inference for a test of nonequality based on a confidence interval. The hypotheses $H_0\colon \mu_T - \mu_R = 0$ versus $H_A\colon \mu_T - \mu_R \neq 0$ are tested at the α significance level. Each line represents a $100(1-\alpha)\%$ confidence interval for $\mu_T - \mu_R$. In Cases A and C, the confidence interval excludes the null value of 0, and we therefore reject H_0 and conclude $\mu_T - \mu_R \neq 0$ ($\mu_T \neq \mu_R$) at the α significance level. In Case B, we do not reject H_0.

Inference for a one-sided test at significance level α is equivalent to using a $100(1-2\alpha)\%$ confidence interval. For example, inference for a one-sided test at level 0.025 is equivalent to using a 95% confidence interval.

Example 4.2. For a one-sided, two-sample t test with equal variances and equal allocation, we reject the null hypothesis for a test of superiority $H_0\colon \mu_T - \mu_R \leq 0$ in favor of $H_A\colon \mu_T - \mu_R > 0$ at the 0.025 level if

$$\frac{\bar{Y}_T - \bar{Y}_R}{s_p\sqrt{4/N}} > t_{N-2,0.975}$$

which is equivalent to rejecting H_0 if the 95% confidence interval

$$(\bar{Y}_T - \bar{Y}_R) \pm t_{N-2,0.975}\, s_p\sqrt{4/N}$$

lies entirely above the null value of zero.

Figure 4.2 illustrates situations in which we would conclude or not conclude superiority using confidence intervals.

4.4 Test for noninferiority

In some situations, a test treatment may be deemed acceptable even if it slightly underperforms the reference treatment on some outcomes because

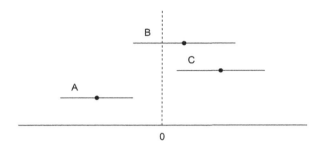

FIGURE 4.2: Inference for a test of superiority based on a confidence interval. Assume that a higher mean represents a better outcome. The hypotheses $H_0: \mu_T - \mu_R \leq 0$ and $H_A: \mu_T - \mu_R > 0$ are tested at the α significance level, one-sided. Each line represents a $100(1-2\alpha)\%$ confidence interval for $\mu_T - \mu_R$. In Case C, the confidence interval lies entirely above the null value of 0, and we therefore reject H_0 and conclude $\mu_T - \mu_R > 0$ ($\mu_T > \mu_R$) at the α significance level, one-sided. In Cases A and B, we do not reject H_0.

it has advantages such as lower risk of adverse events, lower cost or easier adminstration. A common objective in such settings is to show that the test treatment is *not inferior* to the reference treatment, meaning that it might perform slightly worse than the reference treatment on an efficacy outcome, but not by a clinically meaningful amount.

To conduct a **test for noninferiority**, the study investigators need to identify a **margin of noninferiority** m, defined as the smallest difference in mean outcomes that is clinically meaningful. Specifying this value is a clinical issue, not a statistical issue. Then, we set up the hypotheses such that H_A states the conclusion that we seek to reach. Suppose that a higher mean corresponds to a better outcome. Let m be a positive quantity. Then the desired conclusion is $\mu_T > \mu_R - m$. In Figure 4.3, the top right panel shows the range of values of μ_T for which Treatment T is noninferior to Treatment R, assuming that a higher mean corresponds to a better outcome.

The null hypothesis is formulated as the complement of the alternative hypothesis. The hypotheses for a test of noninferiority, when a higher mean corresponds to a better outcome and $m > 0$, are thus

$$H_0: \mu_T \leq \mu_R - m \text{ versus } H_A: \mu_T > \mu_R - m$$

which we could also write as

$$H_0: \mu_T - \mu_R \leq -m \text{ versus } H_A: \mu_T - \mu_R > -m$$

or, putting all of the parameters on one side, we could write

$$H_0: \mu_T - \mu_R + m \leq 0 \text{ versus } H_A: \mu_T - \mu_R + m > 0.$$

Test for noninferiority

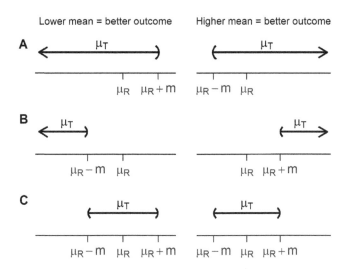

FIGURE 4.3: Relationships between μ_R, μ_T, and m (where $m > 0$) when a lower mean (left side) or a higher mean (right side) corresponds to a better outcome. The figures show the range of values of μ_T for which (A) Treatment T is noninferior to Treatment R; (B) T is superior by a margin to R; (C) T is equivalent to R.

For the situation of a lower mean corresponding to a better outcome, see Section 4.7.

Example 4.3. Suppose that a higher mean corresponds to a better outcome. The margin of noninferiority m is specified to be 3 and the mean under reference treatment μ_R is 10. Then values of μ_T that exceed $\mu_R - m = 7$ imply that the test treatment is noninferior to the reference treatment.

Inference for noninferiority trials often uses confidence intervals. Figure 4.4 shows confidence intervals for $\mu_T - \mu_R$ and the conclusion of a noninferiority test. We can conclude noninferiority of Treatment T to Treatment R for a one-sided test at significance level α if a $100(1 - 2\alpha)\%$ confidence interval falls entirely above $-m$. Inferences for one-sided tests with α of 0.025 will correspond to 95% confidence intervals.

Power and sample size for tests of noninferiority. When higher is better and $m > 0$, noninferiority entails a one-sided, upper-tailed test with $-m$ substituted for Δ_0. This means that the quantity $\Delta_A - \Delta_0$ becomes $\Delta_A + m$. Power and sample size calculations often assume that under the alternative there is no difference in means, that is, $\Delta_A = \mu_T - \mu_R = 0$.

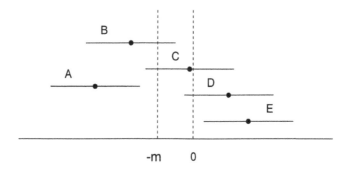

FIGURE 4.4: Inference for a test of noninferiority based on a confidence interval. We assume that a higher mean represents a better outcome. The noninferiority margin is $m > 0$. The hypotheses $H_0\colon \mu_T - \mu_R \leq -m$ versus $H_A\colon \mu_T - \mu_R > -m$ are tested at the α significance level, one-sided. Each line represents a $100(1 - 2\alpha)\%$ confidence interval for $\mu_T - \mu_R$. In Cases D and E, the confidence interval lies entirely above $-m$ and so we reject H_0 and conclude noninferiority of T to R at the α significance level, one-sided. In Case E, we can further conclude superiority, that is, $\mu_T > \mu_R$. For Cases A, B and C, we do not reject H_0 and thus do not conclude noninferiority.

Example 4.4. Nas et al. [166] report a randomized trial testing whether virtual reality cardiopulmonary resuscitation (CPR) training is noninferior to face-to-face training. The primary outcome was CPR quality, including chest compression depth, measured in mm. The investigators chose a noninferiority margin of 5 mm, based in part on studies showing that a decrement greater than 5 mm is associated with lower survival after cardiac arrest. Other specifications are equal allocation, no difference in means under the alternative, an expected standard deviation of 10 mm, a one-sided test with α of 0.05, and power of 90%.

Recall that the `delta` argument in the `ttest.2samp` function takes as input $\Delta_A - \Delta_0$. For this example, $\Delta_A - \Delta_0 = 0 - 5 = -5$.

```
library(powertools)
ttest.2samp(n1 = NULL, delta = -5, sd1 = 10, power = 0.9, sides = 1)
[1] 69.19782
```

Rounding up, we need 70 participants per group.

In a noninferiority trial, is it possible to make a conclusion stronger than noninferiority? In Case E of Figure 4.4, it seems logical to conclude that not only is Treatment T not inferior to Treatment R, it is in fact superior.

Morikawa and Yoshida [163] show that we can come to this conclusion without making adjustments to α for maintaining the overall type I error rate.

4.5 Test for superiority by a margin

In some studies, the objective may be to show that outcomes under Treatment T are not merely better than outcomes under Treatment R, but that they are so much better that Treatment T can be considered superior to Treatment R by a clinically meaningful amount. This is called **superiority by a margin**. Showing superiority by a margin might be the goal when an active treatment is compared to a sham or placebo treatment; in such settings, simply showing nonequality or simple superiority to the sham treatment may be deemed insufficient. Further, showing superiority by a margin might be the aim if the test treatment has some disadvantages, such as a higher risk of adverse effects, and it would only be recommended over the reference treatment if these disadvantages are outweighed by its clinical superiority.

In this setting, and assuming a higher mean is better, we define a **margin of superiority** $m > 0$ and conduct a **test for superiority by a margin**:

$$H_0: \mu_T \leq \mu_R + m \text{ versus } H_A: \mu_T > \mu_R + m$$

By rejecting H_0, we conclude that μ_T exceeds μ_R by a clinically meaningful amount. We can also express the hypotheses as

$$H_0: \mu_T - \mu_R \leq m \text{ versus } H_A: \mu_T - \mu_R > m$$

or putting all of the parameters on one side, we can write this as

$$H_0: \mu_T - \mu_R - m \leq 0 \text{ versus } H_A: \mu_T - \mu_R - m > 0.$$

Some authors call this a "super-superiority" test.

Example 4.5. Suppose that the margin of superiority m is specified to be 5 and the mean under reference treatment μ_R is 20. Then values of μ_T that exceed $\mu_R + m = 25$ imply that the test treatment is superior by a margin to the reference treatment.

Figure 4.5 shows confidence intervals for $\mu_T - \mu_R$ and the conclusions of tests for superiority by a margin. The confidence interval must fall entirely above the superiority margin m in order for Treatment T to be declared superior to Treatment R by the margin m (when a higher mean corresponds to a better outcome).

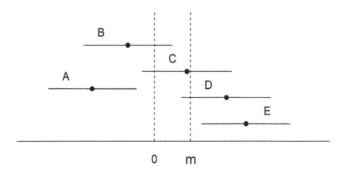

FIGURE 4.5: Inference for a test of superiority by a margin based on a confidence interval. Higher outcomes are assumed to be better. The hypotheses $H_0\colon \mu_T - \mu_R \leq m$ versus $H_A\colon \mu_T - \mu_R > m$ are tested at the α significance level, one-sided. The lines represent $100(1 - 2\alpha)\%$ confidence intervals for $\mu_T - \mu_R$. In Case E, we reject H_0 and conclude superiority by a margin at the α significance level, one-sided. We cannot conclude superiority by a margin in Cases A through D.

Power and sample size for tests of superiority by a margin. When a higher mean indicates a better outcome and $m > 0$, a test for superiority by a margin is a one-sided upper-tailed test with m used for Δ_0. It will usually be supposed that outcomes under Treatment T are indeed superior to those under Treatment R (otherwise why conduct the study?) and calculations will assume that under the alternative, $\mu_T - \mu_R = \Delta_A > m$.

Example 4.6. Sullivan et al. [213] report a trial comparing gastric plication, a weight loss surgery, to a sham procedure in patients with obesity. The efficacy endpoint was percent of total body weight loss (%TBWL). The trial was powered to demonstrate clinical superiority of active over sham treatment with a superiority margin of $m = 3\%$ TBWL. The sample size calculation was based on expected mean TBWL of 11.5% and 3.5% in the active and sham groups, respectively ($\Delta_A = 8\%$), with a common standard deviation of $\sigma = 8.5\%$. The trial used 2:1 allocation to active versus sham. Desired power is 0.9.

The `delta` argument in the `ttest.2samp` function takes as input $\Delta_A - \Delta_0$. For this example, $\Delta_A - \Delta_0 = 8 - 3 = 5$.

```
library(powertools)
ttest.2samp(n1 = NULL, n.ratio = 2, delta = 5, sd1 = 8.5,
    alpha = 0.025, power = 0.9, sides = 1)
[1] 46.53015
```

Rounding up, the calculation indicates that we need 47 in the sham surgery group and $2 \times 47 = 94$ in the active surgery group.

In Example 4.6, percent of total body weight loss was one of two co-primary efficacy endpoints in the trial. The other co-primary efficacy endpoint was a binary outcome defined as $\geq 5\%$ TBWL. In a trial with co-primary endpoints, all such endpoints must be declared significant in order to declare the intervention to be a success. No adjustment for multiple testing is required. This topic is discussed further in Chapter 17.

4.6 Test for equivalence

Another possible study objective is to show that two treatments are clinically equivalent, meaning that neither one is better or worse than the other in a clinically meaningful way. Assume that a higher mean is better and let $m > 0$ represent the smallest difference in means that is clinically meaningful. The hypotheses for a **test of equivalence** are

$$H_0 \colon \mu_T - \mu_R \leq -m \text{ or } \mu_T - \mu_R \geq m \text{ versus } H_A \colon -m < \mu_T - \mu_R < m \quad (4.1)$$

which we can also write as

$$H_0 \colon |\mu_T - \mu_R| \geq m \text{ versus } H_A \colon |\mu_T - \mu_R| < m. \quad (4.2)$$

If we reject H_0, we conclude that $-m < \mu_T - \mu_R < m$, that is, the two treatments do not differ in a clinically meaningful way in either direction. Tests for equivalence are common in **bioequivalence** studies, in which two formulations of a drug are compared with respect to rate and extent of absorption or other pharmacokinetic or pharmacodynamic parameters. Such studies often use crossover designs, discussed in Chapter 12. The design and analysis of bioavailability and bioequivalence studies are discussed in Chow and Liu [32].

Occasionally, the investigators may choose asymmetric lower and upper equivalence bounds m_L and m_U, where $m_L \neq -m_U$, which leads to the more general hypotheses

$$H_0 \colon \mu_T - \mu_R \leq m_L \text{ or } \mu_T - \mu_R \geq m_U \text{ versus } H_A \colon m_L < \mu_T - \mu_R < m_U. \quad (4.3)$$

In this case, m_L is a negative value and m_U is a positive value.

In an equivalence test, the null hypothesis is the union of two sets, $\{(\mu_T, \mu_R) \colon \mu_T - \mu_R \leq m_L \cup \mu_T - \mu_R \geq m_U\}$, and the alternative is an

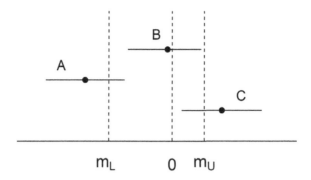

FIGURE 4.6: Inference for a test of equivalence based on a confidence interval. The hypotheses are $H_0: \mu_T - \mu_R \leq m_L$ or $\mu_T - \mu_R \geq m_U$ versus $H_A: m_L < \mu_T - \mu_R < m_U$. The lines represent $100(1-2\alpha)\%$ confidence intervals for $\mu_T - \mu_R$. In Case B, we conclude equivalence at level α; the confidence interval is entirely within the interval (m_L, m_U). Equivalence cannot be concluded in Cases A and C. Often, we have symmetry around zero such that $m_L = -m_U$.

intersection, $\{(\mu_T, \mu_R): \mu_T - \mu_R > m_L \cap \mu_T - \mu_R < m_U\}$. In order to reject the null hypothesis, we must reject both of its components. A common testing approach is the **two one-sided test** (TOST) procedure [199]. The two tests are an upper-tailed test,

$$H_{01}: \mu_T - \mu_R \leq m_L \quad \text{versus} \quad H_{A1}: \mu_T - \mu_R > m_L,$$

and a lower-tailed test,

$$H_{02}: \mu_T - \mu_R \geq m_U \quad \text{versus} \quad H_{A2}: \mu_T - \mu_R < m_U,$$

each at level α. Because the null hypothesis is rejected only if both of the components are rejected, the overall Type I error rate will not exceed α and there is no need for multiplicity adjustment. This follows from the theory of intersection-union tests, discussed in Berger [17, 18].

Operationally, the TOST procedure is the same as constructing a $100(1-2\alpha)\%$ confidence interval for $\mu_T - \mu_R$ and declaring equivalence at the α significance level if the interval falls entirely within (m_L, m_U) [199, 227]. Thus the use of a 90% confidence interval in an equivalence trial corresponds to using α of 0.05 for both tests. Figure 4.6 illustrates the use of confidence intervals for equivalence testing.

Power and sample size for test of equivalence. For simplicity, let $-m_L = m_U = m$ and assume equal variances and equal sample sizes n in each group for a total sample size of $N = 2n$. The two test statistics for the TOST procedure are

$$T_1 = \frac{\bar{Y}_T - \bar{Y}_R + m}{s_p\sqrt{4/N}} \quad \text{and} \quad T_2 = \frac{\bar{Y}_T - \bar{Y}_R - m}{s_p\sqrt{4/N}}. \quad (4.4)$$

We reject the null hypothesis if $T_1 > t_{1-\alpha,N-2}$ and $T_2 < t_{\alpha,N-2}$. These can be combined into one rejection region. Dropping the degrees of freedom on the t quantiles for brevity, the rejection region is

$$t_{1-\alpha}s_p\sqrt{4/N} - m < \bar{Y}_T - \bar{Y}_R < t_\alpha s_p\sqrt{4/N} + m \quad (4.5)$$

Power is the probability that this event occurs given an alternative $\mu_T - \mu_R = \Delta_A$. If this alternative is true, then $(\bar{Y}_T - \bar{Y}_R - \Delta_A)/(\sigma\sqrt{4/N})$ has a standard normal distribution. Subtracting Δ_A and dividing by $\sigma\sqrt{4/N}$ throughout equation (4.5), we obtain that power is equal to

$$1 - \beta = P\left(t_{1-\alpha}\frac{s_p}{\sigma} - \frac{\Delta_A + m}{\sigma\sqrt{4/N}} < Z < t_\alpha \frac{s_p}{\sigma} - \frac{\Delta_A - m}{\sigma\sqrt{4/N}}\right)$$

where $Z \sim \mathcal{N}(0,1)$. In this expression, the pooled estimate of the variance, s_p^2, is a random variable. This complicates the computation of the probability and numerical integration is required [199]. Phillips [180] suggested a method using a bivariate noncentral t distribution for the vector (T_1, T_2). Such computations can be performed using Owen's Q function [178]. This approach can be implemented using the package PowerTOST.

To show that the type I error rate does not exceed α when performing the two one-sided tests at level α, let $\theta = \mu_T - \mu_R$ and let Ω_0 denote the parameter space corresponding to H_0, which is $\Omega_0 = \{(-\infty, -m] \cup [m, \infty)]\}$. A test has significance level α if $P(\text{Reject } H_0 \text{ given } \theta \in \Omega_0) \leq \alpha$. The maximum probability of falsely rejecting H_0 occurs when θ is on one of the boundaries, that is, $\theta = m$ or $\theta = -m$. In this case, the rejection region continues to be defined as in equation (4.5). If we subtract m and then divide by $s_p\sqrt{4/N}$ throughout, we obtain

$$t_{1-\alpha} - \frac{2m}{s_p\sqrt{4/N}} < \frac{\bar{Y}_T - \bar{Y}_R - m}{s_p\sqrt{4/N}} < t_\alpha$$

and the type I error rate is the probability of this event. The middle term has a $t(N-2)$ distribution, and thus it follows that the type I error rate is

$$P\left(t_{1-\alpha} - \frac{2m}{s_p\sqrt{4/N}} < T < t_\alpha\right) \leq P(T < t_\alpha) = \alpha$$

where $T \sim t(N-2)$. See Chow and Liu [32] for more details.

An approximation of required sample size can be found as follows. If σ^2 were known rather than estimated, we would reject H_0 if

$$z_{1-\alpha}\sigma\sqrt{4/N} - m < \bar{Y}_T - \bar{Y}_R < z_\alpha\sigma\sqrt{4/N} + m$$
$$= z_{1-\alpha}\sigma\sqrt{4/N} - m < \bar{Y}_T - \bar{Y}_R < -z_{1-\alpha}\sigma\sqrt{4/N} + m.$$

Subtracting Δ_A and dividing by $\sigma\sqrt{4/N}$ throughout, we find that power in the case of known σ^2 is equal to

$$P\left(-\frac{(m+\Delta_A)}{\sigma\sqrt{4/N}} + z_{1-\alpha} < Z < \frac{m-\Delta_A}{\sigma\sqrt{4/N}} - z_{1-\alpha}\right)$$
$$= \Phi\left(\frac{m-\Delta_A}{\sigma\sqrt{4/N}} - z_{1-\alpha}\right) - \Phi\left(-\frac{(m+\Delta_A)}{\sigma\sqrt{4/N}} + z_{1-\alpha}\right)$$
$$= 1 - \Phi\left(\frac{\Delta_A - m}{\sigma\sqrt{4/N}} + z_{1-\alpha}\right) - \Phi\left(\frac{-\Delta_A - m}{\sigma\sqrt{4/N}} + z_{1-\alpha}\right)$$
$$\approx 1 - 2\Phi\left(\frac{\Delta_A - m}{\sigma\sqrt{4/N}} + z_{1-\alpha}\right)$$

assuming that Δ_A is close to zero, with equality when $\Delta_A = 0$.

To find the sample size that will achieve power of at least $1 - \beta$, we can set up the following inequality and solve for sample size:

$$1 - \beta \leq 1 - 2\Phi\left(\frac{\Delta_A - m}{\sigma\sqrt{4/N}} + z_{1-\alpha}\right)$$
$$\beta/2 \leq \Phi\left(\frac{\Delta_A - m}{\sigma\sqrt{4/N}} + z_{1-\alpha}\right)$$
$$z_{\beta/2} = -z_{1-\beta/2} \leq \frac{\Delta_A - m}{\sigma\sqrt{4/N}} + z_{1-\alpha}$$

Solving for N, we get an approximation for total sample size N under equal allocation as

$$N \geq \frac{4\sigma^2(z_{1-\beta/2} + z_{1-\alpha})^2}{(\Delta_A - m)^2}.$$

This assumes that $m > 0$ and $\Delta_A \geq 0$. Often, Δ_A is set equal to zero, reflecting a presumption of no difference in means, and the approximation becomes

$$N \geq \frac{4\sigma^2(z_{1-\beta/2} + z_{1-\alpha})^2}{m^2}. \tag{4.6}$$

This approximate formula can be helpful for examining how factors affect power and conducting preliminary calculations. For precise results, it is better to use software that uses Owen's Q function.

Example 4.7. The SLEEVEPASS study [193] aimed to compare outcomes from two types of surgery, sleeve gastrectomy and gastric bypass, in patients with morbid obesity. Sleeve gastrectomy was a simpler operation with lower risk of complications compared to gastric bypass, but its long-term outcomes had not been as well studied. An equivalence study was planned to test the hypothesis that the long-term results of sleeve gastrectomy would be equivalent to those of gastric bypass with regard to weight loss and resolution of comorbidities. The primary endpoint was percent excess weight loss at 5 years, defined as (initial weight - follow-up weight)/(initial weight - ideal weight for BMI of 25)×100%. The equivalence limits were prespecified as $(-9\%, 9\%)$. We specify equal allocation, common σ of 20, α of 0.05, power of 90% and no true difference in means ($\Delta_A = 0$). Using the approximate formula (4.6), we calculate:

```
zb2 <- qnorm(p = 1 - 0.1/2)
za <- qnorm(p = 1 - 0.05)
sigma <- 20
m <- 9
N <- 4 * sigma^2 * (zb2 + za)^2 / m^2  ; N
[1] 213.7713
```

This suggests that we need a total of 214 patients, which is 107 per group.

The function `sampleN.TOST` in the `PowerTOST` package performs the calculation using Owen's Q function when specifying `method = "exact"`. The function is designed for use with lognormal data and has an argument `CV` that is used to specify the coefficient of variation when using lognormal data or the standard deviation when using normal data. Users should consult the package documentation for further details.

```
library(PowerTOST)
sampleN.TOST(alpha = 0.05, targetpower = 0.9, logscale = FALSE,
   theta0 = 0, theta1 = -9, theta2 = 9, CV = 20,
   design = "parallel", method = "exact")

+++++++++++ Equivalence test - TOST +++++++++++
            Sample size estimation
---------------------------------------------------
Study design: 2 parallel groups
untransformed data (additive model)

alpha = 0.05, target power = 0.9
BE margins = -9 ... 9
True diff. = 0,  CV = 20

Sample size (total)
 n      power
 216    0.901359
```

The result indicates that we need a total N of 216.

The output from the `sampleN.TOST` function notes that the calculation is for an "additive model". This is referring to the fact that the hypotheses are expressed in terms of a difference in means. This is sometimes called **additive equivalence**. In bioequivalence studies, the data are often positively skewed and log-transformed prior to analysis. As discussed in Section 3.4, when the original data are lognormal, the mean μ on the log-transformed scale equals the logarithm of the geometric mean or median γ on the original scale, $\mu = \log(\gamma)$. The difference of means of the log-transformed data, $\mu_T - \mu_R$, equals the log of the ratio of the medians, $\log(\gamma_T/\gamma_R)$, and hypotheses (4.3) become

$$H_0: \log\left(\frac{\gamma_T}{\gamma_R}\right) \leq m_L \text{ or } \log\left(\frac{\gamma_T}{\gamma_R}\right) \geq m_U \text{ versus } m_L < \log\left(\frac{\gamma_T}{\gamma_R}\right) < m_U.$$

Taking the antilog, we obtain

$$H_0: \frac{\gamma_T}{\gamma_R} \leq \theta_L \text{ or } \frac{\gamma_T}{\gamma_R} \geq \theta_U \text{ versus } H_A: \theta_L < \frac{\gamma_T}{\gamma_R} < \theta_U \tag{4.7}$$

where $\theta_L = \exp(m_L)$ and $\theta_U = \exp(m_U)$. This is referred to as a test of **multiplicative equivalence**, since it focuses on a multiplicative difference between the medians on the original scale of the data.

Power and sample size for test of multiplicative equivalence. Although the multiplicative equivalence hypotheses (4.7) are stated in terms of ratios of medians, the actual test for equivalence is a test for a difference between the two means of the log-transformed data. Thus the underlying sample size and power procedures for tests of additive equivalence and multiplicative equivalence are the same; the test for multiplicative equivalence simply uses log-transformed data. However, many software procedures take the geometric means (medians) and/or their ratio and the CVs of the two populations on the original scale as inputs, rather than means and standard deviations on the log-transformed scale.

United States Food and Drug Administration (FDA) guidance specifies that establishing average bioequivalence involves the calculation of a 90% confidence interval for the ratio of the population geometric means of the measures for the test and reference products, and that the usual bioequivalence limits are 80–125% for the ratio [218]. Note that $0.80 < \gamma_T/\gamma_R < 1.25$ corresponds to $-0.223 < \mu_T - \mu_R < 0.223$, so that the equivalence bounds are symmetric on the log-transformed scale of the data.

Example 4.8. Cho et al. [30] report a randomized trial to assess the pharmacokinetic equivalence of a candidate bevacizumab biosimilar product and two reference products. Primary endpoints were serum bevacizumab area under the concentration–time curve (AUC) and maximum serum concentration (Cmax).

Subjects were randomized 1:1:1 to the three study arms. The biosimilar product was compared to each of the two references using separate tests. The required sample size was estimated when specifying a CV of 30%, true geometric mean ratio of 1.03 for each of the two comparisons, 90% power, α of 0.05 for each of the two one-sided tests, and equivalence bounds of $(\theta_L, \theta_U) = (80\%, 125\%)$.

```
library(PowerTOST)
sampleN.TOST(alpha = 0.05, targetpower = 0.9, logscale = TRUE,
  theta0 = 1.03, theta1 = 0.8, theta2 = 1.25, CV = 0.3,
  design = "parallel", method = "exact")

+++++++++++ Equivalence test - TOST +++++++++++
           Sample size estimation
-----------------------------------------------------
Study design: 2 parallel groups
log-transformed data (multiplicative model)

alpha = 0.05, target power = 0.9
BE margins = 0.8 ... 1.25
True ratio = 1.03,  CV = 0.3

Sample size (total)
  n     power
 84    0.900118
```

The output indicates that for two parallel groups, we need 84 total subjects, or 42 per arm. To repeat the same test comparing the biosimilar product to the second reference, we need an additional 42 subjects, for a total of 126. Anticipating a 10% dropout rate, the target sample size is $N/(1-p) = 126/(1-0.1) = 140$ (see Section 2.8), which, when rounded up to the next multiple of 3, equates to 141 subjects (47 per arm).

We note that the TOST procedure is applicable to testing for *average* bioequivalence. Additional methods have been developed for assessing *population* and *individual* bioequivalence. More coverage of power and sample size for equivalence testing can be found in [32]. Readers may also wish to consult FDA guidance on statistical approaches to establishing bioequivalence for more information [218].

4.7 Hypotheses when a lower mean corresponds to a better outcome

How do we formulate the null and alternative hypotheses for noninferiority, superiority by a margin and equivalence when a lower mean corresponds to a better outcome? To work this out, remember the key principle: **focus on the alternative hypothesis**. H_A represents the conclusion that the investigators hope to reach. Once we have properly expressed H_A, we can express H_0 as its complement.

When a lower mean corresponds to a better outcome, we can conclude that outcomes under Treatment T are noninferior to outcomes under Treatment R so long as μ_T does not exceed $\mu_R + m$, where m, the margin of noninferiority, is positive. The upper left panel of Figure 4.3 shows the relationship between μ_R and m and the range of values of μ_T that would make T noninferior to R. The alternative hypothesis is $H_A: \mu_T < \mu_R + m$, or equivalently,

$$H_A: \mu_T - \mu_R < m$$

and so the null hypothesis is the complement, $H_0: \mu_T - \mu_R \geq m$.

When a lower mean corresponds to a better outcome, we can conclude that outcomes under Treatment T are superior by a margin to outcomes under Treatment R so long as μ_T is lower than $\mu_R - m$, where $m > 0$ is the margin of superiority. The middle left panel of Figure 4.3 shows the relationship between μ_R and m and the range of values of μ_T that would make T superior by a margin to R. The alternative hypothesis is $H_A: \mu_T < \mu_R - m$, or equivalently,

$$H_A: \mu_T - \mu_R < -m$$

and the null hypothesis is the complement, $H_0: \mu_T - \mu_R \geq -m$.

For equivalence hypotheses, no modifications to the hypotheses are needed. The lower left panel of Figure 4.3 shows the range of values of μ_T that would make T equivalent to R.

4.8 Remarks

For simplicity, we have used the same symbol m to denote the margin in noninferiority tests, superiority by a margin tests and equivalence tests. However, it is possible that different margins could be selected for different types of tests, even for the same outcome.

In the literature, the terms "noninferior" and "equivalent" are sometimes used interchangeably, and "noninferior" and "superior" are also sometimes conflated. To resolve confusion, look at the hypotheses, particularly the alternative hypothesis, which generally expresses the objective of the study.

In equivalence and non-inferiority trials, special care is needed for analyzing the study data and interpreting the results, especially with regard to handling withdrawals, missing outcomes and protocol deviations in which participants do not receive their assigned treatment. For superiority trials, investigators often conduct an **intention to treat** (ITT) analysis, in which patients are analyzed in the condition to which they were assigned, regardless of whether or not they actually received that condition. If there are protocol deviations, ITT analysis will tend to make outcomes under the two conditions look more similar. If we are trying to show superiority, this approach will make it less likely that we reject the null hypothesis, which is generally considered conservative. However, for non-inferiority and equivalence trials, ITT analysis may be anticonservative; it may bias the findings toward similarity between conditions. In this situation, a **per protocol** analysis is often recommended; a per protocol analysis analyzes participants in the conditions that they actually received. These issues are discussed further in [110].

5

Analysis of variance for comparing means

5.1 Introduction

Analysis of variance (ANOVA) is a collection of methods used to compare means across different levels of categorical variables, sometimes called "factor" variables. In this chapter, we discuss power and sample size for one-way ANOVA, which is used to compare means across levels of a single factor, and two-way ANOVA, which is used to compare means when the observations are cross-classified according to two factors.

We restrict attention in this chapter to "between-subjects" designs. In a between-subjects design, each participant experiences only one condition and contributes only one outcome measurement, and all observations can be considered independent. In a "within-subjects" design, participants are exposed to more than one treatment or condition; observations made on the same participant are not independent, which needs to be accounted for in sample size and power calculations. We discuss within-subject designs in the context of crossover designs in Chapter 12.

5.2 One-way analysis of variance

Suppose that we have a groups, indexed by i, where group is defined by factor level. We will refer to this factor as Factor A. Within each group, there are n_i observations, indexed by j. The total number of observations is $\sum_{i=1}^{a} n_i = N$. Let Y_{ij} be the value of the outcome variable for individual j in group i. The one-way ANOVA model specifies that observations in group i are normally distributed with mean μ_i and variance σ^2, equal across groups, which can be expressed as $Y_{ij} = \mu_i + \epsilon_{ij}$, where $\epsilon_{ij} \sim \mathcal{N}(0, \sigma^2)$, with all ϵ_{ij} mutually independent. An alternative way to parametrize the model is to express each group mean μ_i as a sum of the mean of the group means, $\mu = \frac{1}{a}\sum_{i=1}^{a} \mu_i$, and a group effect α_i, in which case the model equation becomes

$$Y_{ij} = \mu + \alpha_i + \epsilon_{ij}, \qquad (5.1)$$

where we add the constraint $\sum_i \alpha_i = 0$ so that the values of α_i are uniquely identifiable. Since $\mu_i = \mu + \alpha_i$, we have that $\alpha_i = \mu_i - \mu$.

Example 5.1. Suppose that in a randomized trial with three study arms, the population group means are 5, 10 and 12. Then the mean of the group means can be found as

```
mu1 <- 5
mu2 <- 10
mu3 <- 12
mu <- (mu1 + mu2 + mu3) / 3  ;  mu
[1] 9
```

and the population group effects can be found as

```
alpha1 <- mu1 - mu
alpha2 <- mu2 - mu
alpha3 <- mu3 - mu
alpha1 ;  alpha2 ;   alpha3
[1] -4
[1] 1
[1] 3
```

Note that the group effects sum to zero.

The μ_i's, μ and α_i's are population parameters. The corresponding sample statistics are the sample group means, $\hat{\mu}_i = \bar{Y}_{i\cdot} = \frac{1}{n_i} \sum_{j=1}^{n_i} Y_{ij}$; the mean of the sample group means, $\hat{\mu} = \frac{1}{a} \sum_{i=1}^{a} \bar{Y}_{i\cdot}$; and the sample group effects, $\hat{\alpha}_i = \hat{\mu}_i - \hat{\mu}$. In our notation, a dot "$\cdot$" replacing an index indicates the average over that index.

Another important sample statistic is the overall sample mean, $\bar{Y}_{\cdot\cdot} = \frac{1}{N} \sum_{i=1}^{a} \sum_{j=1}^{n_i} Y_{ij}$, equal to the sum of all observations divided by the total number of observations. The overall mean can also be expressed as a weighted average of the group means, $\bar{Y}_{\cdot\cdot} = \sum_{i=1}^{a} \frac{n_i}{N} \bar{Y}_{i\cdot}$. If the group sizes are equal, then the overall mean will equal the mean of the group means. If the group sizes are not equal, these two values could be different. An ANOVA with equal sized groups is called a **balanced** design and an ANOVA with unequal group sizes is called an **unbalanced** design.

In a one-way ANOVA, the term "grand mean" is sometimes used. This term is sometimes used to refer to the overall mean and sometimes used to refer to the mean of the group means, and these two values could be different when the group sizes are unequal. We avoid using this term to avoid confusion.

Hypothesis testing for a one-way ANOVA involves the **omnibus F test** for any differences among population group means and **contrasts** which test

TABLE 5.1: One-way ANOVA sources of variation table.

Source	SS	df	MS	F
A	$\text{SSA} = \sum_i \sum_j (\bar{Y}_{i\cdot} - \bar{Y}_{\cdot\cdot})^2$	$a - 1$	$\text{MSA} = \frac{\text{SSA}}{a-1}$	$F = \frac{\text{MSA}}{\text{MSE}}$
Error	$\text{SSE} = \sum_i \sum_j (Y_{ij} - \bar{Y}_{i\cdot})^2$	$N - a$	$\text{MSE} = \frac{\text{SSE}}{N-a}$	
Total	$\text{SSTot} = \sum_i \sum_j (Y_{ij} - \bar{Y}_{\cdot\cdot})^2$	$N - 1$		

specific hypotheses about relationships among population group means. We discuss power and sample size for these tests in the following sections.

5.2.1 Omnibus F test

Standard output from fitting a one-way ANOVA model to data includes a sources of variation table, depicted in Table 5.1. We call the two sources of variation in a one-way ANOVA "group" and "error". Other terms for these sources of variation are "between-group" and "within-group". The sum of squares for the factor (SSA) quantifies how much the sample group means, $\bar{Y}_{i\cdot}$, vary from the overall mean, $\bar{Y}_{\cdot\cdot}$. The sum of squares for error (SSE) quantifies how much the individual observations within a group, Y_{ij}, vary from their sample group mean, $\bar{Y}_{i\cdot}$. The total sum of squares (SSTot) quantifies how much the individual observations vary from the overall mean. Each source of variation is associated with a degrees of freedom. Mean squares MSA and MSE are computed as each sum of squares divided by its degrees of freedom. The MSE is an estimate of the error variance σ^2.

The table also includes an F statistic that is used for the omnibus or "overall" F test, which is a test for any differences among group means. The null hypothesis is $H_0: \mu_1 = \ldots = \mu_a$, which is equivalent to all group effects equal to zero, $H_0: \alpha_1 = \ldots = \alpha_a = 0$. The alternative hypothesis is that not all group means are equal, $H_A: \mu_j \neq \mu_k$ for some $j \neq k$, or equivalently, not all group effects are equal to zero. The omnibus test uses the F statistic

$$F = \frac{\text{MSA}}{\text{MSE}} = \frac{\frac{1}{a-1} \sum_{i=1}^{a} \sum_{j=1}^{n_i} (\bar{Y}_{i\cdot} - \bar{Y}_{\cdot\cdot})^2}{\frac{1}{N-a} \sum_{i=1}^{a} \sum_{j=1}^{n_i} (Y_{ij} - \bar{Y}_{i\cdot})^2}. \quad (5.2)$$

To get an expression for power, we need to determine the distribution of the test statistic when H_0 is true and when some alternative is true. To derive these distributions (see [50, 142]), we divide the numerator and denominator of (5.2) by σ^2, obtaining

$$F = \frac{\frac{1}{a-1}\sum_i n_i \left(\frac{\bar{Y}_{i.} - \bar{Y}_{..}}{\sigma}\right)^2}{\frac{1}{N-a}\sum_i \sum_j \left(\frac{Y_{ij} - \bar{Y}_{i.}}{\sigma}\right)^2}. \tag{5.3}$$

Recall that a noncentral F distribution is formed as the ratio of a noncentral chi-squared random variable and a central chi-squared random variable, each divided by its degrees of freedom (see Section 3.1.4.) Here, the numerator of (5.3) has a noncentral chi-square distribution $\chi^2(a-1, \Lambda)$ with

$$\Lambda = \sum_i n_i \left(\frac{\mu_i - \sum_i \frac{n_i}{N}\mu_i}{\sigma}\right)^2 = \sum_i n_i \left(\frac{\alpha_i - \sum_i \frac{n_i}{N}\alpha_i}{\sigma}\right)^2. \tag{5.4}$$

The denominator has a central chi-squared distribution, $\chi^2(N-a)$. Thus $F \sim F(a-1, N-a, \Lambda)$. When all group sizes are equal ($n_i = n$), the noncentrality parameter simplifies to

$$\Lambda = n \sum_i \left(\frac{\mu_i - \mu}{\sigma}\right)^2 = n \sum_i \left(\frac{\alpha_i}{\sigma}\right)^2. \tag{5.5}$$

When H_0 is true, all α_i are equal to zero and so $\Lambda = 0$ and $F \sim F(a-1, N-a)$. H_0 is rejected at level α if $F > f_{1-\alpha, a-1, N-a}$. This is an upper-tailed test. Under an alternative where some $\alpha_i \neq 0$, Λ will be positive. Power for the omnibus F test can be computed as

$$P[F > f_{1-\alpha, a-1, N-a} \mid F \sim F(a-1, N-a, \Lambda)] \tag{5.6}$$
$$= 1 - \mathcal{F}_{a-1, N-a, \Lambda}(f_{1-\alpha, a-1, N-a}).$$

To calculate power, we need to calculate the noncentrality parameter, which requires values for σ, the group sample sizes $(n_1, \ldots, n_a)$, and either the group means $(\mu_1, \ldots, \mu_a)$ or the group effects $(\alpha_1, \ldots, \alpha_a)$. The noncentrality parameter can also be calculated by providing $\alpha_1/\sigma, \ldots, \alpha_a/\sigma$. These **standardized effect sizes for ANOVA** quantify the distance of each group mean from the mean of the group means in units of standard deviation.

Example 5.2. Continuing Example 5.1, for a three-arm study, the population group means are 5, 10 and 12. Suppose there are 40 subjects per group and we expect that the population standard deviation σ is 10. Power for an omnibus F test at $\alpha = 0.05$ can be calculated as follows:

```
library(powertools)
anova1way.F.bal(n = 40, mvec = c(5, 10, 12), sd = 10, power = NULL)
[1] 0.8208967
```

Power is 82%. Note that we can input the vector of effects c(-4, 1, 3) rather than the vector of means, or standardized effect sizes c(-0.4, 0.1, 0.3) with sd = 1, and get the same result. This is because it is only the relative standardized difference between means that matters.

```
anova1way.F.bal(n = 40, mvec = c(-4, 1, 3), sd = 10, power = NULL)
[1] 0.8208967
anova1way.F.bal(n = 40, mvec = c(-0.4, 0.1, 0.3), sd = 1, power = NULL)
[1] 0.8208967
```

Suppose we have an unbalanced design with group sizes 30, 40 and 50. Power for the omnibus F test is:

```
library(powertools)
anova1way.F.unbal(nvec = c(30, 40, 50), mvec = c(5, 10, 12), sd = 10)
[1] 0.7733937
```

The power is lower, even though the total N is the same. In general, power for the omnibus F test is highest when there is equal allocation (assuming equal variance across groups).

Sample size. There is no closed-form expression for the sample size needed to achieve a specified level of power for a one-way ANOVA omnibus F test. The smallest sample size that will achieve a desired level of power can be found using software that solves the power formula for sample size using numerical methods.

Example 5.3. In the study described in Example 5.2, the sample size needed to attain 80% power can be found using the command:

```
library(powertools)
anova1way.F.bal(n = NULL, mvec = c(5, 10, 12), sd = 10, power = 0.8)
[1] 38.07305
```

What factors affect power? To determine what factors affect power, we use the principle that power increases as the magnitude of the noncentrality parameter increases. Examining the noncentrality parameter in equation (5.4), it is clear that power increases as group sizes increases and decreases with higher σ^2. Also, power will be higher when the group effects are larger in magnitude. However, we should think carefully about whether we wish to focus on power for the omnibus F test when planning a study. If we reject the null hypothesis for this test, we conclude that some group means are not equal. This is generally an unsatisfactory conclusion because it does not tell

One-way analysis of variance 93

us *which* means are different. To test for differences among the group means, we need to conduct contrast tests, which are covered in Section 5.2.3.

▶ Rejection of the null hypothesis of the omnibus F test in a one-way ANOVA allows us to conclude that *some* group means are not equal, but more tests will be required to determine *which* means are different. Often it will be better to base power and sample size for a one-way ANOVA on contrast tests that test specific hypotheses of interest rather than the omnibus F test.

Connection to two-sample t test. When there are only two groups, the one-way ANOVA F test is equivalent to a two-sided, two-sample t test with equal group variances. We will have $\alpha_1 = \mu_1 - \mu = \mu_1 - (\mu_1 + \mu_2)/2 = \frac{1}{2}(\mu_1 - \mu_2)$ and $\alpha_1 = -\alpha_2$. Power for a test at significance level α can be calculated as $1 - \mathcal{F}_{1,N-2,\Lambda}(f_{1-\alpha,1,N-2})$, where $N = n_1 + n_2$ and $\Lambda = \frac{n_1 n_2}{N} \frac{(\mu_1 - \mu_2)^2}{\sigma^2}$.

5.2.2 Effect sizes for omnibus tests

Cohen [36] defined two types of effect sizes for ANOVA omnibus tests, the f effect size and the η^2 (eta-squared) effect size. The f effect size is based on quantifying the dispersion of the group means and then standardizing. The dispersion of the group means is quantified using the **standard deviation of the effects**, defined as

$$\sigma_A = \sqrt{\frac{\sum_i (\alpha_i - \bar{\alpha})^2}{a}} = \sqrt{\frac{\sum_i \alpha_i^2}{a}}. \tag{5.7}$$

Note that $\bar{\alpha} = 0$ because $\sum \alpha_i = 0$. Dividing σ_A by σ, we get the f effect size for a one-way ANOVA,

$$f = \frac{\sigma_A}{\sigma}.$$

The f effect size expresses the dispersion of the group means in units of standard deviation of the outcome variable. Cohen proposed $f = 0.1, 0.25$ and 0.4 as small, medium and large effect sizes, respectively [36].

The f effect size is in the same family as the standardized mean difference between two groups, $d = \frac{\mu_1 - \mu_2}{\sigma}$ (see Section 3.2.1). For a two-group ANOVA with means μ_1 and μ_2, $\alpha_1 = \mu_1 - \mu = \frac{\mu_1 - \mu_2}{2}$ and $\alpha_2 = \mu_2 - \mu = -\frac{\mu_1 - \mu_2}{2}$ and the f effect size is $\frac{\mu_1 - \mu_2}{2\sigma} = d/2$. Recall that $d = 0.2, 0.5$ and 0.8 are small, medium and large standardized mean effect sizes (Section 2.4), and thus the definitions of small, medium and large are consistent for one-way ANOVA and a difference between two means.

For a balanced one-way ANOVA, the relationship between the f effect size and the noncentrality parameter is

$$\Lambda = Nf^2, \tag{5.8}$$

where $N = na$, the total sample size. Thus when group sizes are equal, the noncentrality parameter can be computed by specifying only N and f. When group sizes are not equal, we can still compute an f effect size, but Λ needs to be computed using formula (5.4), which requires the values of σ, $\alpha_1, \ldots, \alpha_a$ and $n_1, \ldots, n_a$.

Example 5.4. In Example 5.2, the f effect size can be found as follows:

```
library(powertools)
es.anova.f(means = c(5, 10, 12), sd = 10, v = TRUE)

    Cohen's f effect size calculation for
    one-way analysis of variance

         fA = 0.294392
```

This f value is considered a medium effect size. The `pwr` package uses f effect sizes to conduct power calculations for a one-way ANOVA with equal-sized groups. For example,

```
library(pwr)
pwr.anova.test(k = 3, n = 40, f = 0.294392, power = NULL)

    Balanced one-way analysis of variance power calculation

              k = 3
              n = 40
              f = 0.294392
      sig.level = 0.05
          power = 0.8208967

NOTE: n is number in each group
```

This function does not support calculations involving unequal group sizes. A similar function is available in the `pwr2` package.

Another class of effect sizes in ANOVA are effect sizes based on proportion of variance explained. For the one-way ANOVA model (5.1), we can express the total variance of an observation as the sum of the variance of the means and the error variance, $\sigma_{tot}^2 = \sigma_A^2 + \sigma^2$, where σ_A is the standard deviation of the effects, defined in equation (5.7). This stretches the meaning of the term "variance" since the group means are not considered random variables in a one-way ANOVA. Then the proportion of the total variance of the observations

One-way analysis of variance 95

that is attributable to variance in the group means is

$$\omega^2 = \frac{\sigma_A^2}{\sigma^2 + \sigma_A^2}, \qquad (5.9)$$

pronounced "omega-squared" [121]. This quantity is also called η^2 ("eta-squared") [185]. Dividing the numerator and denominator by σ^2, we can find that $\omega^2 = f^2/(1+f^2)$. We can also find that $f = \sqrt{\omega^2/(1-\omega^2)}$.

Note that the variances in equation (5.9) are population parameters. Output from fitting ANOVA models to data often reports estimates of (5.9) with various names. These include $\hat{\eta}^2 = $ SSA/SSTot, $\hat{\omega}^2 = $ [SSA $-$ ($a-1$)MSE]/(SSTot $+$ MSE) and $\hat{\varepsilon}^2 = $ [SSA $-$ ($a-1$)MSE]/SSTot [7]; typically these are reported without the "hat" notation even though they are estimates. It has been show that $\hat{\eta}^2$ is biased upward [7, 174], that is, it overestimates the true effect size (5.9), especially when sample sizes are small. $\hat{\omega}^2$ and $\hat{\varepsilon}^2$ are preferred as estimates.

5.2.3 Contrast tests

In a one-way ANOVA, the omnibus F test may not answer the most important scientific questions. If the null hypothesis is rejected, we conclude that some of the means are different, but the test gives us no information about which means are different. The purpose of contrast tests is to test specific hypotheses about the relationships among the means. For example, in a three-group study, can we reject H_0: $\mu_1 = \mu_2$? Or H_0: $(\mu_1 + \mu_2)/2 = \mu_3$? Designing a study to have adequate power for specific hypothesis tests of interest is often the most sensible approach.

A **contrast** is a linear combination of the group means of the form

$$\psi = c_1\mu_1 + \ldots + c_a\mu_a = \sum_{i=1}^{a} c_i\mu_i$$

where $\sum_{i=1}^{a} c_i = 0$. The constants $c_1, \ldots, c_a$ are called **contrast coefficients**. Equivalently, contrasts can be specified as linear combinations of the effects, $\psi = \sum_i c_i\alpha_i$ with $\sum_i c_i = 0$.

Contrasts are used to express hypotheses. For example, for a 3-group one-way ANOVA, H_0: $\mu_1 - \mu_2 = 0$ can be expressed using the contrast $\psi = 1\mu_1 - 1\mu_2 + 0\mu_3$, where the contrast coefficient vector is $(c_1, c_2, c_3) = (1, -1, 0)$. Similarly, H_0: $(\mu_1 + \mu_2)/2 = \mu_3$ can be written as H_0: $(\mu_1 + \mu_2)/2 - \mu_3 = 0$ and expressed using $(c_1, c_2, c_3) = (0.5, 0.5, -1)$.

Hypotheses expressed using contrasts can be one- or two-sided. To test a hypothesis expressed as a contrast, for example, H_0: $\sum c_i\mu_i = c_0$ versus H_A: $\sum c_i\mu_i \neq c_0$, where c_0 is some constant, we compute the sample contrast,

$$\hat{\psi} = \sum c_i\hat{\mu}_i = \sum c_i\bar{Y}_{i\cdot}.$$

We can find that $Var(\sum_i c_i \bar{Y}_{i.}) = \sigma^2 \sum_i c_i^2/n_i$ and form the test statistic

$$T = \frac{\sum_i c_i \bar{Y}_{i.} - c_0}{\hat{\sigma}\sqrt{\sum c_i^2/n_i}}.$$

This test statistic has a $t(N-a)$ distribution when H_0 is true and a $t(N-a, \lambda)$ distribution when an alternative is true, with

$$\lambda = \frac{\sum_i c_i \mu_i - c_0}{\sigma\sqrt{\sum c_i^2/n_i}}. \tag{5.10}$$

For one-sided tests at level α, power can be calculated as

Lower-tailed test: $P(T < t_{\alpha, N-a}) = \mathcal{T}_{N-a, \lambda}(t_{\alpha, N-a})$

Upper-tailed test: $P(T > t_{1-\alpha, N-a,}) = 1 - \mathcal{T}_{N-a, \lambda}(t_{1-\alpha, N-a})$

For a two-sided tests, it is convenient to use the squared version of the test statistic,

$$F = T^2 = \frac{(\sum_i c_i \bar{Y}_{i.} - c_0)^2}{\hat{\sigma}^2 \sum c_i^2/n_i}$$

which has an $F(1, N-a, \Lambda)$ distribution, where $\Lambda = \lambda^2$ for λ as given in equation (5.10). Power for a two-sided test at level α can be calculated as

$$P(F > f_{1-\alpha, 1, N-a}) = 1 - \mathcal{F}_{1, N-a, \Lambda}(f_{1-\alpha, 1, N-a}).$$

For example, to test a hypothesis involving the contrast $\mu_1 - \mu_3$, the sample contrast is $\bar{Y}_{1.} - \bar{Y}_{3.}$ and the test statistic is

$$T = \frac{\bar{Y}_{1.} - \bar{Y}_{3.}}{\hat{\sigma}\sqrt{1/n_1 + 1/n_3}}$$

or the squared version for a two-sided test. This test statistic resembles the test statistic for a two-sample t test with pooled variance; see equation (3.12). However, in an ANOVA, $\hat{\sigma}$ is the square root of the MSE, which is obtained from the full sample, not just groups 1 and 3, and the degrees of freedom for the t (or F) distribution come from the MSE and are equal to $N - a$ rather than $n_1 + n_3 - 2$, which they would be for a two-sample t test.

Example 5.5. Continuing Example 5.2, we have 3 groups of size 20, $(\mu_1, \mu_2, \mu_3) = (5, 10, 12)$ and $\sigma = 10$. Suppose we plan to test all three pairwise comparisons among the means, $H_{01}: \mu_1 = \mu_2$, $H_{02}: \mu_1 = \mu_3$ and $H_{03}: \mu_2 = \mu_3$, each at level $0.05/3 = 0.0167$; this is a Bonferroni correction; see Section 5.2.4. The contrast coefficient vectors are $(1, -1, 0)$, $(1, 0, -1)$ and $(0, 1, -1)$. We can calculate the power for these contrasts as follows:

One-way analysis of variance

TABLE 5.2: Counts of the outcomes of m hypothesis tests in terms of whether or not H_0 is true and whether or not H_0 is rejected for each test, with $U + V + T + S = m$.

	Do not reject H_0	Reject H_0	
H_0 true	U	V	m_0
H_0 false	T	S	$m - m_0$
	W	R	m

```
library(powertools)
anova1way.c.bal(n = 40, mvec = c(5, 10, 12), cvec = c(1, -1, 0),
    sd = 10, alpha = 0.0167, power = NULL)
[1] 0.4268012

anova1way.c.bal(n = 40, mvec = c(5, 10, 12), cvec = c(1, 0, -1),
    sd = 10, alpha = 0.0167, power = NULL)
[1] 0.7576748

anova1way.c.bal(n = 40, mvec = c(5, 10, 12), cvec = c(0, 1, -1),
    sd = 10, alpha = 0.0167, power = NULL)
[1] 0.0660835
```

Power is higher when the two means are farther apart.

5.2.4 Multiple comparisons in ANOVA

Testing contrasts in ANOVA brings up the issue of **multiple testing** or **multiple comparisons**. In this section, we briefly discuss multiple testing procedures and then focus on how to estimate power when using such procedures. For more information on multiple testing methodology, see [23, 45, 54]. The related topic of multiple primary endpoints is discussed in Chapter 17.

Suppose that we plan to conduct m hypothesis tests. Table 5.2 shows counts of the outcomes of m tests in terms of whether or not H_0 is true and whether or not H_0 is rejected for each test, with $U + V + T + S = m$. When we test each of m hypotheses at significance level α, e.g., $\alpha = 0.05$, we are controlling the **comparisonwise error rate**, that is, the type I error rate for a single test or comparison. By doing so, we ensure that the proportion of incorrectly rejected null hypotheses will not exceed α. Referring to Table 5.2, this means that $V/m_0 < \alpha$. However, this allows for multiple erroneous rejections of null hypotheses, which may not be considered adequate control of the overall probability of making incorrect decisions. Options for controlling the probability of making incorrect decisions include controlling the familywise error rate or controlling the false discovery rate. The **familywise error rate** (FWER) is the probability of incorrectly rejecting *any* of the null hypotheses, $P(V > 0)$. The **false discovery rate** (FDR) is the expected value of V/R, where V/R is the proportion of "discoveries" (rejections of a null hypothesis) that are false (incorrect).

We can further define **weak control** and **strong control** of the FWER [182]. A procedure that controls the FWER under every scenario in which at least one null hypothesis is true is said to provide strong control of the FWER. A procedure that controls the FWER only under some scenarios (e.g., only when all null hypotheses are true) is said to provide weak control of the FWER.

Many different approaches have been developed to control the FWER or the FDR [54]. These include general methods that can be applied in many different multiple testing scenarios as well as methods that are specifically designed for ANOVA contrast testing. Recall from our discussions of factors affecting power that specifying a higher type I error rate will increase power, but at the expense of allowing for a higher probability of falsely rejecting the null hypothesis. A desirable feature of a FWER or FDR control procedure is that it provide control against type I errors while preserving power as much as possible.

General methods for controlling the FWER include the Bonferroni correction, in which the significance level for m tests is set to α/m for each test. The Bonferroni method can be quite conservative (meaning low power) when the number of tests is large or the test statistics are positively correlated [54]. Less conservative methods include those of Holm [97], Hochberg [95] and Hommel [98]. General methods for controlling the FDR include Benjamini & Hochberg [15] and Benjamini & Yekutieli [16]. Controlling the FDR is a less stringent condition than controlling the FWER, and so FDR control methods are more powerful than FWER control methods. However, in some settings, FDR control is considered inadequate protection against incorrect decisions and strong control of the FWER is expected.

FWER control methods for contrast testing in ANOVA include the following: for a small set of preplanned contrasts: Bonferroni, Šidák-Bonferroni or the Holm, Hochberg or Hommel methods; for comparing multiple treatment conditions to a common control condition: Dunnett's method; for all pairwise comparisons: Tukey's honest significant difference (HSD) method and Student-Neuman-Keuls procedure; for controlling error over the set of all contrasts: Scheffé's method. For more information on these procedures, see general texts such as [50, 121].

In general, if we use a multiple test correction, power will be reduced compared to using only comparisonwise error rate control. It is important to select a multiple comparison method carefully to preserve power. Except for Bonferroni and Šidák-Bonferroni corrections, analytic formulas for power when using these methods are not available and power must be estimated using simulation. The general topic of estimating power using simulation was discussed in Section 2.10.

A useful package for computing power for ANOVA designs using simulation is the Superpower package, which has online resources (https://aaronc aldwell.us/SuperpowerBook/) as well as related publications [133]. We demonstrate the use of this package to simulate power for a one-way ANOVA when using a FWER control method in the following example.

Example 5.6. Using the Superpower package is a two-step process: the first step is to create an ANOVA_design object and the next step is to run simulations to estimate power using the ANOVA_power function. By default, ANOVA_power finds power for the omnibus test and all pairwise contrasts among means. As a first demonstration, we replicate Example 5.5. This is for educational purposes, since power when using a Bonferroni correction can be calculated analytically rather than by simulation. We specify an α level of 0.05 with a Bonferroni correction. We set a seed to make the results reproducible.

```
library(Superpower)
design.3b <- ANOVA_design(design = "3b", n = 40, mu = c(5, 10, 12),
    sd = 10, label_list = list(group = c("A1", "A2", "A3")))
ANOVA_power(design_result = design.3b, alpha_level = 0.05,
    p_adjust = "bonferroni", nsims = 1000, seed = 678)

Power and Effect sizes for ANOVA tests
            power effect_size
anova_group  82.4    0.09473

Power and Effect sizes for pairwise comparisons (t-tests)
                     power effect_size
p_group_A1_group_A2   45.6    0.5125
p_group_A1_group_A3   75.7    0.7061
p_group_A2_group_A3    5.4    0.1926
```

The estimated levels of power for the omnibus test and contrasts are similar to what we found using analytical methods. The effect size displayed for the omnibus test is a partial eta-squared effect size calculated from the simulated data based on the aov_car function in the afex package. The effect sizes displayed for pairwise comparisons are standardized mean effect sizes calculated from the simulated data.

Now we estimate power when using Tukey's HSD for all pairwise comparisons:

```
ANOVA_power(design_result = design.3b, alpha_level = 0.05, emm = "TRUE",
    emm_p_adjust = "tukey", nsims = 1000, seed = 678)
# some output omitted
Power and Cohen's f from estimated marginal means
```

```
                    contrast power cohen_f
p_1 group_A1 - group_A2   47.7 0.21210
p_2 group_A1 - group_A3   77.3 0.29077
p_3 group_A2 - group_A3    5.5 0.09971
```

Tukey's HSD method is more powerful than the Bonferroni method and power is slightly higher for each contrast. The Cohen f effect sizes reported here are 1/2 of the d effect sizes comparing groups pairwise.

Suppose that group 1 is a control condition and our main interest is to compare groups 2 and 3 to group 1. The Dunnett method is designed to control the FWER in this situation. We can estimate power as follows:

```
ANOVA_power(design_result = design.3b, alpha_level = 0.05, emm = "TRUE",
    contrast_type = "trt.vs.ctrl1", emm_p_adjust = "dunnettx",
    nsims = 1000, seed = 678)
# some output omitted
 Power and Cohen's f from estimated marginal means
                    contrast power cohen_f
p_1 group_A2 - group_A1   51.8  0.2121
p_2 group_A3 - group_A1   81.9  0.2908
```

Power for our contrasts of interest is higher than it was when we planned to estimate all pairwise contrasts. By limiting the number of comparisons, we can increase power.

5.3 Two-way analysis of variance

In a two-way ANOVA, subjects are cross-classified according to two factors, which we will call A and B. For example, we may have 2 levels of Factor A and 3 levels of Factor B, for a total of $2 \times 3 = 6$ possible combinations of factor levels. In ANOVA nomenclature, this is referred to as a 2×3 factorial design.

One motivation for using a two-way or higher-order ANOVA design is efficiency: by using a two-way design, we may be able to gain power for detecting the effects of each factor, compared to studying each factor by itself in a one-way design. The efficiency of ANOVA designs is discussed in Section 5.3.4. Another possible motivation is to allow for investigation of interactions between factors. Power for detecting interactions is discussed in Section 5.3.5.

Suppose we have $i = 1, \ldots, a$ levels of Factor A and $j = 1, \ldots, b$ levels of Factor B. Levels of A and B define the rows and columns of an $a \times b$ matrix. Within cell ij, there are n_{ij} observations indexed by k, $k = 1, \ldots, n_{ij}$, with

Two-way analysis of variance 101

N total observations. The two-way ANOVA model can be expressed as

$$Y_{ijk} = \mu_{ij} + \epsilon_{ijk}$$

where μ_{ij} is the mean for cell ij and $\epsilon_{ijk} \sim \mathcal{N}(0, \sigma^2)$ with all ϵ_{ijk} mutually independent. We can express each cell mean μ_{ij} as a sum $\mu_{ij} = \mu + \alpha_i + \beta_j$, where μ is the mean of the cell means ($\mu = \frac{1}{ab}\sum_i \sum_j \mu_{ij}$), α_i is the effect of being at level i of Factor A and β_j is the effect of being at level j of Factor B. The model equation becomes

$$Y_{ijk} = \mu + \alpha_i + \beta_j + \epsilon_{ijk} \qquad (5.11)$$

with the constraints $\sum_i \alpha_i = 0$ and $\sum_j \beta_j = 0$ so that the values of α_i and β_j are identifiable. This model implies that the effect of one factor is the same regardless of the level of the other factor, meaning there are no interactions. To allow for interactions, we write the model as

$$Y_{ijk} = \mu + \alpha_i + \beta_j + (\alpha\beta)_{ij} + \epsilon_{ijk} \qquad (5.12)$$

with the additional constraints $\sum_i (\alpha\beta)_{ij} = 0$ for all j and $\sum_j (\alpha\beta)_{ij} = 0$ for all i. The term $(\alpha\beta)_{ij}$ represents the interaction effect associated with the combination of the ith level of A and jth level of B. This term quantifies how much the mean of cell ij differs from the mean that would be expected if the effects of A and B were additive.

Tests of interest for a two-way ANOVA include tests for the main effects of the factors, that is, whether cell means differ by levels of Factor A or by levels of Factor B; test for an interaction between A and B; and contrast tests. As we will see, these tests and the power and sample size procedures for them are extensions of the methods for one-way ANOVA.

5.3.1 Solving for the factor effects (no interaction model)

The factor effects play an important role in power calculations. In the following example, we show how to start with a set of cell means for a two-way ANOVA model with no interactions and solve for the factor effects.

Example 5.7. A randomized trial will use a 2 × 3 factorial design to assess the effectiveness of two intervention strategies to improve diabetes control in patients with poorly controlled type 2 diabetes: a behavioral skills intervention with two levels (no and yes) and an educational intervention with 3 levels (none, 3 sessions and 6 sessions). The primary outcome is hemoglobin A1c level at 12-month follow-up. The expected mean A1c without any interventions is 9.3%. The behavioral skills intervention is expected to reduce mean A1c by 0.6 percentage points. Three sessions of education is expected to reduce mean A1c by 0.4 and 6 sessions is expected to reduce it by 0.8 percentage points. The effects of the two interventions are expected to be additive, i.e., not interact. The cell means are thus:

	None	3 sessions	6 sessions
No	$\mu_{11} = 9.3$	$\mu_{12} = 8.9$	$\mu_{13} = 8.5$
Yes	$\mu_{21} = 8.7$	$\mu_{22} = 8.3$	$\mu_{23} = 7.9$

We can find the values of the effects α_1, α_2 and $\beta_1, \beta_2, \beta_3$ given the cell means using the following logic. In a 2×3 ANOVA with no interactions, the cell means are parametrized as:

	B1	B2	B3
A1	$\mu + \alpha_1 + \beta_1$	$\mu + \alpha_1 + \beta_2$	$\mu + \alpha_1 + \beta_3$
A2	$\mu + \alpha_2 + \beta_1$	$\mu + \alpha_2 + \beta_2$	$\mu + \alpha_2 + \beta_3$

where $\sum_i \alpha_i = 0$ and $\sum_j \beta_j = 0$. If we subtract μ from each cell, we will obtain

	B1	B2	B3
A1	$\alpha_1 + \beta_1$	$\alpha_1 + \beta_2$	$\alpha_1 + \beta_3$
A2	$\alpha_2 + \beta_1$	$\alpha_2 + \beta_2$	$\alpha_2 + \beta_3$

The next step is to calculate the marginal row and column means:

	B1	B2	B3	Marginal means
A1	$\alpha_1 + \beta_1$	$\alpha_1 + \beta_2$	$\alpha_1 + \beta_3$	α_1
A2	$\alpha_2 + \beta_1$	$\alpha_2 + \beta_2$	$\alpha_2 + \beta_3$	α_2
Marginal means	β_1	β_2	β_3	

The simple forms of the marginal means occur because of the zero-sum constraints $\sum_i \alpha_i = 0$ and $\sum_j \beta_j = 0$. For example, the marginal mean for the first row is $(3\alpha_1 + \sum_j \beta_j)/3 = \alpha_1$.

Applying this procedure to our example, the mean of the cell means is $\mu = (\sum_i \sum_j \mu_{ij})/6 = 8.6$. Subtracting μ from each entry and calculating the marginal means, we obtain

	None	3 sessions	6 sessions	Marginal means
No	0.7	0.3	-0.1	$\alpha_1 = 0.3$
Yes	0.1	-0.3	-0.7	$\alpha_2 = -0.3$
Marginal means	$\beta_1 = 0.4$	$\beta_2 = 0$	$\beta_3 = -0.4$	

Thus we have determined the values of the factor effects that are implied by the values of the cell means. Note that they satisfy the zero-sum constraints.

Two-way analysis of variance 103

TABLE 5.3: Sources of variation table for a two-way ANOVA with only main effects.

Source	SS	df	MS	F
A	$\text{SSA} = \sum_i \sum_j \sum_k (\bar{Y}_{i..} - \bar{Y}_{...})^2$	$a-1$	$\text{MSA} = \frac{\text{SSA}}{a-1}$	$F_A = \frac{\text{MSA}}{\text{MSE}}$
B	$\text{SSB} = \sum_i \sum_j \sum_k (\bar{Y}_{\cdot j \cdot} - \bar{Y}_{...})^2$	$b-1$	$\text{MSB} = \frac{\text{SSB}}{b-1}$	$F_B = \frac{\text{MSB}}{\text{MSE}}$
Error	$\text{SSE} = \sum_i \sum_j \sum_k (Y_{ijk} - \bar{Y}_{ij\cdot})^2$	$N-a-b+1$	$\text{MSE} = \frac{\text{SSE}}{N-a-b+1}$	
Total	$\text{SSTot} = \sum_i \sum_j \sum_k (Y_{ijk} - \bar{Y}_{...})^2$	$N-1$		

5.3.2 Tests for main effects

Table 5.3 displays a sources of variation table for a two-way ANOVA with main effects only. SSA quantifies how much the row means $\bar{Y}_{i..}$ differ from the overall mean $\bar{Y}_{...}$, SSB quantifies how much the column means $\bar{Y}_{\cdot j \cdot}$ differ from the overall mean and SSE quantifies how observations within cell ij differ from $\bar{Y}_{ij\cdot}$, their cell mean.

A test for a main effect of a factor in a two-way ANOVA is similar to an omnibus F test in one-way ANOVA. The test proceeds as if we are testing for an effect of Factor A ignoring Factor B, or the effect of B ignoring A. The test for the main effect of A has the null hypothesis H_0: $\alpha_i = 0$ for all i; the alternative hypothesis is H_A: $\alpha_i \neq 0$ for some i. The test statistic is

$$F_A = \frac{\text{MSA}}{\text{MSE}} = \frac{\frac{1}{a-1}\sum_{i=1}^{a}\sum_{j=1}^{b}\sum_{k=1}^{n_{ij}}(\bar{Y}_{i..} - \bar{Y}_{...})^2}{\frac{1}{N-a-b+1}\sum_{i=1}^{a}\sum_{j=1}^{b}\sum_{k=1}^{n_{ij}}(Y_{ijk} - \bar{Y}_{ij\cdot})^2}.$$

When H_0 is true, $F_A \sim F(a-1, N-a-b+1)$. H_0 is rejected at level α if $F_A > f_{1-\alpha, a-1, N-a-b+1}$. When H_0 is false, F_A has a noncentral F distribution, $F_A \sim F(a-1, N-a-b+1, \Lambda_A)$, where

$$\Lambda_A = \sum_i \sum_j \left(\frac{\alpha_i}{\sigma/\sqrt{n_{ij}}}\right)^2. \tag{5.13}$$

When all cell sizes are equal to n, this simplifies to $\Lambda_A = (nb/\sigma^2)\sum_i \alpha_i^2$. Power is $P(F_A > f_{1-\alpha, a-1, N-a-b+1}) = 1 - \mathcal{F}_{a-1, N-a-b+1, \Lambda_A}(f_{1-\alpha, a-1, N-a-b+1})$. Similarly, to test H_0: $\beta_j = 0$ for all j versus H_A: $\beta_j \neq 0$ for some j, we use the test statistic

$$F_B = \frac{\text{MSB}}{\text{MSE}} = \frac{\frac{1}{b-1}\sum_i \sum_j \sum_k (\bar{Y}_{\cdot j \cdot} - \bar{Y}_{...})^2}{\frac{1}{N-a-b+1}\sum_i \sum_j \sum_k (Y_{ijk} - \bar{Y}_{ij\cdot})^2},$$

which is distributed as $F(b-1, N-a-b+1, \Lambda_B)$, where

$$\Lambda_B = \sum_j \sum_i \left(\frac{\beta_j}{\sigma/\sqrt{n_{ij}}}\right)^2. \tag{5.14}$$

This simplifies to $\Lambda_B = (na/\sigma^2) \sum_j \beta_j^2$ when all cell sizes are equal to n. Power can be found as $1 - \mathcal{F}_{b-1, N-a-b+1, \Lambda_B}(f_{1-\alpha, b-1, N-a-b+1})$.

Example 5.8. Continuing Example 5.7, suppose that the common standard deviation is 2 and we have 30 participants per cell. We can compute power for the two tests of main effects in a balanced two-way ANOVA, each at level 0.05, using the anova2way.F.bal function. As an initial step, we create a matrix with the cell means.

```
library(powertools)
mmat <- matrix(c(9.3, 8.9, 8.5, 8.7, 8.3, 7.9), nrow = 2, byrow = TRUE)
anova2way.F.bal(n = 30, mmatrix = mmat, sd = 2, alpha = 0.05, v = TRUE)

    Balanced two-way analysis of variance
    omnibus F test power calculation

              n = 30
        mmatrix = 9.3, 8.9, 8.5
                  8.7, 8.3, 7.9
             sd = 2
 f effect size = 0.1500, 0.1633
          alpha = 0.05
          power = 0.5166, 0.4796
```

Note that the levels of power for the two main effects are different. The output includes f effect sizes, which are discussed in Section 5.3.3. To find the sample size to achieve 80% power for each main effect, we can use the following code:

```
anova2way.F.bal(n = NULL, mmatrix = mmat, sd = 2, alpha = 0.05,
    power = 0.8, v = F)

       nA       nB
 58.4634  60.7203
```

To attain 80% power for the main effect of A, we need 59 per cell; for 80% power for the main effect of B, we need 61 per cell. To ensure at least 80% power for both, we need 61 per cell, for a total of $N = 6 \times 61 = 366$.

5.3.3 Effect sizes

In a two-way ANOVA, we can define f effect sizes for each main effect that are standardized versions of the standard deviations of the effects [36], analogous to a one-way ANOVA f effect size (Section 5.2.2). The standard deviations of the effects are defined as

$$\sigma_A = \sqrt{\frac{\sum_i \alpha_i^2}{a}} \quad \text{and} \quad \sigma_B = \sqrt{\frac{\sum_j \beta_j^2}{b}}$$

from which we can compute the f effect sizes for each factor as

$$f_A = \frac{\sigma_A}{\sigma} \quad \text{and} \quad f_B = \frac{\sigma_B}{\sigma}.$$

The benchmarks are the same as for one-way ANOVA: $0.1, 0.25$ and 0.4 are considered small, medium and large f effect sizes, respectively [36].

For a balanced two-way ANOVA (equal cell sizes), we can express the noncentrality parameters for the main effects tests using f effect sizes:

$$\Lambda_A = N f_A^2 = nab f_A^2 \quad \text{and} \quad \Lambda_B = N f_B^2 = nab f_B^2.$$

For an unbalanced two-way ANOVA (unequal cell sizes), the values of the factor effects, $\alpha_1, \ldots, \alpha_a$ and $\beta_1, \ldots, \beta_b$, are needed to calculate the noncentrality parameters according to formulas (5.13) and (5.14). The following example derives the f effect sizes for a two-way balanced ANOVA and uses them in a power calculation.

Example 5.9. We continue with Examples 5.7 and 5.8. The factor effects were $(\alpha_1, \alpha_2) = (0.3, -0.3)$ and $(\beta_1, \beta_2, \beta_3) = (0.4, 0, -0.4)$. The standard deviations of the effects are

```
sigmaA <- sqrt((0.3^2 + (-0.3)^2) / 2)
sigmaB <- sqrt((0.4^2 + 0^2 + (-0.4)^2) / 3)
sigmaA  ;  sigmaB
[1] 0.3
[1] 0.3265986
```

Given $\sigma = 2$, the f effect sizes are

```
sd <- 2
fA <- sigmaA / sd
fB <- sigmaB / sd
fA  ; fB
[1] 0.15
[1] 0.1632993
```

These are considered "small" effect sizes. The function es.anova.f computes the f effect sizes based on the matrix of cell means:

```
library(powertools)
mmat <- matrix(c(9.3, 8.9, 8.5, 8.7, 8.3, 7.9), nrow = 2, byrow = TRUE)
es.anova.f(means = mmat, sd = 2, v = TRUE)

    Cohen's f effect size calculation for
    two-way analysis of variance

          fA = 0.15
          fB = 0.1632993
         fAB = 0
```

fAB is the effect size for the interaction between the two factors. Interactions in a two-way ANOVA are discussed in Section 5.3.5. There is no interaction between factors in this example and this effect size is thus zero.

The `pwr.2way` function in the `pwr2` package computes power using f effect sizes. With 30 in each cell, power is:

```
library(pwr2)
pwr.2way(a = 2, b = 3, alpha = 0.05, size.A = 30, size.B = 30,
    f.A = fA, f.B = fB)

Balanced two-way analysis of variance power calculation
# some output omitted
          power.A = 0.5165924
          power.B = 0.4795865
            power = 0.4795865

NOTE: power is the minimum power among two factors
```

The power matches what we calculated in Example 5.8. The output identifies overall power as the minimum power among the two factors.

5.3.4 Two-way ANOVA designs: efficiency and other considerations

As mentioned earlier, one motivation for using a two-way or higher order ANOVA design is efficiency. In a two-way ANOVA, the main effect of Factor A is estimated ignoring Factor B, that is, it is calculated as if Factor B did not exist. Similarly, the main effect of Factor B is calculated ignoring Factor A. Each observation serves double duty, as an observation for Factor A and an observation for Factor B. As a result, if interaction effects are absent or small, then a two-way ANOVA will require fewer observations to attain the same power to detect the main effects of the two factors, compared to conducting two separate one-way studies, one for each factor. The following example illustrates the potential efficiency gains:

Example 5.10. For the 2×3 design in Example 5.8, we found that we needed a total N of 366 to achieve at least 80% power to detect the main effects of both factors. Suppose that instead of a two-way ANOVA, we conduct two separate one-way ANOVA studies. How many participants will we need in total?

We find the sample sizes for two one-way ANOVAs, one for each factor. Note that we can use a vector of effects in a calculation, rather than a vector of means; this was discussed in Example 5.2:

```
library(powertools)
anova1way.F.bal(n = NULL, mvec = c(0.3, -0.3), sd = 2, power = 0.8)
[1] 175.3847

anova1way.F.bal(n = NULL, mvec = c(0.4, 0, -0.4), sd = 2, power = 0.8)
[1] 121.4378
```

For balanced one-way designs, for Factor A, we will need $2 \times 176 = 352$ participants and for Factor B, we will need $3 \times 122 = 366$ participants, for a total of $352 + 366 = 718$. Using the two-way design, we need only 366. Essentially, the two-way design gives us the test for the main effect of Factor A for "free" – as long as there are no interactions among the factors. This may or may not be realistic to expect, depending on the particular study.

The greatest efficiency occurs when the effect sizes of the two factors are similar. If the effect sizes are different, then to attain adequate power for both factors, the study will need to have sufficient observations to provide power for the smaller effect size; but this larger number of observations will "overpower" the other factor.

The theoretical efficiency gains of a higher-order ANOVA design are not always realized in practice. In particular, the presence of interaction effects can decrease the power to detect main effects. When the no-interaction assumption is not justified, one could consider using instead a one-way multiple-arm design or a factorial design with alternative testing approaches, for example, tests for contrasts and simple effects, discussed Section 5.3.6. For further discussion and recommendations, see [71, 126].

> ▶ When the assumption of no interaction between factors cannot be justified, a two-way ANOVA design that relies on tests for main effects may not be the best choice. Alternative approaches include a one-way multi-arm design or a factorial design with a different analysis approach.

TABLE 5.4: Sources of variation table for a two-way ANOVA with an interaction between the two factors.

Source	SS	df	MS	F
A	$\sum\sum\sum(\bar{Y}_{i..} - \bar{Y}_{...})^2$	$a-1$	$\text{MSA} = \frac{\text{SSA}}{a-1}$	$F_A = \frac{\text{MSA}}{\text{MSE}}$
B	$\sum\sum\sum(\bar{Y}_{.j.} - \bar{Y}_{...})^2$	$b-1$	$\text{MSA} = \frac{\text{SSB}}{b-1}$	$F_B = \frac{\text{MSA}}{\text{MSE}}$
AB	$\sum\sum\sum(\bar{Y}_{ij.} - \bar{Y}_{i..} - \bar{Y}_{.j.} + \bar{Y}_{...})^2$	$(a-1)(b-1)$	$\text{MSAB} = \frac{\text{SSAB}}{(a-1)(b-1)}$	$F_{AB} = \frac{\text{MSAB}}{\text{MSE}}$
Error	$\sum\sum\sum(Y_{ijk} - \bar{Y}_{ij.})^2$	$N-ab$	$\text{MSE} = \frac{\text{SSE}}{N-ab}$	
Total	$\sum\sum\sum(Y_{ijk} - \bar{Y}_{...})^2$	$N-1$		

5.3.5 Test for interaction

The two-way ANOVA model with interactions between the two factors is

$$Y_{ijk} = \mu_{ij} + \epsilon_{ijk} = \mu + \alpha_i + \beta_j + (\alpha\beta)_{ij} + \epsilon_{ijk}, \quad (5.15)$$

$\epsilon_{ijk} \sim \mathcal{N}(0, \sigma^2)$, with constraints $\sum_i \alpha_i = 0, \sum_j \beta_j = 0$ and $\sum_i (\alpha\beta)_{ij} = 0$ for all j and $\sum_j (\alpha\beta)_{ij} = 0$ for all i. The constraints on the interaction terms mean that the interaction effects sum to zero over each row and over each column. The term $(\alpha\beta)_{ij}$ represents the interaction effect associated with the combination of the ith level of A and jth level of B, that is, the amount by which mean for cell ij differs from the mean that would be expected if the effects of Factors A and B were additive. Note that the cell means are parametrized as $\mu_{ij} = \mu + \alpha_i + \beta_j + (\alpha\beta)_{ij}$ and thus the interaction effects are $(\alpha\beta)_{ij} = \mu_{ij} - (\mu + \alpha_i + \beta_j)$.

Table 5.4 displays the sources of variation table for a two-way ANOVA model with an interaction between the factors. The table includes the AB interaction as a source of variation, with an accompanying sum of squares, degrees of freedom, mean square and F statistic. The test for any interaction between Factors A and B has hypotheses $H_0: (\alpha\beta)_{ij} = 0$ for all ij versus H_A: not all $(\alpha\beta)_{ij} = 0$ and uses the test statistic

$$F_{AB} = \frac{\text{MSAB}}{\text{MSE}} = \frac{\frac{1}{(a-1)(b-1)} \sum_i \sum_j \sum_k (\bar{Y}_{ij.} - \bar{Y}_{i..} - \bar{Y}_{.j.} + \bar{Y}_{...})^2}{\frac{1}{N-ab} \sum_i \sum_j \sum_k (Y_{ijk} - \bar{Y}_{ij.})^2}.$$

The numerator involves the differences between each cell mean $\bar{Y}_{ij.}$ and an estimate of its expected value under no interaction, $\bar{Y}_{...} + (\bar{Y}_{i..} - \bar{Y}_{...}) + (\bar{Y}_{.j.} - \bar{Y}_{...})$. The test proceeds in the same manner as tests for the main effects. The test statistic has an F distribution with noncentrality parameter

$$\Lambda_{AB} = \sum_i \sum_j \left[\frac{(\alpha\beta)_{ij}}{\sigma/\sqrt{n_{ij}}} \right]^2. \quad (5.16)$$

Two-way analysis of variance 109

When all cell sizes are equal to n, this simplifies to

$$\Lambda_{AB} = \frac{n}{\sigma^2} \sum_i \sum_j [(\alpha\beta)_{ij}]^2.$$

Power can be calculated as $1 - \mathcal{F}_{(a-1)(b-1), N-ab, \Lambda_{AB}}(f_{1-\alpha,(a-1)(b-1),N-ab})$.

An effect size for the interaction can be computed as the standard deviation of the effects divided by the error standard deviation, $f_{AB} = \sigma_{AB}/\sigma$, where σ_{AB} is computed as

$$\sigma_{AB} = \sqrt{\frac{\sum_i \sum_j [(\alpha\beta)_{ij}]^2}{ab}}.$$

When there are n observations in each cell, we can compute the noncentrality parameter for the interaction test as $\Lambda_{AB} = nabf_{AB}^2 = Nf_{AB}^2$.

The interaction effects are important for calculating power for detecting the interaction. The following example illustrates how interaction and other effects as well as effect sizes can be calculated from a table of means when an interaction is present.

Example 5.11. We modify Example 5.7 to include an interaction. Suppose that we expect the combination of the behavioral intervention and the 6-session education to have an effect that is greater than additive and reduce mean A1c to 7.3. Thus we expect the following cell means:

	None	3 sessions	6 sessions
No	9.3	8.9	8.5
Yes	8.7	8.3	7.3

We use the table of means to solve for all effects and obtain effect sizes. The means follow the parametrization:

	B1	B2	B3
A1	$\mu + \alpha_1 + \beta_1 + (\alpha\beta)_{11}$	$\mu + \alpha_1 + \beta_2 + (\alpha\beta)_{12}$	$\mu + \alpha_1 + \beta_3 + (\alpha\beta)_{13}$
A2	$\mu + \alpha_2 + \beta_1 + (\alpha\beta)_{21}$	$\mu + \alpha_2 + \beta_2 + (\alpha\beta)_{22}$	$\mu + \alpha_2 + \beta_3 + (\alpha\beta)_{23}$

where $\sum_i \alpha_i = 0, \sum_j \beta_j = 0$ and $\sum_i (\alpha\beta)_{ij} = 0 \ \forall j$ and $\sum_j (\alpha\beta)_{ij} = 0 \ \forall i$. If we subtract μ from each cell and then obtain the marginal means (row and column means), we get

	B1	B2	B3	
A1	$\alpha_1 + \beta_1 + (\alpha\beta)_{11}$	$\alpha_1 + \beta_2 + (\alpha\beta)_{12}$	$\alpha_1 + \beta_3 + (\alpha\beta)_{13}$	α_1
A2	$\alpha_2 + \beta_1 + (\alpha\beta)_{21}$	$\alpha_2 + \beta_2 + (\alpha\beta)_{22}$	$\alpha_2 + \beta_3 + (\alpha\beta)_{23}$	α_2
	β_1	β_2	β_3	

These values for the marginal means occur because of the zero-sum constraints. For example, the marginal mean for row A1 is $[3\alpha_1 + \sum_j \beta_j +$

$\sum_j (\alpha\beta)_{1j}]/3 = \alpha_1$ because $\sum_j \beta_j = 0$ and $\sum_j (\alpha\beta)_{1j} = 0$. To find the interaction effects, we subtract α_i and β_j from each cell, which gives

	B1	B2	B3	
A1	$(\alpha\beta)_{11}$	$(\alpha\beta)_{12}$	$(\alpha\beta)_{13}$	α_1
A2	$(\alpha\beta)_{21}$	$(\alpha\beta)_{22}$	$(\alpha\beta)_{23}$	α_2
	β_1	β_2	β_3	

Now we apply this procedure to our example. We could use `es.anova.f` to get the effects, but we go through each step for instructional purposes. In our example, $\mu = (9.3 + 8.9 + 8.5 + 8.7 + 8.3 + 7.3)/6 = 8.5$. Subtracting 8.5 from each cell and then calculating the marginal means, we obtain

	None	3 sessions	6 sessions	
No	0.8	0.4	0	$\alpha_1 = 0.4$
Yes	0.2	-0.2	-1.2	$\alpha_2 = -0.4$
	$\beta_1 = 0.5$	$\beta_2 = 0.1$	$\beta_3 = -0.6$	

To find the interaction effects, we subtract α_i and β_j from each cell in the above table, which gives us

	None	3 sessions	6 sessions	
No	$(\alpha\beta)_{11} = -0.1$	$(\alpha\beta)_{12} = -0.1$	$(\alpha\beta)_{13} = 0.2$	$\alpha_1 = 0.4$
Yes	$(\alpha\beta)_{21} = 0.1$	$(\alpha\beta)_2 = 0.1$	$(\alpha\beta)_{23} = -0.2$	$\alpha_2 = -0.4$
	$\beta_1 = 0.5$	$\beta_2 = 0.1$	$\beta_3 = -0.6$	

It is easy to verify that the effects satisfy all of the zero-sum constraints. We are now able to calculate σ_A, σ_B and σ_{AB} as

```
sigmaA <- sqrt( (0.4^2 + (-0.4)^2) / 2 )
sigmaB <- sqrt( ((0.5)^2 + (0.1)^2 + (-0.6)^2) / 3 )
sigmaAB <- sqrt( ((-0.1)^2 + (-0.1)^2 + (0.2)^2 + (0.1)^2
             + (0.1)^2 + (-0.2)^2) / 6 )
sigmaA  ;  sigmaB  ;  sigmaAB
[1] 0.4
[1] 0.4546061
[1] 0.1414214
```

Dividing by $\sigma = 2$, we obtain the f effect sizes,

```
sd <- 2
fA <- sigmaA / sd
fB <- sigmaB / sd
fAB <- sigmaAB / sd
fA  ;   fB   ;  fAB
[1] 0.2
[1] 0.227303
[1] 0.07071068
```

Two-way analysis of variance   111

The interaction effect is "small" while the main effects are "medium". Interaction effects are often smaller than main effects. Power for the main and interaction effects when each cell has 30 observations can be calculated as follows:

```
library(powertools)
mmat <- matrix(c(9.3, 8.9, 8.5, 8.7, 8.3, 7.3), nrow = 2, byrow = TRUE)
anova2way.F.bal(n = 30, mmatrix = mmat, sd = 2, alpha = 0.05, v = T)
```

```
    Balanced two-way analysis of variance
    omnibus F test power calculation with interaction

              n = 30
        mmatrix = 9.3, 8.9, 8.5
                  8.7, 8.3, 7.3
             sd = 2
  f effect size = 0.2000, 0.2273, 0.0707
          alpha = 0.05
          power = 0.7607, 0.7775, 0.1225
```

NOTE: The 3rd value for f and power or n is for the interaction

With 30 observations in each cell, power to detect each main effect is close to 80%, while power to detect the small interaction effect is very low. If detecting an interaction effect is an important study objective, the sample size will need to be much larger.

5.3.6 Contrasts

As discussed for one-way ANOVA, it is often sensible to design a study to have adequate power for tests of contrasts that reflect specific study hypotheses. We discuss two types of contrasts for a two-way ANOVA: contrasts among the levels of one of the factors (for example, $\beta_1 - \beta_2$) and contrasts among cell means (for example, $\mu_{11} - \mu_{12}$).

A contrast involving levels of Factor A or levels of Factor B has the form

$$\psi = \sum_i c_i \alpha_i \text{ or } \psi = \sum_j c_j \beta_j$$

where the contrast coefficients sum to zero. Such contrasts can be estimated as $\hat{\psi} = \sum_i c_i \bar{Y}_{i..}$ or $\hat{\psi} = \sum_j c_j \bar{Y}_{.j.}$, where $\bar{Y}_{i..}$ is the marginal mean for level i of Factor A and $\bar{Y}_{.j.}$ is the marginal mean for level j of Factor B. To conduct a contrast test and to compute power, the approach is the same as described in Section 5.2.3 for contrasts in one-way ANOVA. For example, for a contrast involving levels of Factor B, we can use the test statistic

$$T = \frac{\sum_j c_j \bar{Y}_{\cdot j}}{\hat{\sigma}\sqrt{\sum c_j^2/n_{\cdot j}}}$$

where $n_{\cdot j}$ is the total number of observations at level j of Factor B. This test statistic has a t distribution with degrees of freedom equal to those for error ($N - a - b + 1$ for two-way ANOVA with main effects only, and $N - ab$ for two-way ANOVA with an interaction) and noncentrality parameter

$$\lambda = \frac{\sum_j c_j \beta_j}{\sigma\sqrt{\sum c_j^2/n_{\cdot j}}}. \tag{5.17}$$

This T statistic can be used for one- or two-sided tests. For a two-sided test, we can also use the F statistic,

$$F = \frac{\left(\sum_j c_j \bar{Y}_{\cdot j}\right)^2}{\hat{\sigma}^2 \sum c_j^2/n_{\cdot j}}$$

which has a F distribution with numerator degrees of freedom of 1 and denominator degrees of freedom equal to those for error. The noncentrality parameter is $\Lambda = \lambda^2$, where λ is given in (5.17).

Example 5.12. For the interaction scenario presented in Example 5.11, suppose we plan to test $H_0: \beta_1 - \beta_3 = 0$ with two-sided significance level 0.05. This corresponds to testing whether six-session education has a different effect on mean A1c level at follow-up compared to no education sessions. The test statistic is

$$F = \left(\frac{\bar{Y}_{\cdot 1} - \bar{Y}_{\cdot 3}}{\hat{\sigma}\sqrt{1/n_{\cdot 1} + 1/n_{\cdot 3}}}\right)^2$$

where $n_{\cdot 1}$ and $n_{\cdot 3}$ are the total numbers of participants who will receive no education and six-session education, respectively. Power can be calculated as:

```
library(powertools)
mmat <- matrix(c(9.3, 8.9, 8.5, 8.7, 8.3, 7.3), nrow = 2, byrow = TRUE)
anova2way.c.bal(n = 30, mmatrix = mmat, cvec = c(1, 0, -1),
    factor = "b", sd = 2, alpha = 0.05)
[1] 0.8498625
```

Power is about 0.85.

Two-way analysis of variance

A contrast can also be formed as a linear combination of the cell means,

$$\psi = \sum_i \sum_j c_{ij} \mu_{ij}$$

with $\sum_i \sum_j c_{ij} = 0$. A common use of such cell-to-cell contrasts is to test for **simple effects**. A simple effect is a contrast between levels of one factor for a given level of the other factor. Simple effects are often of interest when there is an interaction, which implies that the effect of one factor on the outcome depends on the level of the other factor. For such tests, we can use the test statistic

$$T = \frac{\sum_i \sum_j c_{ij} \bar{Y}_{ij\cdot}}{\hat{\sigma}\sqrt{\sum_i \sum_j c_{ij}^2/n_{ij}}}.$$

The degrees of freedom are equal to those for error and the noncentrality parameter is

$$\lambda = \frac{\sum_i \sum_j c_{ij} \mu_{ij}}{\sigma\sqrt{\sum_i \sum_j c_{ij}^2/n_{ij}}}.$$

For a two-sided test, one can use an F statistic equal to T^2, which will have a noncentrality parameter equal to $\Lambda = \lambda^2$, and do an upper-tailed test. The numerator degrees of freedom are 1 and the denominator degrees of freedom are those for error.

Example 5.13. For the 2 × 3 ANOVA with interaction in Example 5.11, suppose we plan to test whether the behavioral skills intervention is effective in the absence of the educational intervention. For the outcome A1c, lower is better. To conduct the test, we use the hypotheses $H_0: \mu_{21} - \mu_{11} \geq 0$ versus $H_A: \mu_{21} - \mu_{11} < 0$. If we reject H_0, we conclude that, when there is no educational intervention, mean A1c levels are lower for the behavioral skills intervention compared to the control condition. We set a 0.025 significance level. Power can be calculated as:

```
library(powertools)
mmat <- matrix(c(9.3, 8.9, 8.5, 8.7, 8.3, 7.3), nrow = 2, byrow = TRUE)
cmat <- matrix(c(-1, 0, 0, 1, 0, 0), nrow = 2, byrow = TRUE)
anova2way.se.bal(n = 30, mmatrix = mmat, cmatrix = cmat, sd = 2,
    alpha = 0.025)
[1] 0.2105612
```

The power is low, about 0.21. This contrast test involves comparing two groups of size 30 when there is a standardized mean difference of magnitude $|8.7 - 9.3|/2 = 0.3$, which is relatively small.

Power for contrasts in factorial ANOVA designs can also be estimated using the `Superpower` package. This package allows for the use of multiple comparison corrections; see Section 5.2.4.

5.4 Analysis of covariance

An ANOVA model that includes covariates is called an analysis of covariance (ANCOVA) model. The term "ANCOVA" is sometimes used to refer more specifically to studies in which the outcome variable is measured at both a baseline and a follow-up time point, and the outcome analysis adjusts for the baseline measurement using a linear regression model. ANCOVA is a common modeling technique and can substantially increase power, as we discuss in this section.

ANOVA and ANCOVA models are types of multiple linear regression models. Power for multiple linear regression models is discussed in Section 10.3. The reader may wish to refer to that section for additional background.

To understand how adding covariates to an ANOVA model impacts power, one needs to focus on the error variance. Recall that the one-way ANOVA model is

$$Y_{ij} = \mu + \alpha_i + \epsilon_{ij}, \quad \epsilon_{ij} \sim \mathcal{N}(0, \sigma^2)$$

where $\sum_i \alpha_i = 0$. In this model, σ^2 is the variance of Y within groups, or in other words, the variance of Y conditional on group membership. We could use new notation to express this more explicitly, writing

$$Y_{ij} = \mu + \alpha_i + \epsilon_{ij}, \quad \epsilon_{ij} \sim \mathcal{N}\left(0, \sigma^2_{Y|A}\right) \quad (5.18)$$

where $\sigma^2_{Y|A}$ is the variance of Y conditional on group as defined by the levels of Factor A. As predictors are added to a linear regression model, the error variance changes. In particular, if we add a covariate that helps to explain variation in Y beyond the variation explained by variables that are already in the model, the error variance can be expected to decrease. Thus if we add a covariate X, taking value X_{ij} for individual j in group i, the model becomes

$$Y_{ij} = \mu + \alpha_i + \gamma X_{ij} + \epsilon_{ij}, \quad \epsilon_{ij} \sim \mathcal{N}\left(0, \sigma^2_{Y|A,X}\right) \quad (5.19)$$

where the error variance is now $\sigma^2_{Y|A,X}$ and is expected to be lower than $\sigma^2_{Y|A}$ if X explains variance in Y beyond that explained by Factor A. In particular, if $Corr(X,Y) = \rho$ and X is not correlated with Factor A, then $\sigma^2_{Y|A,X} = \sigma^2(1-\rho^2)$; that is, the error variance is reduced by a factor of $1-\rho^2$ by adding X to the model (see Chapter 15 in [121]).

How does reducing the error variance affect power? Recall that the error variance is estimated by the MSE, that is, MSE = $\hat{\sigma}^2$, where for simplicity we have dropped the subscripts indicating what terms are in the model. All test statistics for omnibus and contrast tests include the MSE in the denominator, for example, F_A = MSA/MSE. Thus if the error variance is reduced due to a covariate, the magnitude of the test statistic is likely to be higher and the probability of rejecting the null hypothesis will also be higher. Thus power is increased for all tests.

To account for the covariate in power calculations, in the noncentrality parameter, σ^2 is multiplied by $1 - \rho^2$. For example, when adding a covariate to a one-way ANOVA F test, the noncentrality parameter becomes (assuming groups are all of size n)

$$\Lambda = \frac{n}{\sigma^2(1-\rho^2)} \sum_i \alpha_i^2. \tag{5.20}$$

In addition, each covariate reduces the error degrees of freedom by 1. This tends to reduce power and can partially offset the power gains due to the error variance reduction. However, if N is large, the impact will be minimal.

It is important to note that the full power gains due to adding a covariate will only accrue if the covariate is not correlated with the factors. Randomization to groups will, on average, create this lack of correlation. If the study is not randomized or the randomization is compromised, there may be correlation between covariates and factors, and adding covariates may not increase power, although it may be important for other reasons, such as reducing bias.

▶ Adding covariates to an ANOVA model can increase power **if** the covariates are highly correlated with the outcome variable Y **and** they are not correlated with the factors **and** the sample sizes are not small (total N is at least 30 or so).

Continuous covariates in an ANCOVA model are often centered at their mean. Thus a one-way ANCOVA model with a single continuous covariate X_{ij} is often formulated as $Y_{ij} = \mu + \alpha_i + \gamma(X_{ij} - \bar{X}_{..}) + \epsilon_{ij}$, where $\bar{X}_{..}$ is the overall mean of X. Centering covariates changes the interpretation of μ but has no impact on power or model fit. The parameter μ is now the expected mean of the group means when the covariate takes its mean value.

Including more than one covariate. When a set of covariates C is added to an ANOVA model, the error variance is reduced by a factor $1 - \rho_{Y|C}^2$, where $\rho_{Y|C}^2$ is the squared multiple correlation coefficient from regressing Y on the set C. A squared multiple correlation coefficient is the population analogue of a model R^2, which is the proportion of the total variation in Y that is explained by its linear relationship with the covariates; see Section 10.3. In formulas for noncentrality parameters, the error variance σ^2 is replaced by $\sigma^2(1 - \rho_{Y|C}^2)$. When k covariates are added, the error degrees of freedom are reduced by k. The covariates can be continuous or categorical; continuous predictors are often more effective in reducing error variance.

We illustrate the impact of including covariates in an ANOVA in the following example.

Example 5.14. We continue the one-way ANOVA from Example 5.2. The sample size required to achieve 80% power for the omnibus F test with no covariates can be found as

```
library(powertools)
anova1way.F.bal(n = NULL, mvec = c(5, 10, 12), sd = 10, power = 0.8)
[1] 38.07305
```

Suppose that we will adjust for a baseline covariate in the analysis. The correlation between the covariate and outcome measurement is expected to be in the range of 0.4 to 0.6. How does this affect the required sample size?

The ANOVA functions in the powertools package include the parameter Rsq to account for covariates. Rsq is the value of R^2 expected from regressing Y on the covariate(s). For a single X with $Corr(X, Y) = \rho$, this value is ρ^2. The default value of Rsq is zero. We also need to specify a value for ncov, the number of covariates, to properly account for the impact on the error degrees of freedom. Code for calculating power when $\rho = 0.4$ is:

```
anova1way.F.bal(n = NULL, mvec = c(5, 10, 12), sd = 10, Rsq = 0.4^2,
   ncov = 1, power = 0.8)
[1] 32.15828
```

The table below displays required n per group to achieve 80% power when there are no covariates and when there is one covariate with correlation of 0.4, 0.5 or 0.6, and the percent change in required sample size compared to having no covariates:

	No covariates	$\rho = 0.4$	$\rho = 0.5$	$\rho = 0.6$
n per group	38.07	32.16	28.83	24.76
% change		−15.5%	−24.3%	−35.0%

The drop in required sample size due to adding a covariate increases as ρ increases and can be substantial. The reductions in sample size are close to the expected reductions in error variance, which are $16\%, 25\%$ and 36%, but slightly lower due to the loss of one degree of freedom.

Power is sensitive to the value of ρ. This parameter is a good target for a sensitivity analysis.

5.5 Additional resources

Superpower is a comprehensive simulation-based package for estimating power for single factor and factorial ANOVA designs. The package can handle designs with both between-subjects and within-subjects factors. We demonstrated the use of this package in several examples in this chapter. Further information on this package is available at https://cran.r-project.org/web/packages/Superpower/vignettes/intro_to_superpower.html and in Lakens and Caldwell [133].

The pwrss package offers various functions for power and sample size for ANOVA that take as inputs eta-squared or f^2 effect sizes.

6

Proportions: large sample methods

6.1 Preliminaries

In this section, we review the binomial distribution, the distribution of the sample proportion, and the normal approximations to these distributions. These distributions are foundational for the large sample distributions of test statistics for proportions.

Let Y_i denote a Bernoulli random variable taking values 1 ("success") or 0 ("failure") with probabilities p and $1-p$, respectively. Let $X = \sum_{i=1}^{N} Y_i$ denote the sum of N independent Bernoulli random variables, that is, the number of successes that occur out of N independent Bernoulli trials. Then X has a binomial distribution, denoted $X \sim Bin(N, p)$. X can take values $0, 1, \ldots, N$. The probability of each outcome is given by the probability mass function

$$P(X = k) = \binom{N}{k} p^k (1-p)^{N-k} \text{ for } k = 0, \ldots, N.$$

The mean and variance of X are $E(X) = Np$ and $Var(X) = Np(1-p)$.

If we standardize a binomial random variable by subtracting its mean and dividing by its standard deviation, the standardized random variable has approximately a standard normal distribution,

$$\frac{X - Np}{\sqrt{Np(1-p)}} \overset{\cdot}{\sim} \mathcal{N}(0, 1).$$

The approximation is reasonably good when $Np(1-p) \geq 10$ [189].

Suppose we are interested in inference regarding a population proportion p. We can estimate p using the sample proportion, $\hat{p} = \frac{1}{N} \sum_{i=1}^{N} Y_i = X/N$. The sample proportion has mean $E(\hat{p}) = E(X/N) = p$ and variance $Var(\hat{p}) = Var(X/N) = p(1-p)/N$. Note that the variance of $\hat{p}$ depends on the value of p. This means that the precision with which we can estimate a proportion depends on the value of the proportion itself. For a fixed N, a proportion of $p = 0.5$ has the highest variance; the variance decreases as p moves away from 0.5 toward 0 or 1; see Figure 6.1. The important implication is that power will generally be lowest when the true proportion(s) in a study are near 0.5 and higher when proportions are closer to 0 or 1.

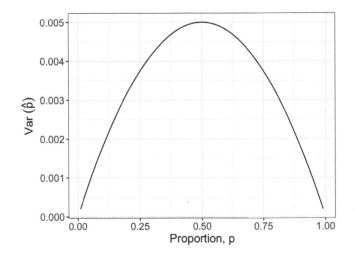

FIGURE 6.1: Variance of the sample proportion $\hat{p}$ as a function of p. Sample size $N = 50$.

▶ The variance of a sample proportion depends on the true value of the proportion. The variance is highest and therefore power is lowest when $p = 0.5$.

If we standardize the sample proportion by subtracting its mean p and dividing by its standard deviation $\sqrt{p(1-p)/N}$, or by $\sqrt{\hat{p}(1-\hat{p})/N}$, the resulting quantity has approximately a standard normal distribution,

$$\frac{\hat{p}-p}{\sqrt{\frac{p(1-p)}{N}}} \stackrel{.}{\sim} \mathcal{N}(0,1) \quad \text{and} \quad \frac{\hat{p}-p}{\sqrt{\frac{\hat{p}(1-\hat{p})}{N}}} \stackrel{.}{\sim} \mathcal{N}(0,1).$$

The normal approximation can be improved by using a continuity correction, which is discussed in many textbooks.

6.2 One-sample proportion test

In the context of a clinical trial with a binary outcome, we will refer to participants with "success" as responders and participants without a success as non-responders. Consider a one-sample study design in which we wish to compare the proportion of responders to some reference proportion p_0,

$$H_0: p = p_0 \text{ versus } H_A: p \neq p_0.$$

For example, we may want to test whether the proportion of patients responding to a new treatment is different from the proportion known to respond to a reference treatment. In Section 7.1, we discuss "exact" power and sample size calculations for a test of one proportion using the binomial distribution. In this section, we discuss using the normal approximation to the binomial for the calculations. There are several different options for approaching the approximation. We consider one common approach and then discuss variations.

For a sample of size N, the test can be conducted using the test statistic

$$Z = \frac{\hat{p} - p_0}{\sqrt{\frac{\hat{p}(1-\hat{p})}{N}}}.$$

When H_0 is true and $p = p_0$, the test statistic has approximately a standard normal distribution. When some alternative is true and $p = p_A$,

$$Z \stackrel{.}{\sim} \mathcal{N}\left(\frac{p_A - p_0}{\sqrt{\frac{p_A(1-p_A)}{N}}}, 1\right).$$

For a two-sided test at level α, power is approximately

$$1 - \beta \approx \Phi\left(\frac{\sqrt{N}|p_A - p_0|}{\sqrt{p_A(1 - p_A)}} - z_{1-\alpha/2}\right) \tag{6.1}$$

and the sample size needed to achieve power of $1 - \beta$ can be approximated as

$$N \geq \frac{(z_{1-\alpha/2} + z_{1-\beta})^2 p_A(1 - p_A)}{(p_A - p_0)^2}. \tag{6.2}$$

For a one-sided test at level α, use $z_{1-\alpha}$.

Example 6.1. An experimental therapy will be considered promising if the proportion of patients responding to it exceeds 0.2. If the true proportion of responders is 0.3, how many patients are needed to achieve 80% power, with a one-sided test at α of 0.05?

The study entails an upper tailed test of $H_0: p \leq 0.2$ versus $H_A: p > 0.2$. We can find N as follows:

```
library(powertools)
prop.1samp(N = NULL, p0 = 0.2, pA = 0.3, power = 0.8, sides = 1)
[1] 129.8337
```

Rounding up, we need 130 patients.

One-sample proportion test

What factors affect power? By inspecting power formula (6.1), we can infer that power increases as sample size N increases and as the difference between the null and alternative values of the proportions, $|p_A - p_0|$, increases. Further, due to the term $p_A(1 - p_A)$, which is the variance of the sample proportion, power is lowest when p_A is equal to 0.5 and increases for values of p_A closer to 0 or 1, all else being equal.

The following example illustrates how required sample size depends not just on the difference of proportions, $|p_A - p_0|$, but also the value of p_A.

Example 6.2. In Example 6.1, when $p_0 = 0.2$ and $p_A = 0.3$, we needed 130 patients to achieve 80% power. Suppose that we have $p_0 = 0.4$ and $p_A = 0.5$. The difference of proportions that we wish to detect, $|p_A - p_0|$, equals 0.1, and is the same. Will we need the same N?

```
library(powertools)
prop.1samp(N = NULL, p0 = 0.4, pA = 0.5, power = 0.8, sides = 1)
[1] 154.5639
```

We need 155 patients. Why is it different? The sample size formula includes the term $p_A(1 - p_A)$, which appears because $Var(\hat{p}_A) = p_A(1 - p_A)/N$. As discussed in Section 6.1, the variance of a sample proportion is highest when the true population proportion equals 0.5. Here, we have $p_A = 0.5$. Thus we need more patients to achieve 80% power, even though the difference in proportions is the same.

There are several variations of the one-sample proportion test statistic. One variation is to condition on the null being true to construct the standard error, which leads to the test statistic

$$Z' = \frac{\hat{p} - p_0}{\sqrt{\frac{p_0(1-p_0)}{N}}}. \tag{6.3}$$

When $H_0: p = p_0$ is true, $Z' \stackrel{.}{\sim} \mathcal{N}(0, 1)$. When an alternative $p = p_A$ is true,

$$Z' \stackrel{.}{\sim} \mathcal{N}\left(\frac{p_A - p_0}{\sqrt{\frac{p_0(1-p_0)}{N}}}, \frac{p_A(1-p_A)}{p_0(1-p_0)}\right).$$

For a two-sided test at level α, power is approximately

$$1 - \beta \approx \Phi\left(\frac{\sqrt{N}|p_A - p_0| - z_{1-\alpha/2}\sqrt{p_0(1-p_0)}}{\sqrt{p_A(1-p_A)}}\right) \tag{6.4}$$

Solving this equation for N leads to a required sample size of

$$N \geq \frac{\left[z_{1-\beta}\sqrt{p_A(1-p_A)} + z_{1-\alpha/2}\sqrt{p_0(1-p_0)}\right]^2}{(p_A - p_0)^2} \quad (6.5)$$

A further variation is to use a continuity correction. This leads to test statistics

$$Z_c = \frac{\hat{p} - p_0 + c}{\sqrt{\frac{\hat{p}(1-\hat{p})}{N}}} \quad \text{and} \quad Z'_c = \frac{\hat{p} - p_0 + c}{\sqrt{\frac{p_0(1-p_0)}{N}}}$$

where $c = -\frac{1}{2N}$ if $\hat{p} > p_0$ and $c = \frac{1}{2N}$ if $\hat{p} < p_0$. We do not provide explicit formulas for power and sample size in the case of using continuity corrections. Rather, we note that accuracy can be further improved by using an exact binomial calculation (see Section 7.1).

6.2.1 Application to vaccine efficacy trials

In this section, we show how one sample proportion methods can be applied to finding the required sample size for a vaccine efficacy trial. Although we might think to use a comparison of two proportions (Section 6.3) to compare outcomes in vaccinated and unvaccinated groups, the incidence of disease cases in a vaccine efficacy trial is typically very low and the conventional comparison of two proportions can break down. Hence there is a need for alternative approaches. This exposition draws on Chow et al. [33].

Suppose that disease cases occur in vaccinated and unvaccinated populations with probabilities π_V and π_U, respectively. The risk ratio is defined as the ratio of these probabilities, RR = $\frac{\pi_V}{\pi_U}$. Vaccine efficacy (VE) is traditionally measured as VE = $1 - $ RR = $\frac{\pi_U - \pi_V}{\pi_U}$. We interpret vaccine efficacy as the proportionate reduction in the probability of disease due to the vaccine.

Example 6.3. If the probabilities of disease in vaccinated and unvaccinated populations are $\pi_V = 0.002$ and $\pi_U = 0.008$, then the risk ratio is RR = $\frac{\pi_V}{\pi_U} = 0.25$ and vaccine efficacy is VE = $1 - $ RR = 0.75. The vaccine reduces the probability of disease by 75%.

Denote the numbers of individuals in the vaccinated and unvaccinated groups as n_V and n_U and let $r = n_U/n_V$ be the ratio of group sizes, i.e., the allocation ratio. Let X_V and X_U be random variables denoting the numbers of disease cases in the vaccinated and unvaccinated groups. These counts are assumed to be binomial distributed with $X_V \sim \text{Bin}(n_V, \pi_V)$ and $X_U \sim \text{Bin}(n_U, \pi_U)$. Let x_V and x_U denote the observed numbers of cases in a trial. Given a total number of cases $x_{tot} = x_V + x_U$ occurring during the trial, the

One-sample proportion test

number occurring in the vaccinated group is distributed as Binomial(x_{tot}, p) where p, the probability that a case is in the vaccinated group, is

$$p = \frac{E(X_V)}{E(X_V) + E(X_U)} = \frac{n_V \pi_V}{n_V \pi_V + n_U \pi_U} = \frac{\text{RR}}{\text{RR} + r} = \frac{1 - \text{VE}}{1 - \text{VE} + r}. \quad (6.6)$$

To go from the third term to the fourth term, we divided the numerator and denominator by $n_U \pi_U$. These relationships allow us to translate hypotheses involving vaccine efficacy into hypotheses involving a single proportion p.

Typically, the goal is to conclude that vaccine efficacy exceeds a certain value, VE_0. This corresponds to the hypotheses

$$H_0 : \text{VE} \le \text{VE}_0 \quad \text{versus} \quad H_A : \text{VE} > \text{VE}_0.$$

By defining $p_0 = \frac{1 - \text{VE}_0}{1 - \text{VE}_0 + r}$, we can equate this to testing $H_0 : p \ge p_0$ versus $H_A : p < p_0$. Thus the test becomes a one sample proportion test. The proportion of interest is the proportion of the total observed cases that occurred in the vaccinated group, estimated as $\hat{p} = \frac{x_V}{x_V + x_U}$.

Power for a given sample size can be estimated using equation (6.1) and sample size to achieve a desired level of power can be estimated using equation (6.2). When using this approach, the sample size is the total number of observed cases, $x_V + x_U$, which is called the target number of events (TNE). We demonstrate this calculation in the next example.

Example 6.4. A two-arm vaccine efficacy trial aims to find that the efficacy of a vaccine exceeds 30%. What is the target number of events (TNE) needed to have at least 90% power to reject $H_0 : \text{VE} \le 30\%$ with α of 0.025 when the true probabilities of events (cases) in the vaccinated and unvaccinated groups are 0.0032 and 0.0080? Allocation will be 1:1.

First, we find the true vaccine efficacy that is implied by the given parameters:

```
piV <- 0.0032  ;  piU <- 0.0080
veA <- 1 - piV / piU  ;  veA
[1]   0.6
```

Thus $\text{VE}_A = 0.6$ or 60%. Next, we find the values p_0 and p_A that are implied by the vaccine efficacy values of $\text{VE}_0 = 0.3$ and $\text{VE}_A = 0.6$:

```
ve0 <- 0.3  ;  veA <- 0.6  ;  r <- 1
p0 <- (1 - ve0) / (1 - ve0 + r)
pA <- (1 - veA) / (1 - veA + r)
p0 ; pA
[1] 0.4117647
[1] 0.2857143
```

Based on these values, we can calculate the TNE:

```
library(powertools)
prop.1samp(N = NULL, p0 = p0, pA = pA, alpha = 0.025, power = 0.9,
    sides = 1)
[1] 134.962
```

Rounding up, the target number of events is 135.

Based on the TNE, the allocation ratio r and the expected probability of being a case in each group, π_U and π_V, the required total number of individuals to enroll can be calculated. In particular, we have

$$TNE = n_V \pi_V + n_U \pi_U = n_V \pi_V + n_V r \pi_U = n_V (\pi_V + r \pi_U).$$

Solving for n_V, we obtain

$$n_V = \frac{TNE}{\pi_V + r \pi_U}$$

and the total sample size needed is $N = n_V(1+r)$. The sample size may need to be adjusted due to additional considerations such as expected attrition.

Example 6.5. Continuing Example 6.4, for equal allocation, we find that the sample size needed in each group is

```
n <- 135 / (piV + piU)  ; n
[1] 12053.57
```

We need over 12,000 in each group and over 24,000 in total. Vaccine efficacy trials can require very large sample sizes.

6.3 Test of two independent proportions

6.3.1 Test for nonequality

Now we consider study designs that compare outcome proportions in two independent groups. Suppose we wish to test for nonequality using the hypotheses

$$H_0 \colon p_1 - p_2 = 0 \text{ versus } H_A \colon p_1 - p_2 \neq 0.$$

Similar to the case of one proportion designs, there are several ways to calculate a test statistic. We discuss commonly used normal approximation approaches in this section. The test can also be conducted using exact methods (Section 7.3) or a chi-square test (Section 8.2).

Test of two independent proportions

Suppose we have group sizes n_1 and n_2 and sample proportions $\hat{p}_1$ and $\hat{p}_2$. The test can be conducted using the test statistic

$$Z = \frac{\hat{p}_1 - \hat{p}_2}{\sqrt{\frac{\hat{p}_1(1-\hat{p}_1)}{n_1} + \frac{\hat{p}_2(1-\hat{p}_2)}{n_2}}}. \tag{6.7}$$

Under the null, $Z \stackrel{.}{\sim} \mathcal{N}(0,1)$. Under an alternative that the true proportions are p_1 and p_2, power for a two-sided test at level α is approximately

$$1 - \beta \approx \Phi\left(\frac{|p_1 - p_2|}{\sqrt{\frac{p_1(1-p_1)}{n_1} + \frac{p_2(1-p_2)}{n_2}}} + z_{\alpha/2}\right). \tag{6.8}$$

Total sample size N for a two-sided test when $n_2 = rn_1$ is approximately

$$N \geq \frac{1+r}{r} \frac{(z_{1-\alpha/2} + z_{1-\beta})^2 [rp_1(1-p_1) + p_2(1-p_2)]}{(p_1 - p_2)^2}. \tag{6.9}$$

For a one-sided test at level α, replace $\alpha/2$ with α.

Example 6.6. A randomized trial will compare two treatments on a binary outcome. The expected outcome proportions are $p_1 = 0.6$ and $p_2 = 0.8$. For equal allocation, how many participants are needed to achieve 90% power to test $H_0: p_1 \geq p_2$ versus $H_A: p_1 < p_2$ at $\alpha = 0.025$?

We use the `prop.2samp` function from the `powertools` package. In this function, `n1` is the sample size in group 1 and the default is equal allocation (`n.ratio = 1`).

```
library(powertools)
prop.2samp(n1 = NULL, p1 = 0.6, p2 = 0.8, alpha = 0.025, power = 0.9,
    sides = 1)
[1] 105.0742
```

Rounding up, we find that we need 106 per arm.

An alternative approach is to calculate the standard error conditioning on the null hypothesis that $p_1 = p_2$ and using a pooled estimate of the common proportion, $\hat{p}_c = \frac{n_1 \hat{p}_1 + n_2 \hat{p}_2}{n_1 + n_2}$. The test statistic is

$$Z' = \frac{\hat{p}_1 - \hat{p}_2}{\sqrt{\left(\frac{1}{n_1} + \frac{1}{n_2}\right)\hat{p}_c(1-\hat{p}_c)}}. \tag{6.10}$$

Under this approach, the required sample size is approximately

$$N \geq \frac{1+r}{r} \frac{[z_{1-\alpha/2}\sqrt{(1+r)p_c(1-p_c)} + z_{1-\beta}\sqrt{rp_1(1-p_1) + p_2(1-p_2)}]^2}{(p_1 - p_2)^2} \tag{6.11}$$

where $p_c = (rp_1 + p_2)/(1+r)$.

Whether to choose the pooled or the unpooled approach is not always clear, because it is not the case that one is always more powerful than the other [33]. A drawback of the pooled approach is that it is difficult to generalize to tests of inferiority, superiority by a margin and equivalence [33].

Example 6.7. Power calculations based on the pooled proportion test statistic (6.10) are implemented by the power_prop_test function in the MESS package. We repeat Example 6.6 using this function:

```
library(MESS)
power_prop_test(n = NULL, p1 = 0.6, p2 = 0.8, power = 0.9,
  sig.level = 0.025, alternative = "one.sided")

    Two-sample comparison of proportions power calculation

              n = 108.2355
             p1 = 0.6
             p2 = 0.8
      sig.level = 0.025
          power = 0.9
    alternative = one.sided

NOTE: n is number in *each* group
```

Using this approach, we need 108.2355 per arm.

6.3.2 Effect size for difference of two proportions

In Chapter 3, we discussed the standardized effect size for the difference between two means, defined as $d = (\mu_1 - \mu_2)/\sigma$. We also saw that to calculate power or sample size, we could specify only d rather than all three parameters μ_1, μ_2 and σ. Is there a similar standardized effect size for the difference between two proportions?

Developing an effect size for a difference in proportions is complicated by the fact that the variance of a sample proportion depends on the value of the proportion, so we cannot vary the value of a proportion and its variance independently. Cohen [36] proposed an effect size for the difference between two proportions using the arcsine square root transformation, $\arcsin(\sqrt{p})$. This transformation is a variance stabilizing transformation for a proportion [10], because $Var[\arcsin(\sqrt{\hat{p}})] \approx 1/(4N)$, which depends on sample size but not p. Cohen defined an h effect size for the difference in proportions as

$$h = 2\arcsin(\sqrt{p_1}) - 2\arcsin(\sqrt{p_2}). \tag{6.12}$$

Test of two independent proportions 127

Differences in proportions with the same h have similar detectability. Benchmarks for h effect sizes are the same as for d effect sizes: $0.2, 0.5$ and 0.8 are "small", "medium" and "large". The following pairs of proportions correspond to h of 0.2: (0.05, 0.10), (0.20, 0.29), (0.40, 0.50), (0.50, 0.60), (0.71, 0.80), (0.90, 0.95). These differences in proportions range from 0.05 (when proportions are closer to 0 or 1) to 0.10 (when proportions are close to 0.5). For more information, see Cohen [36], Section 6.2.

Example 6.8. In Example 6.6, the h effect size is

```
library(powertools)
es.h(p1 = 0.6, p2 = 0.8)

    Cohen's h effect size calculation for two proportions

              p1 = 0.8
              p2 = 0.6
               h = -0.4421432
```

This is a medium effect size.

Sample size requirements can be approximated using h effect sizes. For a two-sided, one-sample test of proportion at level α,

$$N \geq \frac{(z_{1-\alpha/2} + z_{1-\beta})^2}{h^2} \tag{6.13}$$

where $h = 2\arcsin(\sqrt{p_0}) - 2\arcsin(\sqrt{p_A})$. For a two-sided, two-sample test of proportions at level α with equal allocation,

$$N = 2n \geq \frac{2(z_{1-\alpha/2} + z_{1-\beta})^2}{h^2}. \tag{6.14}$$

The pwr package has functions for power and sample size for one or two proportions that use h effect sizes. The use of h effect sizes may be useful at early stages of planning a study. However, for final calculations, it is usually preferable to use a method that specifies the anticipated values of the two proportions and reflects the planned method of analysis.

6.3.3 Tests for noninferiority and superiority by a margin

In Chapter 4, we discussed tests of noninferiority and superiority by a margin for comparing two means. We discuss such tests for comparing two proportions in this section. Section 6.3.4 discusses tests of equivalence for two proportions.

Suppose that a lower outcome proportion is better. When testing for noninferiority of an outcome proportion between a test treatment and a reference treatment, we hope to conclude that $p_T < p_R + m$, where $m > 0$, i.e., the proportion of participants with the outcome under test treatment is not higher than the proportion under reference treatment plus a small margin. Remember the tip from Chapter 4 that *the alternative hypothesis is typically the conclusion that the investigators would like to reach, and thus communicates the objective of the study*. This tip helps us to formulate the null and alternative hypotheses properly. Moving all of the parameters to the left-hand side of the inequality yields H_A, and H_0 is its complement:

$$H_0: p_T - p_R - m \geq 0 \text{ versus } H_A: p_T - p_R - m < 0. \qquad (6.15)$$

When a lower outcome proportion is better and we want to test whether the test treatment is superior by a margin to the reference, we hope to conclude that $p_T < p_R - m$, where $m > 0$. Taking this as H_A leads to the hypotheses

$$H_0: p_T - p_R + m \geq 0 \text{ versus } H_A: p_T - p_R + m < 0. \qquad (6.16)$$

When a higher outcome proportion is better, for a noninferiority test, we hope to conclude that $p_T > p_R - m$, which leads to the hypotheses

$$H_0: p_T - p_R + m \leq 0 \text{ versus } H_A: p_T - p_R + m > 0 \qquad (6.17)$$

where $m > 0$; and for a test of superiority by a margin, we hope to conclude that $p_T > p_R + m$ and the hypotheses are

$$H_0: p_T - p_R - m \leq 0 \text{ versus } H_A: p_T - p_R - m > 0. \qquad (6.18)$$

Tests for noninferiority and superiority by a margin both involve null hypotheses that specify a nonzero difference between two proportions. For such tests, we can use the methods in Section 6.3 with the addition or subtraction of m from the difference of proportions. Under this approach, power for a two-sided test at level α is approximately

$$1 - \beta \approx \Phi \left(\frac{|p_T - p_R \pm m|}{\sqrt{\frac{p_T(1-p_T)}{n_T} + \frac{p_R(1-p_R)}{n_R}}} + z_{\alpha/2} \right) \qquad (6.19)$$

and total sample size N for a two-sided test when $n_R = r n_T$ is approximately

$$N \geq \frac{(z_{1-\alpha/2} + z_{1-\beta})^2 (r+1)[r p_T 1(1-p_T) + p_R(1-p_R)]}{r(p_T - p_R \pm m)^2}, \qquad (6.20)$$

where we use $+m$ or $-m$ ($m > 0$) according to the hypotheses (6.15) – (6.18).

Example 6.9. Under reference treatment, 25% of patients experience a relapse in 30 days. An experimental treatment is easier to administer and will be considered noninferior if relapses are not increased by more than 10 percentage points compared to reference treatment. To calculate sample size for a noninferiority test, we assume the true proportions are $p_R = p_T = 0.25$ and want 80% power for a one-sided test at $\alpha = 0.025$ with equal allocation. What is the required sample size?

For lower-is-better and a test of noninferiority, the hypotheses are as given in (6.15), with $H_A\colon p_T - p_R - m < 0$. The prop.2samp function assumes that margin will be subtracted from p1 - p2; we specify margin = 0.1 so that the numerator of the test statistic will be of the form p1 - p2 - margin.

```
library(powertools)
prop.2samp(n1 = NULL, p1 = 0.25, p2 = 0.25, margin = 0.1, alpha = 0.025,
   power = 0.8, sides = 1)
[1] 294.333
```

This calculation suggests 295 per arm.

Farrington and Manning [67] have noted problems estimating the null variance when using this approach, and other difficulties sometimes arise. They propose a maximum likelihood estimation approach. Their test statistic is

$$Z_{FM} = \frac{\hat{p}_T - \hat{p}_R \pm m}{\sqrt{\frac{\tilde{p}_T(1-\tilde{p}_T)}{n_T} + \frac{\tilde{p}_R(1-\tilde{p}_R)}{n_R}}} \quad (6.21)$$

where $\tilde{p}_T$ and $\tilde{p}_R$ are maximum likelihood estimates of the proportions under the restriction $\tilde{p}_T - \tilde{p}_R = m$. Formulas are given in [67]. This approach tends to give results similar to using power equation (6.19), as illustrated in the following example.

Example 6.10. We repeat Example 6.9 using the Farrington-Manning approach. The nBinomial function in the gsDesign package implements this method. The default is a one-sided test and the output is total sample size.

```
library(gsDesign)
nBinomial(p1 = 0.25, p2 = 0.25, delta0 = 0.1, alpha = 0.025, beta = 0.2)
[1]    590.1882
```

Rounding up to the next multiple of 2 gives us 592 (296 per arm).

Power and sample size for tests of superiority by a margin use the same approach as tests for noninferiority. For such tests we will usually assume that under the alternative, the test treatment is superior to the reference treatment.

6.3.4 Test for equivalence

In a test for the equivalence of two proportions, the hypotheses are

$$H_0: |p_T - p_R| \geq m \text{ versus } |p_T - p_R| < m \quad (6.22)$$

where $m > 0$. If we reject H_0, we conclude that $-m < p_T - p_R < m$, i.e., the outcome proportions under the two treatments do not differ in a clinically meaningful way in either direction.

As described for means in Section 4.6, a test for equivalence can be performed using a two one-sided test (TOST) procedure: we test $H_{01}: p_T - p_R \leq -m$ versus $H_{A1}: p_T - p_R > -m$ and $H_{02}: p_T - p_R \geq m$ versus $H_{A2}: p_T - p_R < m$, each at level α. Because the null is rejected only if both hypotheses are rejected, the overall Type I error rate will not exceed α and a multiplicity adjustment is not needed. Following the same logic as in Section 4.6, a large sample approximation of power for a test of equivalence of two proportions is given by (see [33])

$$1 - 2\Phi\left(z_{1-\alpha} - \sqrt{N\frac{r}{(1+r)}} \frac{m - |p_T - p_R|}{\sqrt{rp_T(1-p_T) + p_R(1-p_R)}}\right) \quad (6.23)$$

where N is the total sample size and $r = n_R/n_T$. An approximation for total N is given by

$$N \geq \frac{(z_{1-\beta/2} + z_{1-\alpha})^2}{(m - |p_T - p_R|)^2} \frac{(1+r)}{r} [rp_T(1-p_T) + p_R(1-p_R)]. \quad (6.24)$$

Example 6.11. In an equivalence trial, the expected outcome proportions are $p_R = p_T = 0.5$ and the equivalence margin is $m = 0.1$. What is the required sample size, if we want 80% power with α of 0.05 for each one-sided test?

```
library(powertools)
prop.test.equiv(n1 = NULL, p1 = 0.5, p2 = 0.5, margin = 0.1,
    alpha = 0.05, power = 0.8)
[1] 428.1924
```

We find that we need 429 in each group. This function can also support unequal allocation with the n.ratio argument.

6.3.5 Test of relative risk

In some studies, we may be interested in the **relative risk**, also called the **risk ratio**, defined as $\text{RR} = p_2/p_1$, rather than the difference of proportions. A relative risk measures the multiplicative difference in the outcome probabilities between groups. For example, a RR of 2 indicates that the probability of the outcome is twice as high in group 2 compared to group 1. Relative risks were discussed earlier in this chapter in the context of vaccine efficacy studies, with vaccine efficacy (VE) is defined as $1 - \text{RR}$; see Section 6.2.1.

Denote the sample proportions as $\hat{p}_1 = x_1/n_1$ and $\hat{p}_2 = x_2/n_2$. The distribution of the sample relative risk, $\widehat{\text{RR}} = \hat{p}_2/\hat{p}_1$, is skewed. However, $\log(\widehat{\text{RR}})$ is approximately normal with approximate mean $\log(\text{RR}) = \log(p_2/p_1)$ and approximate variance (see Katz et al. [119])

$$Var(\log(\widehat{\text{RR}})) \approx \frac{1-\hat{p}_1}{n_1\hat{p}_1} + \frac{1-\hat{p}_2}{n_2\hat{p}_2} = \frac{1}{x_1} - \frac{1}{n_1} + \frac{1}{x_2} - \frac{1}{n_2}.$$

We can test H_0: $\text{RR} = \text{RR}_0$ using the test statistic

$$z = \frac{\log(\widehat{\text{RR}}) - \log(\text{RR}_0)}{\sqrt{\frac{1}{x_1} - \frac{1}{n_1} + \frac{1}{x_2} - \frac{1}{n_2}}}.$$

Power for a two-sided test at level α can be approximated as (Blackwelder [20])

$$\Phi\left(\frac{|\log(\text{RR}) - \log(\text{RR}_0)|}{\sqrt{\left(\frac{1+r}{N}\right)\left(\frac{1-p_1}{p_1} + \frac{1-p_2}{rp_2}\right)}} + z_{\alpha/2}\right); \quad (6.25)$$

for a one-sided test, use α rather than $\alpha/2$. Solving for N, we obtain

$$N \geq \frac{(z_{1-\alpha/2} + z_{1-\beta})^2 (1+r)\left(\frac{1-p_1}{p_1} + \frac{1-p_2}{rp_2}\right)}{[\log(\text{RR}) - \log(\text{RR}_0)]^2} \quad (6.26)$$

where $r = n_2/n_1$. Several other approaches, including using likelihood score tests and a Poisson approximation, are discussed in Blackwelder [20], who reported that the score test has highest power and type I error rates closest to nominal rates but that the score and log methods are comparable for large studies. The log transformation approach is also used in precision analysis for a relative risk; see Section 9.4.

Example 6.12. A cohort study is planned in which the probability of the outcome in the unexposed group is 0.1. The ratio of unexposed to exposed subjects is about 6. What sample size is needed to detect a relative risk of 2, with α of 0.05 two-sided and power of 80%?

If we label the unexposed subjects as group 1 and the exposed subjects as group 2, then $r = n_2/n_1 = 1/6$ and $RR = p_2/p_1 = 2$ so $p_2 = p_1 RR = 0.2$.

```
library(powertools)
relrisk(n1 = NULL, n.ratio = 1/6, p1 = 0.1, p2 = 0.2, power = 0.8,
  v = TRUE)

    Relative risk power calculation 

          n1, n2 = 539.10169, 89.85028
          p1, p2 = 0.1, 0.2
         RR, RR0 = 2, 1
           alpha = 0.05
           power = 0.8
           sides = 2
```

The result suggests that having 90 in the exposed group and 540 in the unexposed group will provide sufficient power.

Another approach is to use a sample size formula for the difference between two proportions and make the substitution $p_2 = p_1 RR$. This approach is used by Schlesselman [195] and Woodward [235] using formula (6.11). For H_0: $RR = 1$, an expression for sample size for a two-sided test at level α is

$$N = \frac{r+1}{r(RR-1)^2 p_1^2} \qquad (6.27)$$
$$\times \left[z_{1-\alpha/2} \sqrt{(r+1)p_c(1-p_c)} + z_{1-\beta} \sqrt{RR p_1(1-p_1) + r p_1(1-p_1)} \right]^2$$

where $r = n_2/n_1$ and $p_c = \frac{p_1(rRR+1)}{r+1}$, equal to $(p_1 + p_2)/2$ when $n_1 = n_2$. For a one-sided test, use α rather than $\alpha/2$. Methods for odds ratios (which they call relative risks) are discussed in Chow et al. [33], with functions in the TrialSize package.

6.4 Test for two correlated proportions

In some study designs, a binary outcome is measured on the same subjects under two different conditions. Paired binary data also arise in matched case-control studies. Paired binary outcome data are often analyzed using McNemar's test [35, 154]. In this section, we describe power for the large sample McNemar's test as proposed by Connor [39]. We describe power for exact McNemar tests in Section 7.4. For additional power methods, see Lachin [129].

TABLE 6.1: Data set-up and notation for two correlated proportions.

		Condition B outcome		
		No	Yes	
Condition A outcome	No	$\frac{n_{00}}{N} = \hat{p}_{00}$	$\frac{n_{01}}{N} = \hat{p}_{01}$	$\frac{n_{00}+n_{01}}{N} = \hat{p}_{0+}$
	Yes	$\frac{n_{10}}{N} = \hat{p}_{10}$	$\frac{n_{11}}{N} = \hat{p}_{11}$	$\frac{n_{10}+n_{11}}{N} = \hat{p}_{1+}$
		$\frac{n_{00}+n_{10}}{N} = \hat{p}_{+0}$	$\frac{n_{01}+n_{11}}{N} = \hat{p}_{+1}$	

Table 6.1 represents data from a study that assessed binary outcomes on the same N subjects under two conditions, A and B, resulting in N paired responses. Each subject has one of four possible paired responses, $\{(00),(01),(10),(11)\}$, where the first number indicates "success" (1) or "failure" (0) for outcome A and the second indicates outcome B. Responses (00) and (11) are called **concordant pairs** and responses (01) and (10) are called **discordant pairs**. The numbers of paired responses in the four cells are n_{00}, n_{01}, n_{10} and n_{11} with $n_{00} + n_{01} + n_{10} + n_{11} = N$. The observed proportions in each cell are $\hat{p}_{00}, \hat{p}_{01}, \hat{p}_{10}$ and $\hat{p}_{11}$, and they sum to 1. $\hat{p}_{0+}, \hat{p}_{1+}, \hat{p}_{+0}$ and $\hat{p}_{+1}$ are the marginal proportions. Most notably, $\hat{p}_{1+} = \hat{p}_{10} + \hat{p}_{11}$ is the proportion with "success" under condition A and $\hat{p}_{+1} = \hat{p}_{01} + \hat{p}_{11}$ is the proportion with "success" under condition B.

The typical null hypothesis is that the proportion of successes under conditions A and B are the same, $H_0: p_{1+} = p_{+1}$. Subtracting p_{11} from both sides, we can express the null hypothesis as $H_0: p_{10} = p_{01}$, which states that the proportions of each type of discordant pair are equal. Further dividing both sides by $p_{10} + p_{01}$, the total proportion of pairs that are discordant, we have

$$H_0: \frac{p_{10}}{p_{10}+p_{01}} = \frac{p_{01}}{p_{10}+p_{01}} = 0.5.$$

That is, the null hypothesis states that conditioning on the probability of being discordant, the probabilities of the response pairs (01) and (10) are equal. In order for these two proportions to be equal, they must both equal 0.5, since they must sum to 1.

When H_0 is true and conditioning on the observed number of discordant pairs $n_{10} + n_{01}$, the count in either discordant cell is distributed as binomial, n_{01} or $n_{10} \sim \text{Bin}(n_{10} + n_{01}, 0.5)$. Without loss of generality, we focus on n_{10}. Since $E(n_{10}) = (n_{10}+n_{01})/2$ and $Var(n_{10}) = (n_{10}+n_{01})/4$, using the normal approximation to the binomial distribution, we have that

$$\frac{n_{10} - (n_{10} + n_{01})/2}{\sqrt{(n_{10} + n_{01})/4}} = \frac{n_{10} - n_{01}}{\sqrt{n_{10} + n_{01}}} \stackrel{.}{\sim} \mathcal{N}(0,1).$$

This leads to the use of the test statistic

$$Z = \frac{n_{10} - n_{01}}{\sqrt{n_{10} + n_{01}}}$$

which has approximately a $\mathcal{N}(0,1)$ distribution under H_0. We obtain the same test statistic by conducting a one-sample test of proportion $H_0: p = 0.5$, where $p = p_{10}/(p_{10} + p_{01})$ using equation (6.3).

What is the distribution of Z under an alternative that $p_{01} \neq p_{10}$? For fixed N, $n_{10} - n_{01}$ has $E(n_{10} - n_{01}) = N(p_{10} - p_{01})$ and $Var(n_{10} - n_{01}) = Var(n_{10}) + Var(n_{01}) - 2Cov(n_{10}, n_{01}) = N[p_{10} + p_{01} - (p_{10} - p_{01})^2]$; the covariance can be found using the multinomial distribution. Thus power can be approximated as

$$\Phi\left(\frac{\sqrt{N}(p_{10} - p_{01}) - z_{1-\alpha/2}\sqrt{p_{10} + p_{01}}}{\sqrt{p_{10} + p_{01} - (p_{10} - p_{01})^2}}\right) \quad (6.28)$$

and the total required sample size is approximately

$$N \geq \frac{\left(z_{1-\alpha/2}\sqrt{p_{01} + p_{10}} + z_{1-\beta}\sqrt{p_{10} + p_{01} - (p_{10} - p_{01})^2}\right)^2}{(p_{10} - p_{01})^2} \quad (6.29)$$

where N is the total number of subjects, who provide a total of $2N$ observations.

Formulas (6.28) and (6.29) require the user to specify expected values for the discordant proportions p_{01} and p_{10}, which can be difficult. There are several ways to reparametrize these proportions so that it is easier to specify inputs for calculations. If we define the **discordant proportion ratio** as DPR $= p_{01}/p_{10}$ and the proportion of observations that are discordant as $p_{\text{disc}} = p_{01} + p_{10}$, we can express the sample size as

$$N \geq \frac{\left[z_{1-\alpha/2}(\text{DPR} + 1) + z_{1-\beta}\sqrt{(\text{DPR} + 1)^2 - (\text{DPR} - 1)^2 p_{\text{disc}}}\right]^2}{(\text{DPR} - 1)^2 p_{\text{disc}}}. \quad (6.30)$$

Another option is to specify the marginal proportions p_{1+} and p_{+1}, which are the probabilities of success under conditions A and B, and ϕ, the phi coefficient. The **phi coefficient** is a measure of association between two binary variables defined as

$$\phi = \frac{p_{00}p_{11} - p_{01}p_{10}}{\sqrt{p_{1+}(1 - p_{1+})p_{+1}(1 - p_{+1})}}.$$

Test for two correlated proportions

The phi coefficient is equivalent to the Pearson correlation coefficient; however, its values are constrained due to dependencies among the proportions [48]. In particular, for two proportions $p_2 \geq p_1$,

$$\phi_{\max} = \sqrt{\frac{p_1(1-p_2)}{p_2(1-p_1)}};$$

see Ferguson [69]. Together, p_{1+}, p_{+1} and ϕ allow us to compute p_{01} and p_{10} as

$$p_{01} = p_{+1}(1-p_{1+}) - \phi\sqrt{(1-p_{1+})p_{1+}(1-p_{+1})p_{+1}} \qquad (6.31)$$
$$p_{10} = p_{01} + p_{1+} - p_{+1}$$

Example 6.13. The sensitivity of a test is the proportion of positive tests that are true positives. Suppose we plan to compare the sensitivity of a new test and a standard test for detecting the presence of a contaminant in a specimen. Specimens will be split and assessed using each test. The standard test has sensitivity of 0.8 and we expect the new test to have sensitivity of 0.9. What sample size is needed to achieve 90% power to reject the null of no difference in sensitivity, with two-sided α of 0.05?

We are given the marginal proportions, 0.8 and 0.9. The phi coefficient is not known, but cannot exceed $\phi_{\max} = \sqrt{\frac{0.8(1-0.9)}{0.9(1-0.8)}} = 0.667$. We calculate N for $\phi = 0, 0.1, 0.2$. For $\phi = 0$,

```
library(powertools)
prop.paired(N = NULL, p1 = 0.8, p2 = 0.9, phi = 0, power = 0.9,
    sides = 2)
[1] "NOTE: N is the number of pairs"
[1] 269.0142
```

For $\phi = 0.1$, we get $N = 243.7938$ and for $\phi = 0.2$, we get $N = 218.5729$. The required sample size decreases as ϕ increases. The function can also take as inputs the discordant proportion ratio and the smaller of the two discordant proportions.

To get a sense of the various interrelated quantities, we calculate the discordant cell proportions and discordant proportion ratio when p1 = 0.8, p2 = 0.9 and phi = 0.2:

```
p1 <- 0.8  ;  p2 <- 0.9  ;  phi <- 0.2
p01 <- p1 * (1 - p2) - phi * sqrt((1 - p2) * p1 * (1 - p1) * p2) ; p01
[1] 0.056
p10 <- p01 + p2 - p1 ; p10
[1] 0.156
p_disc <- p01 + p10  ; p_disc
[1] 0.212
```

```
dpr <- p10 / p01  ;  dpr
[1] 2.785714
```

Note that when 21.2% of the cells are expected to be discordant, for a sample size of 219, the expected number of discordant cells is about $219 \times 0.212 \approx 46$.

What factors affect power? McNemar's test is conducted by conditioning on the number of pairs in the two discordant cells and then performing a one-sample proportion test comparing the proportion $p_{10}/(p_{01} + p_{10})$ (or $p_{01}/(p_{01} + p_{10})$) to a null value of 0.5. Thus the factors that affect power are in essence the same as those for a one-sample test of proportion, discussed on page 121. Increasing the total sample size N increases the expected number of pairs in discordant cells, which thus increases power. As $p_{10}/(p_{01} + p_{10})$ gets closer to 0 or 1, its variance decreases and so power is higher. Given that $p_{10} = p_{01} + p_{1+} - p_{+1}$, a greater difference between the marginal proportions $p_{1+} - p_{+1}$ leads to a greater difference between p_{10} and p_{01} and thus values of $p_{10}/(p_{01} + p_{10})$ closer to 0 or 1, which increases power. For the same reason, power will be higher when the DPR diverges from 1 in either direction because this indicates greater difference between p_{10} and p_{01}. Power tends to increase as the phi coefficient ϕ increases.

7
Exact methods for proportions

7.1 One proportion: exact binomial test

A one-sample test of a proportion arises when we want to test whether the proportion of individuals responding to a new treatment is different from the proportion known to respond to a reference treatment, for example. Such single arm study designs may be used in the early stages of clinical testing of a new treatment. Such studies often involve small sample sizes and so exact methods are used for statistical analysis rather than large-sample methods. The exact binomial test is one such method.

7.1.1 Test procedure

Suppose that in a single-arm study, we want to compare the population proportion p to a reference proportion p_0 using the one-sided hypotheses

$$H_0: p \leq p_0 \quad \text{versus} \quad H_A: p > p_0.$$

An exact binomial test for these hypotheses is conducted as follows. For a sample of size N, when H_0 is true, the number of successes, X, is distributed as $Bin(N, p_0)$. Suppose that we observe x successes. We can compute an exact p-value as the probability that we observe x or more successes when the probability of success is p_0,

$$P[X \geq x | X \sim Bin(N, p_0)] = \sum_{i=x}^{N} \binom{N}{i} p_0^i (1-p_0)^{N-i}.$$

We then compare the exact p-value to the significance level α to decide whether or not to reject H_0. We illustrate in the following example.

Example 7.1. Suppose we want to test $H_0: p \leq 0.4$ versus $H_A: p > 0.4$. From a sample of 20 patients, we observed 12 responders ("successes"). The exact p-value is calculated as $P[X \geq 12 | X \sim Bin(20, 0.4)]$. We can calculate this probability in R but need to use some care. When working with discrete distributions such as the binomial, we must be careful about what values are included in the calculation. The R function `pbinom` computes $P(X \leq x)$ when `lower.tail = T` and $P(X > x)$ when `lower.tail = F`, so to get the correct calculation, we need to calculate $1 - P(X \leq 11)$ or $P(X > 12) + P(X = 12)$:

```
1 - pbinom(11, 20, 0.4, lower.tail = T)
[1] 0.05652637
pbinom(12, 20, 0.4, lower.tail = F) + dbinom(12, 20, 0.4)
[1] 0.05652637
```

Would we reject H_0 in Example 7.1? That depends on what we specified as the type I error rate and the corresponding critical value. Because binomial random variables take discrete values, we typically cannot find a critical value that will achieve a type I error rate of exactly α. Rather, the usual approach is to specify a critical value that will lead to a type I error rate that does not exceed α. For an upper-tailed test, the critical value is the integer c such that

$$P[X \geq c | X \sim Bin(N, p_0)] \leq \alpha \text{ and } P[X \geq c - 1 | X \sim Bin(N, p_0)] > \alpha.$$

We reject H_0 if the observed number of successes is c or higher, and the actual type I error rate will be $P[X \geq c | X \sim Bin(N, p_0)]$. For a lower-tailed test, the critical value is c such that

$$P[X \leq c | X \sim Bin(N, p_0)] \leq \alpha \text{ and } P[X \leq c + 1 | X \sim Bin(N, p_0)] > \alpha.$$

We reject H_0 if x is c or lower, and the actual type I error rate is $P[X \leq c | X \sim Bin(N, p_0)]$.

Example 7.2. Suppose that we wish to test $H_0: p \leq 0.4$ versus $H_A: p > 0.4$ with 12 subjects and a type I error rate not exceeding 0.05. What is the appropriate critical value and what is the actual type I error rate?

Below, we list probabilities for the null distribution, $Bin(12, 0.4)$:

x	$P(X = x)$	$P(X \leq x)$	$P(X \geq x)$
0	0.002177	0.002177	1.000000
1	0.017414	0.019591	0.997823
2	0.063852	0.083443	0.980409
3	0.141894	0.225337	0.916557
4	0.212841	0.438178	0.774663
5	0.227030	0.665209	0.561822
6	0.176579	0.841788	0.334791
7	0.100902	0.942690	0.158212
8	0.042043	0.984733	0.057310
9	0.012457	0.997190	0.015267
10	0.002491	0.999681	0.002810
11	0.000302	0.999983	0.000319
12	0.000017	1.000000	0.000017

We find that $P(X \geq 9) = 0.0153 \leq 0.05$ and $P(X \geq 8) = 0.0573 > 0.05$. Therefore we should use $c = 9$ as the critical value, rejecting the null if $x \geq 9$, and the actual type I error rate is 0.0153.

If we were testing $H_0\colon p \geq 0.4$ versus $H_A\colon p < 0.4$ with a type I error rate not exceeding 0.05, we would choose $c = 2$ as the critical value, rejecting the null if $x \leq 2$, and the actual type I error rate would be 0.0196.

7.1.2 Power

When the true probability of success is p_A, the power to reject H_0 for an upper-tailed test is

$$P[X \geq c | X \sim Bin(N, p_A)] = \sum_{i=c}^{N} \binom{N}{i} p_A^i (1 - p_A)^{N-i}.$$

Similarly, the power to reject H_0 for a lower-tailed test is

$$P[X \leq c | X \sim Bin(N, p_A)] = \sum_{i=0}^{c} \binom{N}{i} p_A^i (1 - p_A)^{N-i}.$$

Example 7.3. In the previous example, we found that to test $H_0\colon p \leq 0.4$ versus $H_A\colon p > 0.4$ with 12 subjects and α not exceeding 0.05, we should use $c = 9$ and reject the null if $x \geq 9$. If the true proportion is 0.6, what is the power?

Either of the following R commands will find the correct answer:

```
# Compute 1 - P(X <= 8) = P(X >= 9):
1 - pbinom(8, 12, 0.6, lower.tail = T)
[1] 0.2253373
# Compute P(X > 9) + P(X = 9) = P(X >= 9):
pbinom(9, 12, 0.6, lower.tail = F) + dbinom(9, 12, 0.6)
[1] 0.2253373
```

Power can also be calculated using the power_binom_test function from the MESS package:

```
library(MESS)
power_binom_test(n = 12, p0 = 0.4, pa = 0.6, sig.level = 0.05,
    power = NULL, alternative = "greater")

    One-sample exact binomial power calculation

        n = 12
```

```
              p0 = 0.4
              pa = 0.6
       sig.level = 0.05
           power = 0.2253373
     alternative = greater
```

7.1.3 Sample size

To find the smallest sample size that will achieve a desired level of power with type I error rate no greater than α, we need to find the set (N, c) that satisfies

$$P[X \geq c | X \sim Bin(N, p_0)] \leq \alpha \text{ and} \qquad (7.1)$$
$$P[X \geq c | X \sim Bin(N, p_A)] \geq 1 - \beta$$

and has the smallest N. This requires a search for sets (N, c) that meet these criteria, and then we can choose a design from among these sets.

Example 7.4. Suppose we plan a single arm study that will test $H_0: p \leq 0.65$ versus $H_A: p > 0.65$. We specify $\alpha \leq 0.1$ and want power of at least 90% to reject H_0 when $p_A = 0.8$. What is the smallest N that will be sufficient, and what is the corresponding critical value?

We can find the solution using the `ph2single` function from the `clinfun` package. The parameters for this function are the null proportion `pu`, the proportion under the alternative `pa`, the type I error rate (α) `ep1` and the type II error rate (β) `ep2`. The function assumes that a response is a good outcome and that `pa` is greater than `pu`. The user can specify the number of solutions to return using the `nsoln` argument. We ask for five solutions:

```
library(clinfun)
ph2single(pu = 0.65, pa = 0.8, ep1 = 0.1, ep2 = 0.1, nsoln = 5)

   n  r  Type I error  Type II error
1 61 44   0.09452507     0.08791504
2 62 45   0.08080580     0.09949301
3 64 46   0.09773883     0.07496547
4 65 47   0.08394028     0.08504523
5 66 48   0.07179469     0.09596497
```

In this output, we reject H_0 if more than r responses are observed. Of these solutions, the one with the smallest sample size requires 61 patients, and we reject H_0 if we observe more than 44 responses, that is, 45 or more. In the set-up in equations (7.1), the set (N, c) with smallest N is $(61, 45)$.

As illustrated in this example, there is typically more than one design that will meet our type I error and power specifications. We listed five designs, but there are infinitely many more, with larger sample sizes. Section 7.2 has more discussion about criteria for selecting among possible designs.

7.2 Two-stage designs for single arm trials

Many clinical trials have multistage designs. In a multistage design, data are collected on an initial set of individuals and an analysis is performed. Depending on the result, the trial either stops or proceeds to next stage. Multistage designs can be advantageous from an ethical standpoint; if the experimental treatment is harmful or not efficacious, it is better to stop the trial early. If a treatment is efficacious, it is also better to stop the trial early so that we can proceed more quickly with the next stages. Multistage designs can also help to minimize the patient sample size.

In this section, we discuss two-stage designs that are focused on a test of a single proportion, $H_0: p \leq p_0$ versus $H_A: p > p_0$. At Stage 1, n_1 patients are treated and x_1 responses observed. If the response rate is insufficient, the trial is stopped for futility. Otherwise, the trial proceeds to Stage 2 in which an additional n_2 patients are treated. At the end of Stage 2, the full sample size is analyzed and a decision of whether or not to reject the null hypothesis is made. Such designs are often used to screen potential cancer therapies for efficacy. A patient with a positive outcome, e.g., shrinkage in tumor size, is called a "responder". We will use this setting and assume that a higher response proportion is better.

A classic example of a two-stage design in Simon's two-stage design [112, 113, 204]. Simon's two-stage design has the following procedure:

- Stage 1: Treat n_1 patients. Let the observed number of responders be x_1. If $x_1 \leq a_1$, where a_1 is set as the threshold signifying an insufficient response, terminate the trial for futility. Otherwise, continue to Stage 2.

- Stage 2: Treat an additional n_2 patients, for a total of $N = n_1 + n_2$. Let the observed number of responders in this additional set of patients be x_2. If the total number of responders $x = x_1 + x_2 \leq a$, where a is set as the Stage 2 threshold signifying an insufficient response, fail to reject the null; if $x > a$, reject the null and conclude $p > p_0$.

To design such a trial, the objective is to find an appropriate set of values $(a_1/n_1, a/N)$ such that the type I error rate is less than α and the power is at least $1 - \beta$ for specified values of p_0 and p_A. To find such designs, we need to consider that there are two ways in which H_0 can fail to be rejected; we can stop the trial at Stage 1, or we can continue the trial to Stage 2 completion but then fail to reject H_0. The probability of stopping at Stage 1 is

$$P[X_1 \leq a_1 | X_1 \sim Bin(n_1, p)], \tag{7.2}$$

which is called the **probability of early termination** (PET), and the probability of continuing to Stage 2 but not having enough responders at Stage 2 to exceed a total of a responders is

$$\sum_{x_1 = a_1 + 1}^{min(n_1, a)} P[X_1 = x_1 | X_1 \sim Bin(n_1, p)] P[X_2 \leq a - x_1 | X_2 \sim Bin(n_2, p)]. \tag{7.3}$$

The sum of (7.2) and (7.3) is the probability that we fail to reject H_0 for a given proportion p; we denote this probability as $f(p)$. Thus $1 - f(p)$ is the probability that we reject H_0 when the proportion is p. We want to find designs $(a_1/n_1, a/N)$ such that

$$1 - f(p_0) \leq \alpha \text{ and}$$
$$1 - f(p_A) \geq 1 - \beta.$$

Example 7.5. Continuing Example 7.4, suppose we plan a single arm study to test $H_0: p \leq 0.65$ versus $H_A: p > 0.65$. We believe that the true proportion of responders is $p_A = 0.8$. What two-stage designs, $(a_1/n_1, a/N)$, will achieve power of at least 90% with $\alpha \leq 0.1$?

Such designs can be found using `ph2simon` command in the `clinfun` package.

```
library(clinfun)
ph2simon(pu = 0.65, pa = 0.8, ep1 = 0.1, ep2 = 0.1, nmax = 100)

Simon 2-stage Phase II design

Unacceptable response rate:  0.65
Desirable response rate:  0.8
Error rates: alpha =  0.1 ; beta =  0.1

        r1 n1  r  n  EN(p0) PET(p0)
Optimal 20 30 45 63  41.80  0.6425
Minimax 22 33 43 60  42.64  0.6430
```

In this output, the trial is stopped early if `r1` or fewer responses are seen in Stage 1 and H_0 is rejected if more than `r` responses are observed in the full sample after both stages. For example, in the design labeled "Optimal", Stage 1 enrolls 30 patients and we stop the trial early if 20 or fewer responses are observed. If we observe 21 or more responses, we continue to Stage 2 and collect data from 33 more patients, for a total of 63. At that point, we reject H_0 if more than 45 responses are observed in the total sample. The PET is 0.6425.

There is often more than one design that will meet our type I error and power specifications. What criteria might we use to select among them? Simon defined "minimax" and "optimal" two-stage designs [204]. The minimax design is the design that minimizes the maximum sample size, N. In Example 7.5, the minimax design has total N of 60. The optimal design is the design that minimizes the expected sample size under the null, denoted $E_N(p_0)$, which is calculated as

$$E_N(p_0) = PET(p_0)n_1 + [1 - PET(p_0)]N. \qquad (7.4)$$

In Example 7.5, the optimal design has $E_N(p_0) = 41.80$.

In practice, there are other considerations beyond just minimizing N or $E_N(p_0)$, and investigators may wish to consider other aspects of a design. The ph2simon function in the clinfun package only shows the optimal and minimax designs. Other software programs are available that show more options. For example, an online calculator is available at http://cancer.unc.edu/biostatistics/program/ivanova/SimonsTwoStageDesign.aspx. Some references also provide tables of designs, for example, Jung [112]. Investigators will typically choose from among the minimax design, optimal design and other designs that have similar N or $E_N(p_0)$. They may prefer a design that trades off aspects of the optimal and minimax designs, or that ensures that Stage 1 involves some minimal number of patients, for example.

7.3 Two proportions: Fisher exact test

Power for comparing two proportions when using the normal approximation to the binomial was discussed in Section 6.3. This approximation can be poor for small samples. An alternative is the Fisher exact test [70, 239]. The Fisher exact test can also be used for a test of association in a 2×2 contingency table when a chi-squared test (Section 8.2) is not valid due to small expected cell counts.

Cell counts, row and column totals and total sample size for a 2×2 table are shown in Table 7.1. Such a table might arise from comparing proportions for two independent groups, labeled as $T = 0$ and $T = 1$, with sample proportions $\hat{p}_0 = a/(a+c)$ and $\hat{p}_1 = b/(b+d)$, or when a sample of size N is cross-classified on two dichotomous factors T and Y.

TABLE 7.1: Counts for a 2×2 table.

	$T = 0$	$T = 1$	Row totals
$Y = 1$	a	b	$a + b$
$Y = 0$	c	d	$c + d$
Column totals	$a + c$	$b + d$	$N = a + b + c + d$

The Fisher exact test uses the **hypergeometric distribution** to calculate the probability of observing a particular configuration of counts in a 2×2 table. The hypergeometric distribution arises as follows:

Hypergeometric Distribution

Suppose a finite population of size N contains exactly K successes and $N - K$ failures. We draw a sample of size n without replacement from this population. Let X denote the number of successes in the sample. Then X has a hypergeometric distribution, $X \sim \text{Hypergeo}(N, K, n)$, with probability mass function

$$P(X = k) = \frac{\binom{K}{k}\binom{N-K}{n-k}}{\binom{N}{n}}, \quad k = 0, \ldots, K.$$

The Fisher exact test conditions on the total sample size and the observed number of successes to create the setting of a finite population of size N that contains exactly $a + b$ ($= K$) successes and $c + d$ ($= N - K$) failures. If no association between T and Y exists, then the probability that a sample of size $a + c$ ($= n$), selected without replacement, will contain exactly a ($= k$) successes can be calculated as

$$P(X = a) = \frac{\binom{a+c}{a}\binom{b+d}{b}}{\binom{N}{a+b}} = \frac{(a+b)!\,(c+d)!\,(a+c)!\,(a+d)!}{a!\,b!\,c!\,d!\,N!}.$$

This approach is used to compute a p-value as the probability of observing a table that represents equal or greater deviation from independence than the observed table, given N and $a + b$. Possible tables are ordered by a measure of dependence such as the difference in proportions.

There is no closed-form formula for power or sample size for a Fisher exact test. An approximation based on a corrected χ^2 approach is given by Casagrande et al. [28]. This approach is used by the `fedesign` functions in the `clinfun` package. These functions can also find the exact solution using searches starting with the approximate solution. The `power.fisher.test` function in the `statmod` package uses simulation to calculate power.

Two correlated proportions: exact test 145

Example 7.6. A randomized trial will compare two treatment groups on a binary outcome and test $H_0\colon p_0 \geq p_1$ versus $H_0\colon p_0 < p_1$ at $\alpha = 0.05$. For expected outcome proportions $p_0 = 0.5$ and $p_1 = 0.8$, what is the power if we have 25 participants in each group?

As shown below, using simulation, we estimate power as 0.6414. Exact power is 0.6378. Using the Casagrande approximation method then searching to find the sample size needed for 80% power, we obtain 37 per group by the approximation method and 36 per group by the exact method search.

```
# simulation-based power calculation
library(statmod)
set.seed(2345)
power.fisher.test(p1 = 0.5, p2 = 0.8, n1 = 25, n2 = 25, alpha = 0.05,
    nsim = 10000, alternative = "less")
[1] 0.6414

# exact power calculation
library(clinfun)
# d is difference p2 - p1
# two-sided test is assumed so use alpha = 0.1
fe.power(p1 = 0.5, d = 0.3, n1 = 25, n2 = 25, alpha = 0.1)
    p2     power
   0.8 0.6378199

# sample size by approximation and exact methods:
# npm: range in which to search for exact solution; here, +/- 5
# mmax: maximum group size for the search
fe.ssize(p1 = 0.5, p2 = 0.8, alpha = 0.1, power = 0.8, npm = 5,
    mmax = 50)
              Group 1 Group 2 Exact Power
CPS                37      37   0.8230717
Fisher Exact       36      36   0.8086832
```

7.4 Two correlated proportions: exact test

Power for the large sample McNemar test was discussed in Section 6.4. When sample sizes are small (i.e., the number of discordant pairs is less than 20–25), an exact McNemar test can provide better accuracy.

Various types of exact tests and exact power calculations for correlated proportions are discussed in the literature [59, 198, 212]. Duffy [59] presents the following approach. Assuming a one-sided test of $H_0\colon p_{1+} \leq p_{+1}$ versus $H_A\colon p_{1+} > p_{+1}$, exact power at significance level α is given by

$$P\left[\frac{n_{10} - n_{01}}{\sqrt{n_{10} + n_{01}}} > z_{1-\alpha}\right]$$

where this probability is computed exactly using binomial distributions rather than approximated. In particular, the binomial distribution is used to compute the probability of observing $n_{10} + n_{01}$ discordant cells when the total number of pairs is N, using $n_{10} + n_{01} \sim Bin(N, p_{10} + p_{01})$. When H_0 is true and conditioning on the observed number of discordant pairs $n_{10} + n_{01}$, the count in either discordant cell is distributed as binomial, n_{01} or $n_{10} \sim \text{Bin}(n_{10} + n_{01}, 0.5)$. When the alternative is true, $n_{01} \sim Bin(n_{10} + n_{01}, \frac{p_{01}}{p_{10}+p_{01}})$, $n_{10} \sim Bin(n_{10} + n_{01}, \frac{p_{10}}{p_{10}+p_{01}})$ and $n_{10} + n_{01} \sim Bin(N, p_{10} + p_{01})$. This method is implemented using the `method = "exact"` option in the `power_mcnemar_test` function in the MESS package. This package also implements a `"cond.exact"` method. The exact method is more computationally intensive, especially for large sample sizes. Other software, such as the SAS POWER procedure, also implement an exact power method that uses the exact binomial distributions of the total number of discordant pairs and the two types of discordant pairs. These three methods give similar but not identical power calculations.

Schork and Williams [198] published a formula which provides the exact results for the unconditional case using multinomial enumeration of all possible outcomes. However, we are not aware of an R implementation of this approach.

Example 7.7. The `power_mcnemar_test` function in the MESS package conducts power and sample size calculations for the McNemar test using both asymptotic and exact methods. The option `method = exact` uses the unconditional exact approach and `method = cond.exact` uses a conditional exact method, the derivation of which is not entirely clear. The function takes as input information on the discordant cell proportions. `paid` is the smaller of the two discordant proportions and `psi` is the discordant proportion ratio, calculated with the smaller discordant proportion in the denominator so that $\psi > 1$. These quantities can be computed from the phi coefficient and the marginal proportions using formulas (6.31).

In Example 6.13, we had $p_1 = 0.8$ and $p_2 = 0.9$. When $\phi = 0.2$, we calculated that the smaller discordant proportion was 0.056 and the discordant proportion ratio was 2.785714. We calculate power when we have 50 pairs of observations:

```
library(MESS)
power_mcnemar_test(n = 50, paid = 0.056, psi = 2.785714, power = NULL,
    alternative = "two.sided", method = "exact")

    McNemar paired comparison of proportions exact unconditional
```

```
     power calculation 

             n = 50
          paid = 0.056
           psi = 2.785714
     sig.level = 0.05
         power = 0.3125074
   alternative = two.sided

NOTE: n is number of pairs
```

Power is about 0.31.

8
Categorical variables

8.1 Chi-square goodness-of-fit test

The goodness-of-fit test compares the distribution of a categorical variable to some reference distribution. Let X_i denote the categorical response of individual i, which takes one of the values $k = 1, \ldots, K$. The X_i's are assumed to be independent and identically distributed. Let $p_k = P(X_i = k)$ be the probability that X_i takes value k. Suppose that we collect responses from a total of N individuals, and the observed frequency counts in the K categories are $n_1, \ldots, n_K$ with $n_1 + \cdots + n_K = N$. The observed response proportions are $\hat{p}_k = n_k/N$ for $k = 1, \ldots, K$.

The goodness-of-fit test has the null hypothesis that the response proportions have a specified reference distribution,

$$H_0: p_k = p_{k0} \text{ for all } k,$$

where the p_{k0}, for $k = 1, \ldots, K$, are the proportions in each response category for the hypothesized reference distribution, with $\sum_{k=1}^{K} p_{k0} = 1$. The alternative hypothesis is that $p_k \neq p_{k0}$ for some k. Table 8.1 presents the set up and notation.

The test statistic for the goodness-of-fit test compares the observed frequency counts, $n_1, \ldots, n_K$, to the expected counts when the null hypothesis is true. The expected counts are $Np_{10}, \ldots, Np_{K0}$. The test statistic is

$$X = \sum_{k=1}^{K} \frac{(n_k - Np_{k0})^2}{Np_{k0}} = N \sum_{k=1}^{K} \frac{(\hat{p}_k - p_{k0})^2}{p_{k0}}. \tag{8.1}$$

When H_0 is true, X has a chi-square distribution with $K - 1$ degrees of freedom. H_0 is rejected at significance level α when $X > x^2_{1-\alpha, K-1}$, which is an upper-tailed test.

When a specific alternative regarding the values of the proportions, $p_1 = p_{1A}, \ldots, p_K = p_{KA}$, is true, the test statistic (8.1) has a noncentral chi-square distribution with $K - 1$ degrees of freedom and noncentrality parameter

$$\Lambda = N \sum_{k=1}^{K} \frac{(p_{kA} - p_{k0})^2}{p_{k0}}.$$

DOI: 10.1201/9780429488788-8

Chi-square goodness-of-fit test

TABLE 8.1: Notation for chi-square goodness-of-fit test. N is the total sample size, $N = \sum_{k=1}^{K} n_k$.

	Response categories			
	1	2	$\cdots$	K
Frequency count	n_1	n_2	$\cdots$	n_K
Observed proportion	$\hat{p}_1 = \frac{n_1}{N}$	$\hat{p}_2 = \frac{n_2}{N}$	$\cdots$	$\hat{p}_K = \frac{n_K}{N}$
Null hypothesis proportion	p_{10}	p_{20}	$\cdots$	p_{K0}
Alternative proportion	p_{1A}	p_{2A}	$\cdots$	p_{KA}

Power can be calculated as $1 - \mathcal{X}^2_{K-1,\Lambda}(x^2_{1-\alpha, K-1})$. The noncentral chi-square distribution is described in Section 3.1.4.

Cohen [36] defined an effect size for a chi-square test of goodness-of-fit as

$$w = \sqrt{\sum_{k=1}^{K} \frac{(p_{kA} - p_{k0})^2}{p_{k0}}}. \tag{8.2}$$

Thus the noncentrality parameter can be expressed as

$$\Lambda = Nw^2.$$

The w effect size increases as the differences between the proportions under the null and alternative, $p_{kA} - p_{k0}$, increase. Because the two sets of proportions must each sum to 1, w will not necessarily increase as the number of categories K increases. Cohen defined small, medium and large w effect sizes as $w = 0.1, 0.3$ and 0.5, respectively [36]. These benchmarks can be helpful but may not be appropriate for all contexts.

Example 8.1. A study will collect data on a sample of adults, and they will be categorized as never, past or current tobacco users. In the past, this population had proportions of never, past and current tobacco users of 0.5, 0.3 and 0.2, and we wish to test whether the proportions in the current population differ from these historical values. The investigators expect that the true proportions are 0.7, 0.2 and 0.1. What is the effect size and the power for a chi-square goodness-of-fit test if we have a sample of 50 individuals?

The calculation can be conducted using the `chisq.gof` function:

```
library(powertools)
chisq.gof(p0vec = c(0.5, 0.3, 0.2), p1vec = c(0.7, 0.2, 0.1), N = 50,
    v = TRUE)
```

TABLE 8.2: Notation for chi-square test of independence for an $r \times c$ table.

		Column variable				Row totals
		1	2	$\cdots$	c	
Row variable	1	n_{11}	n_{12}	$\cdots$	n_{1c}	n_{1+}
	2	n_{21}	n_{22}	$\cdots$	n_{2c}	n_{2+}
	$\vdots$	$\vdots$	$\vdots$	$\ddots$	$\vdots$	$\vdots$
	r	n_{r1}	n_{r2}	$\cdots$	n_{rc}	n_{r+}
Column totals		n_{+1}	n_{+2}	$\cdots$	n_{+c}	N

```
     Chi-square goodness-of-fit power calculation

         p1vec = 0.7, 0.2, 0.1
         p0vec = 0.5, 0.3, 0.2
w effect size = 0.4041452
             N = 50
         alpha = 0.05
         power = 0.7270295
```

The w effect size is about 0.4, which is medium-to-large. The power is about 0.73.

8.2 Chi-square test of independence

A two-way contingency table is a two-way table in which observations are cross-classified as to their values on two categorical response variables. We will call these two variables the row variable and the column variable. The chi-square test of independence is used to test whether there is an association between the row and column variables. The null hypothesis is that there is no association (i.e., they are independent) and the alternative hypothesis is that there is a relationship (i.e., they are not independent).

The notation that we will use for the chi-square test of independence is presented in Table 8.2. In the table, n_{ij} is the observed frequency count in row i and column j, $n_{i+} = \sum_{j=1}^{c} n_{ij}$ is the sum of the frequency counts in row i, $n_{+j} = \sum_{i=1}^{r} n_{ij}$ is the sum of the frequency counts in column j, and $N = \sum_{1}^{c} \sum_{1}^{r} n_{ij}$ is the overall total number of observations.

Chi-square test of independence

The observed proportion in cell ij is $\hat{p}_{ij} = n_{ij}/N$. The observed proportion in row i is $\hat{p}_{i+} = n_{i+}/N$ and the observed proportion in column j is $\hat{p}_{+j} = n_{+j}/N$. Under the null hypothesis of no association between the row and column variables, the expected proportion in cell ij is the product of the observed row and column proportions, $\hat{p}_{i+}\hat{p}_{+j}$, and the corresponding expected frequency count under the null is $m_{ij} = N\hat{p}_{i+}\hat{p}_{+j}$. The null hypothesis can be tested using the test statistic

$$X = \sum_{i=1}^{r}\sum_{j=1}^{c} \frac{(n_{ij} - m_{ij})^2}{m_{ij}} = \sum_{i=1}^{r}\sum_{j=1}^{c} \frac{N(\hat{p}_{ij} - \hat{p}_{i+}\hat{p}_{+j})^2}{\hat{p}_{i+}\hat{p}_{+j}}. \quad (8.3)$$

When the null hypothesis is true, X has a chi-square distribution with $(r-1)(c-1)$ degrees of freedom. Suppose that under the alternative for which we wish to calculate power, the proportions are p_{ijA} for cell ij. Then the expected row and column proportions under this alternative are $p_{i+A} = \sum_{j=1}^{c} p_{ijA}$ and $p_{+jA} = \sum_{i=1}^{r} p_{ijA}$. When this alternative is true, X has a noncentral chi-square distribution with $(r-1)(c-1)$ degrees of freedom and noncentrality parameter

$$\Lambda = \sum_{i=1}^{r}\sum_{j=1}^{c} \frac{N(p_{ijA} - p_{i+A}p_{+jA})^2}{p_{i+A}p_{+jA}}.$$

The noncentral chi-square distribution is described in Section 3.1.4. Power for a given significance level α can be found as $1 - \mathcal{X}^2_{(r-1)(c-1),\Lambda}(x^2_{1-\alpha,(r-1)(c-1)})$.

The w effect size for a two-way contingency table is calculated in the same manner as for a chi-square goodness-of-fit test (see equation (8.2)). The effect size is

$$w = \sqrt{\sum_{i=1}^{r}\sum_{j=1}^{c} \frac{(p_{ijA} - p_{i+A}p_{+jA})^2}{p_{i+A}p_{+jA}}}$$

and thus we have that $\Lambda = Nw^2$. The benchmarks for small, medium and large w effect sizes are 0.1, 0.3 and 0.5 [36].

Example 8.2. A study is being planned to evaluate an intervention for pregnant women that addresses maternal weight gain. The outcome is a 3-category variable with possible outcomes of lower than recommended, recommended and higher than recommended weight gain. The trial will use equal allocation to the intervention and a control condition. The cell proportions that are expected to be observed in the planned trial are given in the table below:

	Lower	Recommended	Higher	Row proportion
Intervention	0.050	0.350	0.100	0.500
Control	0.075	0.250	0.175	0.500
Column proportion	0.125	0.600	0.275	1.000

Under the null hypothesis of no association, the expected proportions, calculated from the row and column proportions as $p_{ijA} = p_{i+A}p_{+jA}$, are:

	Lower	Recommended	Higher
Intervention	0.0625	0.300	0.1375
Control	0.0625	0.300	0.1375

We can find the sample size required to achieve 80% power with α of 0.05 using the chisq.indep function:

```
library(powertools)
pmatrix <- matrix(c(0.050, 0.350, 0.100, 0.075, 0.250, 0.175), nrow = 2,
    byrow = TRUE)
chisq.indep(pmatrix = pmatrix, N = NULL, power = 0.8, alpha = 0.05,
    v = TRUE)

    Chi-square test of independence power calculation

       pmatrix = 0.05, 0.35, 0.1
                 0.075, 0.25, 0.175
 w effect size = 0.2052345
             N = 228.7372
         alpha = 0.05
         power = 0.8
```

The effect size is small-to-medium. We need at least 229 participants.

There are several indices of association for two-way contingency tables that are related to w and may be more familiar to investigators and also more readily available from prior studies. The **contingency coefficient** is one such measure. The sample contingency coefficient is calculated from the data as $\hat{C} = \sqrt{X/(X+N)}$, where X is the chi-square test statistic (8.3) and N is the total sample size. The population contingency coefficient is $C = \sqrt{w^2/(w^2+N)}$ and thus we have $w = \sqrt{C^2/(1-C^2)}$. Cohen [36] provides more discussion of measures of association in contingency tables. The phi coefficient is another measure of association applicable to a 2×2 table; see Section 6.4.

8.3 Chi-square test for comparing two proportions

The chi-square test of independence can be used to conduct a test of nonequality of two proportions when the proportions are from two independent samples. This provides another method to calculate power and sample size for a comparison between two independent proportions, in addition to the methods described in Section 6.3.

An important difference between the methods in Section 6.3 and the chi-square test for comparing two independent proportions is that the chi-square test considers the frequency counts and proportions in the form of a 2 × 2 contingency table, as in the following example:

Example 8.3. A two-group randomized trial expects outcome proportions of 0.6 and 0.8 in the intervention and control groups. If the trial will have 100 participants in each group, the expected frequency counts are

	Yes	No	Total
Intervention	60	40	100
Control	80	20	100
Total	140	60	200

The expected proportions are

	Yes	No	Total
Intervention	0.3	0.2	0.5
Control	0.4	0.1	0.5
Total	0.7	0.3	1.0

Power can be calculated as follows:

```
library(powertools)
pmatrix <- matrix(c(0.3, 0.2, 0.4, 0.1), nrow = 2, byrow = TRUE)
chisq.indep(pmatrix = pmatrix, N = 200, power = NULL, alpha = 0.05,
    v = TRUE)

    Chi-square test of independence power calculation

        pmatrix = 0.3, 0.2
```

```
                  0.4, 0.1
w effect size = 0.2182179
            N = 200
        alpha = 0.05
        power = 0.8699393
```

Power is about 0.87.

8.4 Ordinal categorical responses

Many studies yield data with an ordered categorical scale. Examples include Likert scales with categories such as very satisfied, satisfied, neither, dissatisfied and very dissatisfied; severity rating scales with categories such as none, mild, moderate and severe; and frequency scales with categories such as never, rarely, sometimes, often and always.

Table 8.3 shows response categories and their probabilities for a two-group study with an ordinal response variable. The variable has response categories $1, 2, \ldots, K$, ordered from "best" (1) to "worst" (K). For the treatment group, let p_{Tk} denote the probability that an individual has a response in category k; the probabilities must sum to one: $p_{T1} + \cdots + p_{TK} = 1$. Let Q_{Tk} denote the probability of an outcome of k or better (i.e., lower). This is a cumulative probability with $Q_{Tk} = p_{T1} + \cdots + p_{Tk}$. Define p_{Ck} and Q_{Ck} similarly for the control group. The odds ratio for being at or below category k for the

TABLE 8.3: Notation for ordinal categorical response model. The p_{Tk} and p_{Ck} values are probabilities of each response category in the treatment and control groups. Q_{Tk} and Q_{Ck} are cumulative response probabilities.

Group	Response categories			
	1	2	$\cdots$	K
Treatment	p_{T1}	p_{T2}	$\cdots$	p_{TK}
	$Q_{T1} = p_{T1}$	$Q_{T2} = p_{T1} + p_{T2}$	$\cdots$	$Q_{TK} = p_{T1} + \cdots + p_{TK} = 1$
Control	p_{C1}	p_{C2}	$\cdots$	p_{CK}
	$Q_{C1} = p_{C1}$	$Q_{C2} = p_{C1} + p_{C2}$	$\cdots$	$Q_{CK} = p_{C1} + \cdots + p_{CK} = 1$
Average	$\bar{p}_1 = \frac{p_{T1}+p_{C1}}{2}$	$\bar{p}_2 = \frac{p_{T2}+p_{C2}}{2}$	$\cdots$	$\bar{p}_K = \frac{p_{TK}+p_{CK}}{2}$

Ordinal categorical responses

treatment group compared to the control group is

$$OR_k = \frac{\frac{Q_{Tk}}{1-Q_{Tk}}}{\frac{Q_{Ck}}{1-Q_{Ck}}}. \tag{8.4}$$

The data collected are the counts in each cell, $n_{T1}, \ldots, n_{TK}$ and $n_{C1}, \ldots, n_{CK}$, with the totals in each group equal to n_T and n_C, with $n_T + n_C = N$.

Such data are often analyzed under a proportional odds assumption. The proportional odds assumption is that all of the odds ratios OR_k are equal to a common value, $OR_1 = \ldots = OR_K = OR$. Data can be analyzed under this assumption using a cumulative logit model [153], which is an extension of the usual logistic regression model, discussed in Section 11.2.

Whitehead [228] presents power and sample size formulas under the proportional odds assumption; see this reference for details of the derivation. Under this approach, power for a test of $H_0 \colon OR = 1$ versus $H_A \colon OR \neq 1$ at level α, under the alternative that the true value of the (proportional) odds ratio is OR_A, can be approximated as

$$1 - \beta = \Phi\left(|\log(OR_A)|\sqrt{V} - z_{1-\alpha/2}\right) \tag{8.5}$$

where

$$V = \frac{Nr}{3(r+1)^2}\left[1 - \sum_{k=1}^{K}\bar{p}_k^3\right]$$

where $r = n_T/n_C$ and the $\bar{p}_k$ are probabilities for response k averaged across treatment and control, $\bar{p}_k = \frac{p_{Tk}+p_{Ck}}{2}$, assuming the alternative is true. Total sample size is given by

$$N \geq \frac{3(r+1)^2(z_{1-\alpha/2}+z_{1-\beta})^2}{r[\log(OR_A)]^2\left[1-\sum_{k=1}^{K}\bar{p}_k^3\right]}. \tag{8.6}$$

To perform a power or sample size calculation, the average probabilities $\bar{p}_k$ are needed. The propodds function, demonstrated below, internally computes these values based on a given set of response probabilities in the control group $(p_{C1}, \ldots, p_{CK})$ and OR_A.

Example 8.4. The following example is based on Whitehead [228]. Suppose that the outcome variable in a trial is a disease progress classification with categories of very good, good, fair and poor, labeled 1 through 4. The response probabilities expected in the control group are:

	1	2	3	4
p_{Ck}	0.2	0.5	0.2	0.1
Q_{Ck}	0.2	0.7	0.9	1

Thus in the control group, the probability of a "very good" is 0.2, the probability of a "good" or better is 0.7, etc. Suppose that the odds ratio under the alternative is $OR_A = 2.5$. What is the power for a two-sided test at significance level of 0.05 when there are 65 individuals in each group?

```
library(powertools)
pC <- c(0.2, 0.5, 0.2, 0.1)
propodds(pC = pC, OR = 2.5, n1 = 65, n.ratio = 1, alpha = 0.05)

    Power calculation for ordinal categorical outcome
    under proportional odds

              n = 65, 65
             pC = 0.2, 0.5, 0.2, 0.1
             pT = 0.385, 0.469, 0.104, 0.043
             OR = 2.5
          alpha = 0.05
          power = 0.7914087
```

The power is about 0.79. The output includes the response probabilities in the treatment group that are implied by the response probabilities in the control group and the odds ratio. The investigators should consider whether these response probabilities are realistic. If they are not, the assumed odds ratio might be adjusted accordingly, or the proportional odds assumption might be abandoned in favor of another approach.

If the proportional odds assumption is not reasonable for a particular study, different approaches might be used. One alternative is a Mann-Whitney-Wilcoxon rank-sum test. This test can be applied to continuous or ordinal data and is discussed in Section 3.7.3.

8.5 Additional resources

The pwrss and TrialSize packages also offers functions for power and sample size for chi-square goodness-of-fit and independence tests.

9

Precision and confidence intervals

9.1 Introduction

Most of the chapters in this book assume that the study objectives will involve conducting hypothesis tests, and power and sample size calculations are conducted with reference to the planned test or tests. However, in some studies the goals may be more focused on estimating parameters with an acceptable level of precision. For example, a pilot study may be planned with the objective of using its data to estimate the effect size of an intervention, or to estimate the proportion of eligible patients willing to enroll in a study, and it is important to have a large enough sample to ensure that these parameters are estimated with an acceptable level of precision.

Precision-based sample size calculations are focused on determining the sample size needed to achieve a certain level of precision in estimating a parameter. In particular, precision-based calculations focus on confidence intervals and their width. All else being equal, a narrower confidence interval means that the parameter is estimated more precisely.

A $100(1-\alpha)\%$ confidence interval (CI) for a parameter θ is an interval (L, U), where the lower and upper endpoints L and U are random variables that satisfy

$$P(L < \theta < U) = 1 - \alpha.$$

The parameter θ could be a single mean or proportion, a difference of two means or proportions, or some other function of parameters such as a relative risk or an odds ratio, which are functions of two proportions.

The width of a confidence interval is the distance between its upper and lower endpoints, $U - L$. Because the endpoints of a confidence interval are random variables, the width of the confidence interval is also a random variable. For precision analysis, we will need to understand the distribution of confidence interval width. In many cases, confidence intervals take the form $\hat{\theta} \pm c(\alpha)\mathrm{SE}(\hat{\theta})$, where $\hat{\theta}$ is a point estimate of the parameter of interest, $c(\alpha)$ is a confidence coefficient, and $\mathrm{SE}(\hat{\theta})$ is the standard error of $\hat{\theta}$. In this case, the width of the confidence interval is $2c(\alpha)\mathrm{SE}(\hat{\theta})$ and its halfwidth is $c(\alpha)\mathrm{SE}(\hat{\theta})$. $\mathrm{SE}(\hat{\theta})$ is a random variable and precision analysis focuses on the distribution of $\mathrm{SE}(\hat{\theta})$, which will depend on sample size and other factors.

9.2 Confidence intervals for means

In this section, we discuss precision analysis for one mean and for a difference between two means from independent populations. The derivations are based largely on Chapter 8 of Julious [111] and the references therein, in particular Grieve [79]. Precision analysis for a difference between two means is also discussed in Liu [142].

9.2.1 One mean

Precision analysis for one mean focuses on finding the sample size needed to obtain a confidence interval for a single mean that is sufficiently narrow. For example, we may wish to determine the sample size needed to estimate the mean symptom score in a certain population with a given level of precision.

We assume that the sample, $Y_1, ..., Y_N$, comes from a normal distribution with mean μ and variance σ^2. We first consider the situation that the value of the variance is known and then consider the more realistic case that the value of the variance is not known and will be estimated from the sample.

9.2.1.1 Variance known

We first consider the case of a confidence interval for a single mean assuming that the variance is known. Suppose we have a sample $Y_1, ..., Y_N$ from a normal distribution with mean μ and known variance σ^2. Then $\frac{\bar{Y}-\mu}{\sigma/\sqrt{N}} \sim \mathcal{N}(0,1)$ and based on the properties of the standard normal distribution, we can write the probability statement

$$P\left(z_{\alpha/2} < \frac{\bar{Y}-\mu}{\sigma/\sqrt{N}} < z_{1-\alpha/2}\right) = 1 - \alpha.$$

Rearranging, we can arrive at

$$P\left[\bar{Y} - z_{1-\alpha/2}\frac{\sigma}{\sqrt{N}} < \mu < \bar{Y} + z_{1-\alpha/2}\frac{\sigma}{\sqrt{N}}\right] = 1 - \alpha.$$

This relationship implies that when we select a random sample $Y_1, ..., Y_N$ and form a confidence interval as

$$\bar{Y} \pm z_{1-\alpha/2}\frac{\sigma}{\sqrt{N}}, \qquad (9.1)$$

there is probability of $1 - \alpha$ that the mean μ lies within the interval.

In precision analysis, our objective is to find the sample size that will enable us to form a confidence interval that has no more than a specified **halfwidth**. In equation (9.1), the halfwidth of the confidence interval is $z_{1-\alpha/2}\,\sigma/\sqrt{N}$. A confidence interval halfwidth is sometimes called the "margin of error". We

Confidence intervals for means

will denote the observed halfwidth as $\tilde{h}$ and the desired halfwidth as h. Some authors and software focus on the width rather than the halfwidth; in equation (9.1), the width is $2z_{1-\alpha/2}\,\sigma/\sqrt{N}$.

To determine the sample size needed to achieve a $100(1-\alpha)\%$ confidence interval with an observed halfwidth $\tilde{h}$ no greater than h for a single mean when the variance is known, we set up the relationship

$$\tilde{h} = z_{1-\alpha/2}\frac{\sigma}{\sqrt{N}} \leq h$$

and solve for N, yielding

$$N \geq \frac{(z_{1-\alpha/2})^2 \sigma^2}{h^2}.$$

We select the lowest whole number N that satisfies this relationship.

It can be convenient to work with a **standardized halfwidth**, which expresses the halfwidth in units of standard deviation:

$$d = \frac{h}{\sigma}.$$

For example, we might plan for a confidence interval that has a halfwidth of 20% of a standard deviation,

$$d = \frac{h}{\sigma} = \frac{0.2\sigma}{\sigma} = 0.2.$$

The sample size formula in terms of a standardized halfwidth, assuming known variance, is

$$N \geq \frac{(z_{1-\alpha/2})^2}{d^2}.$$

We select the lowest whole number N that satisfies this relationship. Note that although we are using d to denote the standardized halfwidth, this is not the same as Cohen's d, i.e., the standardized difference between two means.

Example 9.1. Suppose we would like to determine the sample size needed to obtain a 95% confidence interval for a mean whose halfwidth is no more than one-fourth of a standard deviation. The variance σ^2 is assumed to be known and will not need to be estimated in the planned study. We can calculate the required sample size as follows:

```
za <- qnorm(p = 0.975)
d <- 0.25
N <- za^2 / d^2 ; N
[1]    61.46334
```

We round up to 62 observations to ensure that the halfwidth does not exceed 0.25 standard deviation units.

9.2.1.2 Variance unknown

In most studies, the variance is unknown and will need to be estimated. When we estimate σ using the sample standard deviation, $\hat{\sigma}$, the quantity $\frac{\bar{Y}-\mu}{\hat{\sigma}/\sqrt{N}}$ has a $t(N-1)$ distribution and we form the $100(1-\alpha)\%$ confidence interval using the $100(1-\alpha/2)^{th}$ quantile of the $t(N-1)$ distribution rather than $z_{1-\alpha/2}$ as the confidence coefficient. The confidence limits are given by

$$\bar{Y} \pm t_{1-\alpha/2, N-1} \frac{\hat{\sigma}}{\sqrt{N}}. \tag{9.2}$$

The observed halfwidth of the interval is $\tilde{h} = t_{1-\alpha/2, N-1} \hat{\sigma}/\sqrt{N}$.

The formula for the observed halfwidth includes the random variable $\hat{\sigma}$, and thus the value of the observed halfwidth will vary randomly due to the sampling variability of $\hat{\sigma}$. In any particular sample, $\hat{\sigma}^2$ could be higher or lower than the true population variance, σ^2. To address the fact that the observed halfwidth will vary randomly, following Grieve [79], we take the approach of finding the sample size that will achieve a specified *probability* of obtaining a certain halfwidth. The probability of obtaining an observed halfwidth of no more than h for a $100(1-\alpha)\%$ confidence interval for one mean can be expressed as

$$P\left(\tilde{h} \leq h\right) = P\left(t_{1-\alpha/2, N-1} \frac{\hat{\sigma}}{\sqrt{N}} \leq h\right) = P\left(\hat{\sigma}^2 \leq \frac{N h^2}{(t_{1-\alpha/2, N-1})^2}\right). \tag{9.3}$$

To calculate this probability, we need the sampling distribution of $\hat{\sigma}^2$. For a sample of size N from a normal distribution, $\hat{\sigma}^2$ has a scaled chi-square distribution, with $\frac{(N-1)\hat{\sigma}^2}{\sigma^2} \sim \chi^2(N-1)$. Multiplying the right-hand side of equation (9.3) by $N-1$ and dividing by σ^2, we obtain

$$P\left[\frac{(N-1)\hat{\sigma}^2}{\sigma^2} < \frac{N(N-1)h^2}{\sigma^2 (t_{1-\alpha/2, N-1})^2}\right] = P\left[W < \frac{N(N-1)h^2}{\sigma^2 (t_{1-\alpha/2, N-1})^2}\right] \tag{9.4}$$

where $W \sim \chi^2(N-1)$. The probability of achieving a specified halfwidth or width is sometimes called the **power of a confidence interval**, although it is not technically statistical power.

The probability (9.4) can be computed using the cumulative distribution function of a chi-square random variable with $N-1$ degrees of freedom, which we denote as $\mathcal{X}^2_{N-1}$:

$$\text{Power of CI for one mean} = \mathcal{X}^2_{N-1}\left(\frac{N(N-1)h^2}{\sigma^2 (t_{1-\alpha/2, N-1})^2}\right). \tag{9.5}$$

For a standardized halfwidth, the formula is

$$\text{Power for CI of one mean (standardized)} = \mathcal{X}^2_{N-1}\left(\frac{N(N-1)d^2}{(t_{1-\alpha/2, N-1})^2}\right). \tag{9.6}$$

Confidence intervals for means 161

The probability or "power" is typically set to 0.8 or 0.9. Since we need to specify N in order to get the degrees of freedom of the chi-square distribution to compute this probability, the equation has to be solved iteratively to find the smallest N that achieves the desired probability.

Example 9.2. We continue Example 9.1, which involved finding sample size such that the observed halfwidth of a 95% confidence interval for a single mean will not exceed one-fourth of a standard deviation, but now account for estimation of σ. Suppose that we want at least 80% probability that the observed halfwidth will not exceed one-fourth of a standard deviation; colloquially, we want the "power" of the confidence interval to be at least 80%. We find sample size using the ci.mean function:

```
library(powertools)
ci.mean(N = NULL, halfwidth = 0.25, sd = 1, power = 0.8, v = TRUE)

    Precision analysis for one mean
    using unconditional probability

             N = 72.34771
     halfwidth = 0.25
            sd = 1
         alpha = 0.05
         power = 0.8
```

The results indicate that we need 73 subjects in order to achieve at least 80% "power", i.e., 80% probability that the observed halfwidth will not exceed 0.25 standard deviation units. The output indicates that the result uses "unconditional probability". This issue is discussed in Section 9.2.1.3.

Note that a sample size of 62, which was calculated in Example 9.1 assuming known variance, yields a probability of achieving the desired halfwidth that is considerably lower than our desired probability of 0.8:

```
ci.mean(N = 62, halfwidth = 0.25, sd = 1, power = NULL, v = FALSE)
[1] 0.455492
```

This highlights the importance of considering the sampling variability of $\hat{\sigma}^2$. Note that some R functions for precision analysis for means, such as the prec_mean function in the presize package, do not consider the sampling variability of $\hat{\sigma}$. This function produces results that assume known variance.

9.2.1.3 Variance unknown: conditional probability

There is one more nuance to consider. A confidence interval will sometimes include the true value of the parameter and sometimes not include it. By definition, a 95% confidence interval for a parameter will include the true value 95% of the time and NOT include it 5% of the time. Equations (9.5) and (9.6) compute the *unconditional* probability of obtaining the desired precision, $P(\tilde{h} < h)$, regardless of whether or not the confidence interval includes the true mean. Let I denote the event that the confidence interval includes the true value of the parameter and $\bar{I}$ denote the event that it does not. The unconditional probability is a sum of two conditional probabilities, the probability that $\tilde{h} < h$ when the interval includes the parameter value and the probability that $\tilde{h} < h$ when it does not; specifically,

$$P(\tilde{h} < h) = P(\tilde{h} < h \mid I)P(I) + P(\tilde{h} < h \mid \bar{I})P(\bar{I}).$$

Rather than selecting a sample size to attain the unconditional probability $P(\tilde{h} < h)$, as in equations (9.5) and (9.6), it may be of interest to select a sample size to attain the conditional probability $P(\tilde{h} < h|I)$, because it is not particularly desirable for the interval to be narrow when it does not include the true parameter value [14].

The conditional probability $P(\tilde{h} < h \mid I)$ can be computed using Owen's Q function [178], which has the form

$$Q_\nu(t, \delta; a, b) = \frac{\sqrt{2\pi}}{\Gamma(\frac{\nu}{2})2^{(\nu-2)/2}} \int_a^b \Phi\left(\frac{tx}{\sqrt{\nu}} - \delta\right) x^{\nu-1} \phi(x) dx \qquad (9.7)$$

where Φ is the cumulative standard normal distribution and ϕ is the standard normal density; see [14]. Owen's Q function is a bivariate version of the noncentral t distribution; for further information, see [178, 31]. Owen's Q function is also used in power for equivalence testing; see Section 4.6. Functions for computing Owen's Q function can be found in the OwenQ package and in the PowerTOST package. The conditional probability that a $100(1 - \alpha)\%$ confidence interval for one mean will have observed halfwidth $\tilde{h}$ of no more than h, conditional on the interval containing the true mean, can be computed as

$$P\left(\tilde{h} \leq h \mid I\right) = \frac{2}{1 - \alpha}\left[Q_{N-1}(t_{1-\alpha/2, N-1}, 0; 0, b_1) - Q_{N-1}(0, 0; 0, b_1)\right]$$

where $b_1 = \frac{h\sqrt{N(N-1)}}{\sigma t_{1-\alpha/2, N-1}} = \frac{d\sqrt{N(N-1)}}{t_{1-\alpha/2, N-1}}$, where $d = h/\sigma$ is the standardized halfwidth.

Example 9.3. In Example 9.2, we calculated that we needed 73 subjects to achieve at least 80% unconditional probability for a 95% confidence interval for a single mean to have a halfwidth of no more than 0.25 standard deviation units. We compare the unconditional and conditional probabilities when we have 73 subjects:

Confidence intervals for means

```
library(powertools)
ci.mean(N = 73, halfwidth = 0.25, sd = 1, cond = FALSE)
[1] 0.8167913

ci.mean(N = 73, halfwidth = 0.25, sd = 1, cond = TRUE)
[1] 0.8122032
```

The conditional probability is only slightly lower than the unconditional probability.

As Example 9.3 suggests, the conditional and unconditional probabilities of achieving a certain halfwidth typically do not differ very much. For most practical purposes, there will be little difference and either can be used.

9.2.2 Difference between two means

Procedures for a confidence interval for the difference between two means from independent populations follow the same logic as described for a confidence interval for one mean. We confine our attention to the situation of equal variances in the two populations.

9.2.2.1 Variance known

Suppose that we have samples of sizes n_1 and n_2 from two independent populations, with $N = n_1 + n_2$ and $n_2/n_1 = r$. For a difference between two means, $\mu_1 - \mu_2$, assuming samples from normal distributions with a known common variance σ^2, the $100(1-\alpha)\%$ confidence interval is

$$\bar{Y}_1 - \bar{Y}_2 \pm z_{1-\alpha/2}\sqrt{\frac{\sigma^2}{n_1} + \frac{\sigma^2}{n_2}}$$

or equivalently,

$$\bar{Y}_1 - \bar{Y}_2 \pm z_{1-\alpha/2}\sqrt{\frac{r+1}{r}\frac{\sigma^2}{n_1}}.$$

Setting up the relationship $\widetilde{h} = z_{1-\alpha/2}\sqrt{\frac{r+1}{r}\frac{\sigma^2}{n_1}} \leq h$ and solving for n_1, we can find the sample sizes needed to achieve a specific halfwidth h as

$$n_1 \geq \left(\frac{r+1}{r}\right)\frac{(z_{1-\alpha/2})^2 \sigma^2}{h^2}. \qquad (9.8)$$

For equal allocation, the total sample size N will be

$$N \geq \frac{4(z_{1-\alpha/2})^2 \sigma^2}{h^2} = \frac{4(z_{1-\alpha/2})^2}{d^2} \qquad (9.9)$$

where $d = h/\sigma$ is the standardized halfwidth. As previously noted, this is not the same as Cohen's d, i.e., the standardized mean difference.

The variance is usually not known and must be estimated. We discuss this situation in the next section.

9.2.2.2 Variance unknown

If the population variance is unknown and will be estimated from the sample, we will use a t distribution quantile to construct the confidence interval, and we must account for the sampling variability of our estimate $\hat{\sigma}^2$. The observed halfwidth of the confidence interval takes the form

$$\widetilde{h} = t_{1-\alpha/2,\nu}\sqrt{\frac{r+1}{r}\frac{\hat{\sigma}^2}{n_1}}$$

where $\nu = n_1(r+1) - 2$. The probability that the observed halfwidth does not exceed h can be calculated as

$$P(\widetilde{h} \leq h) = P\left(t_{1-\alpha/2,\nu}\sqrt{\frac{r+1}{r}\frac{\hat{\sigma}^2}{n_1}} \leq h\right) = P\left(\hat{\sigma}^2 \leq \frac{h^2}{(t_{1-\alpha/2,\nu})^2}\frac{n_1 r}{r+1}\right).$$

The sample variance $\hat{\sigma}^2$, which is the pooled sample variance s_p^2 (see Section 3.2.1), has a scaled chi-squared distribution, $\nu\hat{\sigma}^2/\sigma^2 \sim \chi^2(\nu)$. Thus this probability can be calculated using the cumulative distribution function of a chi-square random variable,

$$\text{Power of CI for mean difference} = \mathcal{X}_\nu^2\left(\frac{\nu h^2 n_1 r}{(t_{1-\alpha/2,\nu})^2(r+1)\sigma^2}\right) \qquad (9.10)$$

where $\nu = n_1(r+1) - 2$.

When expressing the allocation between groups in terms of weights, with a proportion w in Group 1 and $1 - w$ in Group 2 and total sample size N, the formula is

$$\text{Power of CI for mean difference} = \mathcal{X}_\nu^2\left(\frac{\nu h^2 N w(1-w)}{(t_{1-\alpha/2,\nu})^2 \sigma^2}\right). \qquad (9.11)$$

For equal allocation ($r = 1$ or $w = 0.5$), this becomes

$$\mathcal{X}_{N-2}^2\left(\frac{N(N-2)h^2}{4(t_{1-\alpha/2,N-2})^2 \sigma^2}\right). \qquad (9.12)$$

To use a standardized halfwidth, set $d^2 = h^2/\sigma^2$.

The probability is typically set to 0.8 or 0.9. As noted in Section 9.2, this probability is referred to as the "power of a confidence interval", although it is not technically statistical power. Since we need to provide information that specifies the total sample size in order to get the degrees of freedom of the

Confidence intervals for means 165

chi-square distribution, the equation must be solved numerically to find the smallest N that will achieve the desired probability, which software can do for us.

Example 9.4. Suppose we plan a randomized trial with equal allocation to two conditions and wish to have 80% probability of achieving a 95% confidence interval with an observed halfwidth of 0.25 standard deviation units for the difference in means. We can use the `ci.meandiff` function as follows:

```
library(powertools)
ci.meandiff(n1 = NULL, halfwidth = 0.25, sd = 1, power = 0.8, v = TRUE)

  Precision analysis for difference between means
    using unconditional probability

             n = 133.0443, 133.0443
     halfwidth = 0.25
            sd = 1
         alpha = 0.05
         power = 0.8
```

Rounding up, we need 134 per group. By default, the function outputs the unconditional probability.

As discussed in Section 9.2.1.3, the unconditional probability of achieving the desired halfwidth does not condition on whether the confidence interval includes the true parameter value or not. Procedures for targeting the conditional probability are discussed in the next section.

It should be noted that some functions for precision analysis in R do not account for the sampling variability of $\hat{\sigma}^2$ but rather give results for the case of known variance. This includes `prec_meandiff` in the `presize` package and `md_prec` in the `pwr2ppl` package.

9.2.2.3 Variance unknown: conditional probability

As discussed in Section 9.2.1.3, the probabilities computed in equations (9.10) and (9.11) are unconditional probabilities that the observed halfwidth $\tilde{h}$ does not exceed a specified length h; the probability is not conditional on whether or not the interval contains the true parameter value, which in this case is the mean difference. We might prefer the conditional probability that the interval includes the true difference in means, denoted as $P(\tilde{h} \leq h \mid I)$, where I denotes the event that the interval includes the true mean difference. The rationale is that it is not particularly desirable for the interval to be narrow if it does not include the true parameter value [14].

The conditional probability $P(\tilde{h} \leq h \mid I)$ can be computed using Owen's Q function [178]; see equation (9.7). The conditional probability that a $100(1-\alpha)\%$ confidence interval for a mean difference will have an observed halfwidth of no more than h, conditional on the interval containing the true mean difference, can be computed as

$$P\left(\tilde{h} \leq h \mid I\right) = \frac{2}{1-\alpha}\left[Q_{N-2}(t_{1-\alpha/2,N-2}, 0; 0, b_2) - Q_{N-2}(0, 0; 0, b_2)\right]$$

where

$$b_2 = \frac{h\sqrt{Nw(1-w)(N-2)}}{\sigma\, t_{1-\alpha/2,N-2}} = \frac{d\sqrt{Nw(1-w)(N-2)}}{t_{1-\alpha/2,N-2}}.$$

If using the allocation ratio $r = n_2/n_1$, substitute $r/(1+r)^2$ for $w(1-w)$.

Example 9.5. In Example 9.4, for the unconditional probability, we found that we needed 134 in each group to have 80% probability of achieving a 95% confidence interval with an observed halfwidth not exceeding 0.25 standard deviation units for a difference in means, with equal allocation. For comparison, we calculate the unconditional and conditional probabilities when using this sample size:

```
library(powertools)
ci.meandiff(n1 = 134, halfwidth = 0.25, sd = 1, alpha = 0.05,
    power = NULL, cond = FALSE)
[1] 0.823769

ci.meandiff(n1 = 134, halfwidth = 0.25, sd = 1, alpha = 0.05,
    power = NULL, cond = TRUE)
[1] 0.8212589
```

The conditional probability is slightly lower than the unconditional probability.

In general, the conditional and unconditional probabilities will tend to be similar and the difference does not matter for most practical purposes.

9.3 Confidence intervals for proportions

In this section, we consider selecting a sample size to achieve a desired level of precision for estimating one proportion, the difference between two independent proportions, a relative risk or an odds ratio.

9.3.1 One proportion

Let X denote the number of successes in a sample of size N from a binomial distribution with success probability p. Then the point estimate for p is $\hat{p} = X/N$, the sample proportion of successes. A common method of forming a $100(1-\alpha)\%$ confidence interval for a single proportion is the Wald method, which forms the interval as

$$\hat{p} \pm z_{1-\alpha/2} \sqrt{\frac{\hat{p}(1-\hat{p})}{N}}.$$

Although the Wald confidence interval is widely used, it has erratic coverage properties, meaning that the actual percentage of instances that the interval covers the true proportion often differs from the nominal coverage rate, especially for small N or when p is near 0 or 1 [24]. Brown et al. [24] recommend other methods, two of which, the Agresti-Coull interval and the Wilson interval, are implemented in the function prec_prop in the presize package. Rather than using $\hat{p}$ as the midpoint of the interval, the Agresti-Coull and Wilson confidence intervals use an adjusted midpoint $\tilde{p}$. The adjusted midpoint is equal to the sample proportion after adding $(z_{1-\alpha/2})^2$ pseudo observations to N, half of which are successes and half failures. Let $\tilde{N}$ denote the adjusted sample size and let $\tilde{X}$ denote the adjusted number of successes,

$$\tilde{N} = N + (z_{1-\alpha/2})^2$$

$$\tilde{X} = X + \frac{1}{2}(z_{1-\alpha/2})^2.$$

The adjusted midpoint is defined as $\tilde{p} = \tilde{X}/\tilde{N}$. A little algebra shows that $\tilde{p}$ is equivalent to a weighted average of $\hat{p}$ and $1/2$,

$$\tilde{p} = \hat{p}\left(\frac{N}{N + (z_{1-\alpha/2})^2}\right) + \frac{1}{2}\left(\frac{(z_{1-\alpha/2})^2}{N + (z_{1-\alpha/2})^2}\right).$$

The Agresti-Coull $100(1-\alpha)\%$ confidence interval is formed using the adjusted sample proportion and adjusted sample size [4, 24],

$$\tilde{p} \pm z_{1-\alpha/2}\sqrt{\frac{\tilde{p}(1-\tilde{p})}{\tilde{N}}}. \tag{9.13}$$

The Wilson $100(1-\alpha)\%$ confidence interval uses a variance that is a weighted average of the variance of a sample proportion when $p = \hat{p}$ and the variance of a sample proportion when $p = 1/2$ [3, 232]:

$$\tilde{p} \pm z_{1-\alpha/2} \times \tag{9.14}$$

$$\sqrt{\frac{1}{N + (z_{1-\alpha/2})^2}\left[\hat{p}(1-\hat{p})\left(\frac{N}{N + (z_{1-\alpha/2})^2}\right) + \left(\frac{1}{4}\right)\left(\frac{(z_{1-\alpha/2})^2}{N + (z_{1-\alpha/2})^2}\right)\right]},$$

which simplifies to

$$\tilde{p} \pm \frac{z_{1-\alpha/2}}{\tilde{N}} \sqrt{N\hat{p}(1-\hat{p}) + \frac{(z_{1-\alpha/2})^2}{4}}. \qquad (9.15)$$

Brown et al. [24] recommend the Wilson interval for $N \leq 40$ and the Agresti-Coull interval for $N > 40$. For $N \leq 40$, they also recommend an equal-tailed interval corresponding to the Jeffreys prior. However, this interval does not have a closed form expression and is not implemented in prec_prop. The prec_prop function also finds sample size to achieve a desired level of precision for an exact binomial confidence interval. Power and sample size for the exact test of a single binomial proportion are discussed in Section 7.1.

Example 9.6. The true value of a proportion is believed to be 0.85 and we wish to have an observed halfwidth for a 95% confidence interval of no more than 0.10. We can find the sample size required for the Wilson and Agresti-Coull methods as follows:

```
library(presize)
# the function input is full width rather than halfwidth:
prec_prop(p = 0.85, n = NULL, conf.width = 0.2, conf.level = 0.95,
  method = "wilson")
# output has been slightly modified for clarity:

sample size for a proportion with Wilson confidence interval

p       padj      n        conf.width  conf.level  lwr      upr
0.85    0.82435   48.585   0.2         0.95        0.72435  0.92435

NOTE: padj is the adjusted proportion, from which the ci is calculated.

prec_prop(p = 0.85, n = NULL, conf.width = 0.2, conf.level = 0.95,
  method = "agresti-coull")

sample size for a proportion with Agresti-Coull confidence
interval

p       padj      n         conf.width  conf.level  lwr      upr
0.85    0.82568   51.4489   0.2         0.95        0.72568  0.92568

NOTE: padj is the adjusted proportion, from which the ci is calculated.
```

The Wilson method is recommended for $N \leq 40$ and the Agresti-Coull method is recommended for larger N. The results suggest that we will need a sample size larger than 40 and so we should use the Agresti-Coull method and will need a sample size of $N = 52$.

The presize package also has functions prec_sens and prec_spec for conducting precision analysis for estimating sensitivity and specificity. Sensitivity and specificity are concerned with the accuracy of a screening test relative to a "gold standard" reference. Sensitivity is defined as the proportion of positive tests that are true positives (N equals the number of positive tests and X equals the number of positive tests that are true positives) and specificity is defined as the proportion of negative tests that are true negatives (N equals the number of negative tests and X equals the number of negative tests that are true negatives). Sensitivity and specificity are one-sample proportions and these functions make an internal call to the prec_prop function.

9.3.2 Difference between two proportions

We now consider precision analysis for the difference between two independent proportions. Denote the true probabilities of success in two populations as p_1 and p_2. Let n_1 and n_2 denote the sample sizes taken from the two populations and let x_1 and x_2 denote the number of successes observed in each sample. The sample proportions are $\hat{p}_1 = x_1/n_1$ and $\hat{p}_2 = x_2/n_2$. The objective is to find the sample sizes that will result in a confidence interval for $p_1 - p_2$ that does not exceed a specified width or halfwidth.

A commonly used $100(1-\alpha)\%$ confidence interval for a difference between two independent proportions is the Wald interval, which is formed as

$$\hat{p}_1 - \hat{p}_2 \pm z_{1-\alpha/2}\sqrt{\frac{\hat{p}_1(1-\hat{p}_1)}{n_1} + \frac{\hat{p}_2(1-\hat{p}_2)}{n_2}}. \quad (9.16)$$

However, literature shows that this interval behaves poorly [3]. We discuss several other methods with superior performance for which precision analysis can be conducted using the prec_riskdiff function in the presize package.

The Agresti-Caffo confidence interval is based on adding two pseudo observations to each group, with one being a success and one a failure, to obtain the estimates $\tilde{p}_1 = (x_1 + 1)/(n_1 + 2)$ and $\tilde{p}_2 = (x_2 + 1)/(n_2 + 2)$. Denoting the adjusted sample sizes as $\tilde{n}_1 = n_1 + 2$ and $\tilde{n}_2 = n_2 + 2$, the $100(1-\alpha)\%$ Agrest-Caffo confidence interval is formed as [3]

$$\tilde{p}_1 - \tilde{p}_2 \pm z_{1-\alpha/2}\sqrt{\frac{\tilde{p}_1(1-\tilde{p}_1)}{\tilde{n}_1} + \frac{\tilde{p}_2(1-\tilde{p}_2)}{\tilde{n}_2}}. \quad (9.17)$$

The Newcombe confidence interval is based on the Wilson method for a single proportion, discussed in Section 9.3.1. The prec_riskdiff function implements the confidence interval from Newcombe [168] equation 10, which has lower and upper limits L and U formed as

$$L = \hat{p}_1 - \hat{p}_2 - \epsilon_L$$
$$U = \hat{p}_1 - \hat{p}_2 + \epsilon_U$$

where

$$\epsilon_L = z_{1-\alpha/2}\sqrt{\frac{\ell_1(1-\ell_1)}{n_1} + \frac{u_2(1-u_2)}{n_2}}$$

$$\epsilon_U = z_{1-\alpha/2}\sqrt{\frac{u_1(1-u_1)}{n_1} + \frac{\ell_2(1-\ell_2)}{n_2}}$$

and ℓ_1 and u_1 are the roots of $|p_1 - \hat{p}_1| = z_{1-\alpha/2}\sqrt{p_1(1-p_1)/n_1}$ and ℓ_2 and u_2 are the roots of $|p_2 - \hat{p}_2| = z_{1-\alpha/2}\sqrt{p_2(1-p_2)/n_2}$. The Agresti-Caffo and Newcombe intervals have similar performance, with the Newcombe interval tending to be slightly less conservative and shorter [3]. The prec_riskdiff function also implements the Miettinen-Nurminen method, which is based on the restricted maximum likelihood estimate [155].

Example 9.7. We wish to select a sample size for a study that will estimate the difference between proportions in two groups. The study will have equal numbers in the two groups. The true proportions are assumed to be $p_1 = 0.25$ and $p_2 = 0.4$. If we wish to have a 95% confidence interval with a halfwidth of no more than 0.1, what sample size should be selected? We obtain results for the Newcombe and Agresti-Caffo methods:

```
library(presize)
# the function inputs full width rather than halfwidth:
prec_riskdiff(p1 = 0.25, p2 = 0.40, n1 = NULL, conf.width = 0.2,
    r = 1, conf.level = 0.95, method = "ac")
# output slightly edited for clarity

sample size for a risk difference with ac confidence interval

p1    p2    n1      n2      ntot     r    delta
0.25  0.4   162.89  162.89  325.79   1    -0.15

    lwr    upr    conf.width  conf.level
    -0.25  -0.05      0.2        0.95

prec_riskdiff(p1 = 0.25, p2 = 0.40, n1 = NULL, conf.width = 0.2,
    r = 1, conf.level = 0.95, method = "newcombe")

sample size for a risk difference with newcombe confidence interval

p1    p2    n1      n2      ntot     r    delta
0.25  0.4   161.60  161.60  323.20   1    -0.15

       lwr        upr      conf.width  conf.level
       -0.247889  -0.047889    0.2        0.95
```

The sample sizes suggested by the two methods are similar. As expected, the Newcombe interval is slightly shorter.

9.4 Confidence intervals for relative risk

In some studies that compare two groups on a binary outcome, it is of interest to estimate a relative risk, also called a risk ratio, defined as $RR = p_2/p_1$. The relative risk measures the multiplicative difference in outcome probabilities between groups. For example, a RR of 1.5 indicates that the probability of the outcome is 50% higher in group 2 compared to group 1. Many different methods have been developed to form confidence intervals for a relative risk. We consider a few of the simpler methods. For a more in-depth discussion, see [66, 73]. We assume that the two groups are independent.

As discussed in Section 6.3.5, the sample relative risk, $\widehat{RR} = \hat{p}_2/\hat{p}_1$, has a skewed distribution but $\log(\widehat{RR})$ is approximately normal with approximate mean $\log(RR) = \log(p_2/p_1)$ and approximate variance (see Katz et al. [119])

$$Var(\log(\widehat{RR})) \approx \frac{1-\hat{p}_1}{n_1\hat{p}_1} + \frac{1-\hat{p}_2}{n_2\hat{p}_2} = \frac{1}{x_1} - \frac{1}{n_1} + \frac{1}{x_2} - \frac{1}{n_2}.$$

Due to the approximate normality,

$$P\left[z_{\alpha/2} \leq \frac{\log(\widehat{RR}) - \log(RR)}{\sqrt{\frac{1}{x_1} - \frac{1}{n_1} + \frac{1}{x_2} - \frac{1}{n_2}}} \leq z_{1-\alpha/2}\right] \approx 1 - \alpha$$

and an approximate $100(1-\alpha)\%$ confidence interval can be formed as

$$\log(\widehat{RR}) \pm z_{1-\alpha/2}\sqrt{\frac{1}{x_1} - \frac{1}{n_1} + \frac{1}{x_2} - \frac{1}{n_2}}$$

The endpoints are exponentiated to backtransform to the relative risk scale. This method can give overly wide intervals [66]. Fagerland et al. [66] recommend using the method of Koopman [125], which is an asymptotic score confidence interval for the ratio of proportions that is consistent with Pearson's chi-squared test. Sample size and power for this method can be computed using the `prec_riskratio` function in the `presize` package.

Example 9.8. In a cohort study, the outcome proportions in exposed and unexposed groups are expected to be 0.2 and 0.1, for a RR of 2. There will be 100 exposed subjects and 300 unexposed subjects. What is the expected width of a 95% confidence interval?

```
library(presize)
# r is n2 / n1
prec_riskratio(p1 = 0.2, p2 = 0.1, n1 = 100, r = 3, conf.width = NULL,
    method = "koopman")
# output slightly edited for clarity

precision for a relative risk with koopman confidence interval

 p1  p2  n1  n2  ntot r  rr   lwr   upr   conf.width conf.level
 0.2 0.1 100 300 400  3  2    1.188 3.316 2.128      0.95
```

The expected confidence interval width is about 2.13. If the assumed proportions are true, the lower and upper limits of the confidence interval are expected to be about $(1.19, 2.13)$.

The function n_risk_ratio in the precisely package also computes sample size for precision analysis for risk ratios. Precision is defined as the ratio of the upper to the lower confidence interval endpoints, which is an alternative way of defining precision for ratio measures such as relative risk. A Shiny app is also available.

9.5 Confidence intervals for odds ratio

The odds of an outcome is the probability that the outcome occurs divided by the probability that it does not occur, that is, $p/(1-p)$. An odds ratio is the ratio of the odds of the outcome in two groups,

$$\text{OR} = \frac{p_2/(1-p_2)}{p_1/(1-p_1)} \tag{9.18}$$

An odds ratio of 1.5 indicates that the odds of the outcome are 50% higher in group 2 compared to group 1.

In a cohort study estimating the proportions of subjects with a disease outcome in an exposed and an unexposed group, the relative risk $\text{RR} = p_2/p_1$ is frequently the parameter of interest, but the odds ratio is also a valid measure of the association between exposure and disease, and may be preferred because it does not suffer from the range restrictions of a relative risk (see Chapter 13 of Rosner [188]). In a case-control study, the relative risk cannot be estimated while the odds ratio can. In this section, we discuss precision analysis for an odds ratio from a cohort design or an unmatched case-control study.

Confidence intervals for odds ratio

TABLE 9.1: Notation for cell counts in a 2 × 2 contingency table from a cohort or unmatched case-control study.

	Disease status		
Risk factor status	Disease	No disease	Total
Exposed	a	b	a + b
Not exposed	c	d	c + d
Total	a+c	b+d	N=a+b+c+d

Table 9.1 shows the notation for cells counts from a cohort or unmatched case-control design. There are a exposed subjects with disease, b exposed subjects without disease, c unexposed subjects with disease and d unexposed subjects without disease. For a cohort study with exposed and unexposed groups, the odds ratio for disease for the exposed versus unexposed groups is estimated as

$$\widehat{OR} = \frac{\frac{a/(a+b)}{b/(a+b)}}{\frac{c/(c+d)}{d/(c+d)}} = \frac{ad}{bc}.$$

In a case-control study, the odds ratio for exposure for the disease versus no-disease groups is estimated as

$$\widehat{OR} = \frac{\frac{a/(a+c)}{c/(a+c)}}{\frac{b/(b+d)}{d/(b+d)}} = \frac{ad}{bc}.$$

Thus the estimates of the odds ratio are the same.

Many methods have been developed for forming confidence intervals for an odds ratio [66]. One of the most popular is based on Woolf [236], who noted that $\log(\widehat{OR})$ is approximately normally distributed with approximate variance (derived using the delta method)

$$Var(\log(\widehat{OR})) \approx \frac{1}{a} + \frac{1}{b} + \frac{1}{c} + \frac{1}{d}.$$

Thus an approximate $100(1-\alpha)\%$ confidence interval can be formed as

$$\log(\widehat{OR}) \pm z_{1-\alpha/2}\sqrt{\frac{1}{a} + \frac{1}{b} + \frac{1}{c} + \frac{1}{d}}$$

The endpoints are exponentiated to backtransform to the odds ratio scale. This interval does not perform well when there are zero or small cell counts.

To address this, the Gart adjusted logit interval [72] is formed in the same way but adds 0.5 to each cell count. The independence smoothed logit interval [2] adds a cell-specific quantity to each cell.

Example 9.9. We repeat the cohort study in Example 9.8 but assume that we wish to estimate the odds ratio rather than the relative risk. The outcome proportions in exposed and unexposed groups are expected to be 0.2 and 0.1, for a RR of 2. There are 100 exposed and 300 unexposed subjects. What is the expected width of a 95% confidence interval for the odds ratio?

The `presize` package has a function `prec_or` for precision analysis for an odds ratio using the Woolf, Gart or independence smoothed logit methods. We show results from the Gart method:

```
library(presize)
# p1 is proportion among exposed, p2 is among unexposed
# r is n2 / n1
prec_or(p1 = 0.2, p2 = 0.1, n1 = 100, r = 3, conf.width = NULL,
    conf.level = 0.95, method = "gart")
# output slightly edited for clarity

precision for an odds ratio with gart confidence interval

p1   p2  n1  n2   ntot  r   or    lwr    upr    conf.width  conf.level
0.2  0.1 100 300  400   3   2.25  1.224  4.167  2.943       0.95
```

The width is expected to be about 2.9. The limits of the confidence interval are expected to be about 1.22 and 4.17.

9.6 Additional resources

The `precisely` package has functions for conducting precision-based sample size calculations that are focused on planning epidemiologic studies. It includes functions for a risk difference, risk ratio, rate difference, rate ratio and odds ratio. The risk difference function is based on the Wald confidence interval, which, as we discussed, can sometimes have poor performance. The package is based on the paper of Rothman and Greenland [190]. The `presize` package has many different functions for precision based sample size calculation. Parameters supported include means, proportions, rates and correlations. The `precisely` and `presize` packages both have Shiny apps.

10
Correlation and linear regression

10.1 Pearson correlation coefficient

In some studies, we may be interested in the strength of association between two variables. A common measure of the strength of the association between two continuous variables is their correlation. The Pearson correlation coefficient between two random variables X and Y is defined as

$$\rho = Corr(X, Y) = \frac{Cov(X, Y)}{\sqrt{Var(X)Var(Y)}}$$

where $Cov(X, Y)$ is the covariance between X and Y. This is the population Pearson correlation coefficient. If we have a sample of subjects on which we have measured both variables, $(X_i, Y_i), i = 1, \ldots, N$, we can estimate ρ using the sample Pearson correlation coefficient, defined as

$$r = \frac{\widehat{Cov}(X, Y)}{\sqrt{\widehat{Var}(X)\widehat{Var}(Y)}} = \frac{\sum_{i=1}^{N}(X_i - \bar{X})(Y_i - \bar{Y})}{\sqrt{\sum_{i=1}^{N}(X_i - \bar{X})^2 \sum_{i=1}^{N}(Y_i - \bar{Y})^2}}. \quad (10.1)$$

In the next sections, we discuss power and sample size for hypothesis tests involving correlation coefficients. In Section 10.1.1, we discuss tests that compare a single correlation coefficient to a reference value, and in Section 10.1.2 we discuss tests that compare two correlation coefficients.

An issue that arises when using the sample correlation coefficient r to conduct inference about the population correlation coefficient ρ is that r does not have a well-behaved distribution. Therefore it is not convenient to use it directly for conducting tests. It is more convenient to first apply the Fisher z transformation, which is a normalizing transformation for the sample correlation coefficient. This transformation is defined as

$$r' = \frac{1}{2} \log\left(\frac{1+r}{1-r}\right).$$

If (X, Y) are bivariate normal with correlation ρ, then r' is approximately normally distributed. Thus it is more convenient to formulate test statistics using r' rather than r, since we can more easily determine their approximate distribution. The Fisher z transformation is also called the arctanh or inverse hyperbolic tangent function. The mean and variance of r', for a sample of size N when the true correlation coefficient is ρ, are

$$E(r') = \frac{1}{2}\log\left(\frac{1+\rho}{1-\rho}\right) + \frac{\rho}{2(N-1)} \qquad (10.2)$$

$$Var(r') = \frac{1}{N-3}$$

The term $\frac{\rho}{2(N-1)}$ is a bias correction factor. Since the mean has a complicated formula that we will need to use again, we define the function $f(\rho)$ as

$$f(\rho) = \frac{1}{2}\log\left(\frac{1+\rho}{1-\rho}\right) + \frac{\rho}{2(N-1)}. \qquad (10.3)$$

Now we have the results that we need to discuss power for tests involving correlation coefficients.

10.1.1 Single correlation coefficient

Suppose we wish to test $H_0\colon \rho = \rho_0$, where ρ_0 is some reference value. After we compute the sample correlation coefficient r and apply the Fisher z transformation to obtain r', we can conduct the test using a test statistic of the form

$$Z = \frac{r' - E(r'|\rho = \rho_0)}{\sqrt{Var(r'|\rho = \rho_0)}} \qquad (10.4)$$

where $E(r'|\rho = \rho_0)$ and $Var(r'|\rho = \rho_0)$ are the mean and variance of r' when $H_0\colon \rho = \rho_0$ is true. The test statistic is

$$Z = \sqrt{N-3}\,[r' - f(\rho_0)].$$

When the true value of the correlation coefficient is ρ_A, Z has approximately a normal distribution with mean ω,

$$\omega = \sqrt{N-3}\left[\frac{1}{2}\ln\left(\frac{1+\rho_A}{1-\rho_A}\right) + \frac{K\rho_A}{2(N-1)} - f(\rho_0)\right]$$

where

$$K = 1 + \frac{5 + \rho_A^2}{4(N-1)} + \frac{11 + 2\rho_A^2 + 3\rho_A^4}{8(N-1)^2}$$

and variance ν,

$$\nu = \frac{N-3}{N-1}\left[1 + \frac{4 - \rho_A^2}{2(N-1)} + \frac{22 - 6\rho_A^2 - 3\rho_A^4}{6(N-1)^2}\right];$$

see [8] and Section 16.33 of [211]. Power can be approximated as:

Upper one-sided test (H_A: $\rho > \rho_0$): $\Phi\left(\dfrac{\omega - z_{1-\alpha}}{\sqrt{\nu}}\right)$ (10.5)

Lower one-sided test (H_A: $\rho < \rho_0$): $\Phi\left(\dfrac{-\omega - z_{1-\alpha}}{\sqrt{\nu}}\right)$

Two-sided test (H_A: $\rho \neq \rho_0$): $\Phi\left(\dfrac{\omega - z_{1-\alpha/2}}{\sqrt{\nu}}\right) + \Phi\left(\dfrac{-\omega - z_{1-\alpha/2}}{\sqrt{\nu}}\right)$

Since both ω and ν are functions of N, there is no closed form expression for sample size. We need to use software to find the sample size needed to achieve a specific level of power by solving the power function numerically.

Example 10.1. Suppose we wish to test H_0: $\rho \leq 0.2$ versus H_0: $\rho > 0.2$ with $N = 100$ at $\alpha = 0.05$. We expect the true value of the correlation coefficient to be $\rho_A = 0.4$. What is the power?

```
library(powertools)
corr.1samp(N = 100, rho0 = 0.2, rhoA = 0.4, sides = 1, power = NULL)
[1] 0.7058707
```

The power is about 0.71.

Effect size for one correlation coefficient. Cohen defined ρ of 0.1, 0.3 and 0.5 as small, medium and large effect sizes for a correlation coefficient [36]. Implicitly, this pertains to comparing the correlation coefficient to zero. Benchmarks for small, medium and large effect sizes should be taken as rough guides only and may not be appropriate in all contexts.

Additional resources. The `pwrss.z.corr` function in the `pwrss` package also computes power and sample size for tests of a single correlation using Fisher's transformation. The `prec_cor` function in the `presize` package performs precision analysis (see Chapter 9) for a single correlation coefficient. The function computes precision (confidence interval width) or sample size needed to obtain a desired level of precision for one Pearson, Spearman, or Kendall correlation coefficient. The null value is assumed to be zero.

10.1.2 Comparing two correlation coefficients

Suppose that we wish to test H_0: $\rho_1 - \rho_2 = 0$ for two independent samples. For samples of sizes n_1 and n_2, we can estimate the sample correlation coefficients r_1 and r_2 and apply the Fisher z transformation to obtain r'_1 and r'_2. When the true values of the correlation coefficients are ρ_1 and ρ_2,

$$r'_1 - r'_2 \sim \mathcal{N}\left[f(\rho_1) - f(\rho_2), \dfrac{1}{n_1 - 3} + \dfrac{1}{n_2 - 3}\right]$$

where the function f is defined in (10.3). We can form the test statistic

$$Z = \frac{r'_1 - r'_2}{\sqrt{\frac{1}{n_1-3} + \frac{1}{n_2-3}}}. \tag{10.6}$$

When H_0 is true, Z has approximately a standard normal distribution. When some alternative is true and $f(\rho_1) - f(\rho_2) = \Delta_A$, then $Z \sim \mathcal{N}(\lambda, 1)$, where $\lambda = \Delta_A / \sqrt{\frac{1}{n_1-3} + \frac{1}{n_2-3}}$. Power can be approximated as:

Upper one-sided test (H_A: $\rho_1 - \rho_2 > 0$): $\Phi(\lambda - z_{1-\alpha})$ (10.7)

Lower one-sided test (H_A: $\rho_1 - \rho_2 < 0$): $\Phi(-z_{1-\alpha} - \lambda)$

Two-sided test (H_A: $\rho_1 - \rho_2 \neq 0$): $\Phi\left(-z_{1-\alpha/2} - \lambda\right) + \Phi\left(\lambda - z_{1-\alpha/2}\right)$

Example 10.2. Suppose that we wish to conduct a test of H_0: $\rho_1 - \rho_2 \leq 0$ versus H_A: $\rho_1 - \rho_2 > 0$ with 250 participants in each group. The true correlation coefficients are assumed to be $\rho_1 = 0.3$ and $\rho_2 = 0.1$. What is the power for a test with $\alpha = 0.05$?

```
library(powertools)
corr.2samp(n1 = 250, rho1 = 0.3, rho2 = 0.1, sides = 1, power = NULL)
[1] 0.7531026
```

The power is about 0.75.

Effect size for comparing two correlation coefficients. Cohen defined a q effect size for comparing two correlation coefficients that uses the difference of the Fisher z-transformed coefficients, $q = |\rho'_1 - \rho'_2|$. Sets of (ρ_1, ρ_2) with equal values of q are equally detectable. Cohen defines q of 0.1, 0.3 and 0.5 as small, medium and large effect sizes for the difference between two correlation coefficients [36].

Example 10.3. The effect size for Example 10.2 can be calculated as follows:

```
library(powertools)
es.q(rho1 = 0.3, rho2 = 0.1)

    Cohen's q effect size calculation for two correlation coefficients

         rho1 = 0.3
         rho2 = 0.1
            q = 0.2091843
```

This is a small-to-medium effect size.

Simple linear regression

Additional resources. The pwrss.z.2corrs function in the pwrss package also performs power and sample size calculations for tests of the difference between two correlations.

10.2 Simple linear regression

In this chapter, we discuss two approaches to power and sample size for the slope coefficient β_1 in a simple linear regression model. In this section, we discuss an approach based on the least squares estimator $\hat{\beta}_1$ and its sampling distribution. It involves more parameters and can be more complicated to implement, but it illustrates some important concepts and may be the preferred method in some situations. In Section 10.3.3, we discuss another approach which involves specifying only the correlation between X and Y. Some of the derivations in this section are based on Liu [142].

The simple linear regression model is

$$Y_i = \beta_0 + \beta_1 x_i + \epsilon_i,$$

$i = 1, ..., N$, where the error terms ϵ_i are independent and identically distributed as $\mathcal{N}(0, \sigma_\epsilon^2)$. In this model, interest usually focuses on estimating the regression coefficient β_1, which represents the change in $E(Y)$ associated with a one unit increase in the covariate X; this is often called the slope coefficient. The least squares estimator for β_1 is

$$\hat{\beta}_1 = \frac{\sum_{i=1}^{N}(x_i - \bar{x})(Y_i - \bar{Y})}{\sum_{i=1}^{N}(x_i - \bar{x})^2}. \tag{10.8}$$

The sampling distribution of $\hat{\beta}_1$ is the distribution of $\hat{\beta}_1$ under repeated sampling when fixing the values of x_i, sampling new values of Y_i and obtaining the least square estimator $\hat{\beta}_1$. In the simple linear regression model, the sampling distribution of $\hat{\beta}_1$ follows a normal distribution,

$$\hat{\beta}_1 \sim \mathcal{N}\left(\beta_1, \frac{\sigma_\epsilon^2}{\sum_{i=1}^{N}(x_i - \bar{x})^2}\right).$$

To test $H_0\colon \beta_1 = \beta_{10}$ versus $H_A\colon \beta_1 \neq \beta_{10}$, we can use the test statistic

$$T = \frac{\hat{\beta}_1 - \beta_{10}}{\sqrt{\frac{\hat{\sigma}_\epsilon^2}{\sum_{i=1}^{N}(X_i - \bar{X})^2}}}$$

where $\hat{\sigma}_\epsilon^2$, commonly called the residual variance or the mean squared error (MSE), is our estimate of σ_ϵ^2. When H_0 is true, $T \sim t(N-2)$. Under an alternative where $\beta_1 = \beta_{1A}$, T has a noncentral t distribution with the same degrees of freedom and noncentrality parameter

$$\lambda = \frac{(\beta_{1A} - \beta_{10})\sqrt{\sum_{i=1}^{N}(x_i - \bar{x})^2}}{\sigma_\epsilon}. \tag{10.9}$$

Thus power can be calculated as the probability that a $t(N-2, \lambda)$ random variable will fall into the rejection region,

Upper one-sided test $(H_A: \beta_{1A} - \beta_{10} > 0)$: $1 - \mathcal{T}_{N-2,\lambda}(t_{1-\alpha,N-2})$ (10.10)
Lower one-sided test $(H_A: \beta_{1A} - \beta_{10} < 0)$: $\mathcal{T}_{N-2,\lambda}(t_{\alpha,N-2})$

For a two-sided test, we can square T and obtain an F statistic,

$$F = \frac{(\hat{\beta}_{1A} - \beta_{10})^2}{\frac{\hat{\sigma}_\epsilon^2}{\sum_{i=1}^{N}(X_i - \bar{X})^2}} \tag{10.11}$$

which has an $F(1, N-2)$ distribution under the null hypothesis and an $F(1, N-2, \Lambda)$ distribution under the alternative, where $\Lambda = \lambda^2$, with λ as given in equation (10.9). This is an upper-tailed test (H_0 is rejected for values of F higher than the critical value). Power can be calculated as

Two-sided test $(H_A: \beta_{1A} \neq \beta_{10}) : 1 - \mathcal{F}_{1,N-2,\Lambda}(f_{1,N-2,1-\alpha})$. (10.12)

What factors affect power? Recall that power increases as the magnitude of the noncentrality parameter increases. Thus power increases as the magnitude of the difference, $|\beta_{1A} - \beta_{10}|$, increases. Power also increases as the term $\sum_{i=1}^{N}(x_i - \bar{x})^2$ increases. This will be higher as the number of observations N increases, or as the distances between the x_i and their mean $\bar{x}$ increase; that is, when the values of X are more dispersed. Increasing the value of the error variance σ_ϵ^2 will decrease power; higher σ_ϵ^2 means more unexplained variation in the observations.

Example 10.4. Investigators are planning a study that will regress Y on X. They plan to collect data from a sample of 100 individuals and test $H_0: \beta_1 \leq 1$ versus $H_A: \beta_1 > 1$. They assume the true value of the slope is $\beta_{1A} = 1.5$. In a pilot study, they found that s_X^2 was 25 and $\hat{\sigma}_\epsilon$ was 10. If these values hold true in the planned study, what is the power, with α of 0.05?

```
library(powertools)
slr(N = 100, beta10 = 1, beta1A = 1.5, var.x = 25, sigma.e = 10,
    sides = 1, power = NULL)
[1] 0.795423
```

Power is close to 0.80.

Simple linear regression 181

10.2.1 Specifying values for parameters

Using power formulas (10.10) or (10.12) requires specifying values for σ_ϵ^2 and $\sum_{i=1}^N (x_i - \bar{x})^2$. In this section, we give some tips for specifying these values.

Specification of $\sum_{i=1}^N (x_i - \bar{x})^2$ depends on whether we have a designed experiment, in which we select the values of X in advance, or we are selecting a random sample of individuals on which we measure both X and Y. If we will select the values of X in advance, then it may be possible to directly compute $\sum_{i=1}^N (x_i - \bar{x})^2$, as in the following example:

Example 10.5. A study plans to estimate the dose-response relationship between a drug and response. The response is a continuous variable and a simple linear regression model will be fit to the data. The study will administer $d = 4$ doses of the drug, 25, 50, 75 and 100 mg, with $m = 10$ subjects at each dose level. For this study, we can directly calculate s_x^2 as follows:

```
m <- 10
d <- 4
X <- c(rep(25, m), rep(50, m), rep(75, m), rep(100, m))
meanX <- rep(mean(X), m * d)
sd.x.sq <- sum((X - meanX)^2) / (m * d - 1)
sd.x.sq
[1] 801.2821
```

Based on the study design, the value of s_x^2 is 801.2821.

Much work has been done in optimal design for regression models, which involves selecting values of the predictors to maximize s_x^2 and thereby minimize $\widehat{Var}(\hat{\beta}_1)$; see O'Brien and Funk [173] for an introduction to this topic.

If we are selecting a random sample of individuals, then note that $\sum_{i=1}^N (x_i - \bar{x})^2$ equals $(N-1)s_x^2$, where s_x^2 is the sample variance of X. In this case, we can replace $(N-1)s_x^2$ with $N\sigma_x^2$, where σ_x^2 is the population variance of X, and obtain

$$\lambda = \frac{(\beta_{1A} - \beta_{10})\sqrt{N\sigma_x^2}}{\sigma_\epsilon}. \tag{10.13}$$

Another helpful approach for estimating the value of a standard deviation is to use the **range rule**. This statistical rule of thumb is that the standard deviation of a sample is approximately equal to one-fourth of the range of the data [219]. Thus s_x can be estimated by making educated guesses for the minimum and maximum values likely to be observed in the sample and computing $s_x \approx (\max - \min)/4$.

We can also use the range rule to obtain a plausible value for σ_ϵ^2. Recall that σ_ϵ is the standard deviation of the error terms. We can reason that the great majority of observations (about 95%) will lie within $\pm 2\sigma_\epsilon$ of the regression line. By specifying a plausible value for the range of Y values at a given value of X, we can estimate $\sigma_\epsilon \approx \text{range}/4$.

Example 10.6. Referring to Example 10.5, suppose that at a dose of 50 mg, we expect that values of Y will range from 100 to 160. Then we can estimate $\sigma_\epsilon \approx (160 - 100)/4 = 15$.

For a two-sided test of H_0: $\beta_1 = 0$ in the simple linear regression model, an alternative to using power equation (10.12) is to compute power for an omnibus F test, which is described in Section 10.3.1. The omnibus F test power approach can be more convenient because it requires the specification of fewer parameters.

10.3 Multiple linear regression

Multiple linear regression models the relationship between an outcome variable Y and a set of predictor variables $X_1, \ldots, X_p$ using the model

$$Y_i = \beta_0 + \beta_1 x_{i1} + \ldots + \beta_p x_{ip} + \epsilon_i$$

where the ϵ_i's are independent and identically distributed as $\mathcal{N}(0, \sigma_\epsilon^2)$. The model posits that the mean of Y is related to the values of the predictor variables as $E(Y) = \beta_0 + \beta_1 x_1 + \ldots + \beta_p x_p$. A model with p predictors has $p+1$ total regression parameters including the intercept.

The regression parameters can be estimated using the method of least squares. The method of least squares finds the values of the parameters that minimizes the sum of the squared residuals, $\sum_{i=1}^{N}[Y_i - (\hat{\beta}_0 + \hat{\beta}_1 x_{i1} + \ldots + \hat{\beta}_p x_{ip})]^2$. Using the estimated regression parameters, we can obtain the fitted (predicted) values of the outcome variable as $\hat{Y}_i = \hat{\beta}_0 + \hat{\beta}_1 x_{i1} + \ldots + \hat{\beta}_p x_{ip}$.

Standard output from fitting a linear regression model includes a sources of variation table, depicted in Table 10.1. The total sum of squares, SSTot $= \sum_i (Y_i - \bar{Y})^2$, quantifies the total variation of the Y's from the sample mean $\bar{Y}$. SSTot equals the sum of the regression sum of squares, SSReg $= \sum_i (\hat{Y}_i - \bar{Y})^2$, which quantifies how much variation in the Y's is explained by the model (that is, by linear relationship between Y and the predictors), and the error sum of squares, SSE $= \sum_i (Y_i - \hat{Y}_i)^2$, which quantifies the variation in Y not explained by the model.

We consider power for two types of tests involving multiple linear regression models. One is the overall F test for any regression relationship between Y

Multiple linear regression

TABLE 10.1: Linear regression model sources of variation table.

Source	SS	df	MS	F
Regression	$\text{SSReg} = \sum_i (\hat{Y}_i - \bar{Y})^2$	p	$\text{MSReg} = \frac{\text{SSReg}}{p}$	$F = \frac{\text{MSReg}}{\text{MSE}}$
Error	$\text{SSE} = \sum_i (Y_i - \hat{Y}_i)^2$	$N - p - 1$	$\text{MSE} = \frac{\text{SSE}}{N-p-1}$	
Total	$\text{SSTot} = \sum_i (Y_i - \bar{Y})^2$	$N - 1$		

and the predictors, discussed in Section 10.3.1. The other is a partial F test of whether one predictor or a set of predictors is significant, controlling for the other predictors, discussed in Section 10.3.7. Some of the derivations here are based on Liu [142].

10.3.1 Overall F test

The overall F test for any regression relationship tests the hypotheses

$$H_0: \beta_1 = 0, \ldots, \beta_p = 0 \quad \text{versus} \quad H_A: \text{not all } \beta_1 = 0, \ldots, \beta_p = 0. \quad (10.14)$$

The test statistic is

$$F = \frac{\text{MSReg}}{\text{MSE}} = \frac{\text{SSReg}/p}{\text{SSE}/(N-p-1)}. \quad (10.15)$$

We reject H_0 at level α if $F > f_{1-\alpha, p, N-p-1}$; this is an upper-tailed test.

To derive an expression for power, we first re-express the test statistic in terms of R^2, the sample coefficient of multiple determination, also called the squared sample multiple correlation coefficient. R^2 is defined as

$$R^2 = \frac{\text{SSReg}}{\text{SSTot}} = 1 - \frac{\text{SSE}}{\text{SSTot}}$$

and is interpreted as the estimated proportion of the total variation in Y that can be explained by the model, that is, by linear relationship between Y and the predictor variables. The value of R^2 depends on which predictors are in the model. We will denote the R^2 corresponding to the model that includes $X_1, \ldots, X_p$ as $R^2_{Y|X_1,\ldots,X_p}$. Given the relationships among R^2, SSE and SSReg, we can rewrite the overall F test statistic (10.15) in terms of $R^2_{Y|X_1,\ldots,X_p}$ as

$$F = \frac{R^2_{Y|X_1,\ldots,X_p}}{1 - R^2_{Y|X_1,\ldots,X_p}} \left(\frac{N - p - 1}{p} \right). \quad (10.16)$$

$R^2_{Y|X_1,\ldots,X_p}$ is a sample statistic calculated from data. We denote the corresponding population parameter, which is the squared population multiple correlation coefficient, as $\rho^2_{Y|X_1,\ldots,X_p}$. Using this population parameter, we can express the hypotheses in (10.14) as

$$H_0: \rho^2_{Y|X_1,\ldots,X_p} = 0 \quad \text{versus} \quad H_A: \rho^2_{Y|X_1,\ldots,X_p} > 0.$$

The null hypothesis states that there is no linear association between Y and the predictors $X_1, \ldots, X_p$, and the alternative states that some linear association exists.

When H_0 is true, test statistic (10.16) has an $F(p, N-p-1)$ distribution. When H_A is true (and also assuming that the values of the predictors are fixed rather than random; see Section 10.3.6), F has a noncentral F distribution, $F(p, N-p-1, \Lambda)$, where the noncentrality parameter is

$$\Lambda = N \frac{\rho^2_{Y|X_1,\ldots,X_p}}{1 - \rho^2_{Y|X_1,\ldots,X_p}}. \tag{10.17}$$

Thus power can be calculated as $1 - \mathcal{F}_{p,N-p-1,\Lambda}(f_{1-\alpha,p,N-p-1})$.

10.3.2 Effect size for overall F test

Cohen [36] defined an f^2 effect size for the overall F test in multiple linear regression as

$$f^2 = \frac{\rho^2_{Y|X_1,\ldots,X_p}}{1 - \rho^2_{Y|X_1,\ldots,X_p}}.$$

Thus we have $\Lambda = Nf^2$, and power calculations can be performed using the f^2 effect size.

Cohen defined small, medium and large effect sizes as $f^2 = 0.02, 0.15$ and 0.35, respectively. Noting that $\rho^2_{Y|X_1,\ldots,X_p} = f^2/(1+f^2)$, we can find that these effect sizes are equivalent to $\rho^2_{Y|X_1,\ldots,X_p}$ of about $0.02, 0.13$ and 0.26, that is, they imply that the predictors explain about 2%, 13% and 26% of the variation in Y. In general, what constitutes a "small" or "large" effect size depends on the subject matter and these benchmarks should be considered only a rough guide.

Example 10.7. We plan a study to determine whether a particular single nucleotide polymorphism (SNP) is associated with serum levels of triglycerides. The SNP has three categories, AA, AG and GG. We plan to assess the association by regressing triglyceride level (Y) on two dummy indicator variables encoding SNP category. If we have a sample of 400 individuals, what is the power to detect $\rho^2_{Y|X_1,X_2} = 0.02$, with α of 0.05?

```
library(powertools)
mlrF.overall(N = 400, p = 2, Rsq = 0.02, power = NULL, v = TRUE)

     Power calculation for a multiple linear regression
     overall F test assuming fixed predictors

            N = 400
            p = 2
          Rsq = 0.02
          fsq = 0.02040816
        alpha = 0.05
        power = 0.7233772
```

The power is about 0.72. The output indicates that this calculation assumes fixed predictors. The issue of fixed versus random predictors is discussed in Section 10.3.6.

10.3.3 Simple linear regression revisited

When there is only one predictor X in a model, the model R^2 is $R^2_{Y|X}$ and it is equal to the square of the sample Pearson correlation coefficient r^2, where r is the correlation between X and Y, $r = r_{XY} = r_{YX}$. The population parameter versions of these sample statistics are $\rho^2_{Y|X}$ and $\rho = \rho_{XY} = \rho_{YX}$. The overall F test involves a single regression parameter,

$$H_0: \beta_1 = 0 \quad \text{versus} \quad H_A: \beta_1 \neq 0.$$

Test statistic (10.16) becomes

$$F = \frac{r^2_{XY}}{1 - r^2_{XY}} \left(\frac{N-2}{1} \right)$$

and the noncentrality parameter (10.17) becomes

$$\Lambda = N \frac{\rho^2_{XY}}{1 - \rho^2_{XY}}.$$

Power can be calculated as $1 - \mathcal{F}_{1,N-2,\Lambda}(f_{1-\alpha,1,N-2})$.

Example 10.8. A study is planned in which a simple linear regression model will be fit to a sample of 70 observations. The correlation between X and Y is expected to be 0.3. What is the power for a two-sided test of $H_0: \beta_1 = 0$ at level $\alpha = 0.05$? We can use the mlrF.overall function with Rsq specified as $\rho^2_{XY} = 0.3^2 = 0.09$.

```
library(powertools)
mlrF.overall(N = 70, p = 1, Rsq = 0.3^2, power = NULL)
[1] 0.7369265
```

Power is about 0.74.

10.3.4 Connection to single correlation coefficient

The estimated regression coefficient $\hat{\beta}_1$ given in equation (10.8) for the simple linear regression model regressing Y on X is related to the sample correlation r between X and Y given in equation (10.1) as

$$\hat{\beta}_1 = r \frac{s_y}{s_x}$$

where s_y and s_x are the sample standard deviations of Y and X, $s_y^2 = \frac{1}{N-1}\sum_{i=1}^{N}(Y_i - \bar{Y})^2$ and $s_x^2 = \frac{1}{N-1}\sum_{i=1}^{N}(x_i - \bar{x})^2$. Thus a test of $H_0: \beta_1 = 0$ in a simple linear regression model is essentially also a test that the correlation between X and Y equals zero.

10.3.5 Impact of number of predictors on power

Power for the overall F test depends not only on N and $\rho^2_{Y|X_1,\ldots,X_p}$ but also on p, the number of predictors in the model, since p impacts the degrees of freedom for the F distribution, which are p and $N-p-1$. All else being equal, a higher number of predictors reduces power for the overall F test. However, if N is large, the number of predictors may have little impact on power. Figure 10.1 provides an illustration. The figure plots power versus number of predictors for an overall F test to detect of $\rho^2_{Y|X_1,\ldots,X_p}$ of 0.2 with α of 0.05 for sample sizes of 50, 75 and 100. For a sample size of 50, power decreases fairly rapidly as the number of predictors increases whereas for a sample size of 100, adding predictors has little impact on power. Thus the impact of number of predictors needs to be considered within the context of the total sample size.

10.3.6 Power when the distribution of predictors is random

The predictors in a multiple linear regression model can be either fixed values or random variables. Whether they are fixed or random depends on the manner in which the data were collected. The predictors are random variables if we select a sample of subjects and then measure both $X_1, \ldots, X_p$ and Y on each subject. The predictors are fixed if we select the values of the predictors and sample values of Y at these predictor values; for example, we select predictor values of 25, 50, 75 and 100 and take 10 observations of Y at each value, as in Example 10.5.

Multiple linear regression

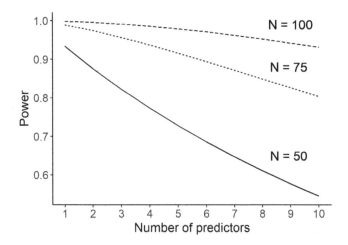

FIGURE 10.1: Power versus number of predictors for an overall F test with a $\rho^2_{Y|X_1,\ldots,X_p}$ of 0.2 and α of 0.05 for sample sizes of 50, 75 and 100.

While the procedures for testing hypotheses about the regression coefficients are the same whether the predictors are random or fixed, the power can be different. The formulas for power in the preceding section assume that the predictors have fixed values. The effect on power of having random predictors will depend on the joint distribution of Y and the predictors. In particular, the distribution of R^2 will depend on the joint distribution of $Y, X_1, \ldots, X_p$. Several authors have considered the distribution of R^2 for the case that $Y, X_1, \ldots, X_p$ have a multivariate normal distribution. The distribution has a complicated form; see Chapter 32 of Johnson et al. [108]. Methods for exact power and sample size calculations in this case are given by Gatsonis and Sampson [74]. These methods are implemented in the SAS power procedure. A number of authors have developed approximations to the distribution of R^2 [108]. We develop a method to calculate approximate power based on an approximation given by Khatri [124].

To simplify notation, we drop subscripts and denote $R^2_{Y|X_1,\ldots,X_p}$ as R^2 and $\rho^2_{Y|X_1,\ldots,X_p}$ as ρ^2. Recall that the test statistic for the overall F test has the form

$$F = \left(\frac{R^2}{1-R^2}\right)\left(\frac{N-p-1}{p}\right);$$

see (10.15). Based on Khatri [124], the quantity

$$\left(\frac{R^2}{1-R^2}\right)\frac{(N-p-1)(1-\rho^2)}{(N-p-1)\rho^2+p}$$

has approximately an F distribution with degrees of freedom u and v given by

$$u = \frac{[(N-p-1)\rho^2 + p]^2}{(N-p-1)\rho^2(2-\rho^2) + p} \quad \text{and} \quad v = N - p - 1. \tag{10.18}$$

Khatri [124] suggested that this approximation is reasonable when $N-p-1 \geq 100$. Using this approximation, we can express power for an overall F test at level α as

$$\text{Power} \approx P(F > f_{1-\alpha,p,N-p-1})$$

$$= P\left[\left(\frac{R^2}{1-R^2}\right)\left(\frac{N-p-1}{p}\right) > f_{1-\alpha,p,N-p-1}\right] \tag{10.19}$$

$$= P\left[\left(\frac{R^2}{1-R^2}\right)\frac{(N-p-1)(1-\rho^2)}{(N-p-1)\rho^2 + p} > \frac{f_{1-\alpha,p,N-p-1}p(1-\rho^2)}{(N-p-1)\rho^2 + p}\right]$$

and the expression on the left-hand side of the inequality has approximately an F distribution with degrees of freedom given by (10.18). Thus power can be approximated as

$$\text{Power} \approx 1 - \mathcal{F}_{u,v}\left(\frac{f_{1-\alpha,p,N-p-1}\,p(1-\rho^2)}{(N-p-1)\rho^2 + p}\right) \tag{10.20}$$

with the degrees of freedom u and v as given in (10.18). This is a "central" F distribution.

Example 10.9. In Example 10.7, we found that with a sample of 400 individuals, the power to detect $\rho^2_{Y|X_1,X_2}$ of 0.02 in a multiple linear regression model with two predictors and α of 0.05 was 0.7233772. That calculation assumed that the values of the predictors were fixed. What would be the power if the predictors were random? We can use the random = TRUE option in mlrF.overall:

```
library(powertools)
mlrF.overall(N = 400, p = 2, Rsq = 0.02, power = NULL, random = TRUE)
[1] 0.721944
```

Power drops slightly compared to assuming that the predictor values are fixed.

Results in the case of joint distributions for $Y, X_1, \ldots, X_p$ other than the multivariate normal are lacking. However, it is probably safe to assume that having random rather than fixed predictors will decrease power, since this introduces additional variance. In the example we considered, however, the impact on power was quite small.

10.3.7 Partial F tests

A partial F test is used when we wish to test whether a certain predictor or set of predictors makes a significant contribution to explaining variation in the outcome Y after the relationship between Y and another set of predictors has already been accounted for. For example, we may wish to test whether an indicator variable for treatment condition is significant after controlling for a set of potential confounders such as age and sex. The methods presented here are based on Maxwell [152].

Denote a set of test predictors as T and a set of control predictors as C. Suppose that we would like to test whether the test predictors will be significant when included in a model with the control predictors. If there are q test predictors and p control predictors, then the test involves comparing the **full model** with all $p+q$ predictors, $E(Y) = \beta_0 + \beta_1 x_1 + \ldots + \beta_p x_p + \beta_{p+1} x_{(p+1)} + \ldots + \beta_{p+q} x_{(p+q)}$, to a **reduced model** with only the control predictors, $E(Y) = \beta_0 + \beta_1 x_1 + \ldots + \beta_p x_p$. The hypotheses can be expressed as

$$H_0: \beta_{p+1} = \ldots = \beta_{p+q} = 0$$
$$H_A: \text{not all } \beta_{p+1}, \ldots, \beta_{p+q} = 0.$$

Equivalently, the hypothesis can be expressed using squared population multiple correlation coefficients as

$$H_0: \rho^2_{Y|TC} = \rho^2_{Y|C} \quad \text{versus} \quad H_A: \rho^2_{Y|TC} > \rho^2_{Y|C}$$

or

$$H_0: \rho^2_{Y|TC} - \rho^2_{Y|C} = 0 \quad \text{versus} \quad H_A: \rho^2_{Y|TC} - \rho^2_{Y|C} > 0.$$

The hypotheses can be tested using a partial F test. The partial F test uses a test statistic that compares the SSReg for the full model including both the T and C predictors and the SSReg for the reduced model including only the C predictors. We denote these as SSReg($Y|TC$) and SSReg($Y|C$). The test statistic is

$$F = \frac{\left(\frac{\text{SSReg}(Y|TC) - \text{SSReg}(Y|C)}{q}\right)}{\left(\frac{\text{SSE}(Y|TC)}{N-p-q-1}\right)}.$$

Note that q is the difference in the number of predictors (and number of regression coefficients) between the two models. The test statistic can also be expressed using the difference of the SSE's, $\text{SSE}(Y|C) - \text{SSE}(Y|TC)$. Using the fact that $R^2_{Y|C} = \frac{\text{SSReg}(Y|C)}{\text{SSTot}}$ and $R^2_{Y|TC} = \frac{\text{SSReg}(Y|TC)}{\text{SSTot}}$, we can rewrite the test statistic as

$$F = \frac{\left(\frac{R^2_{Y|TC} - R^2_{Y|C}}{q}\right)}{\left(\frac{1 - R^2_{Y|TC}}{N-p-q-1}\right)} = \left(\frac{R^2_{Y|TC} - R^2_{Y|C}}{1 - R^2_{Y|TC}}\right)\left(\frac{N-p-q-1}{q}\right). \quad (10.21)$$

When the null hypothesis is true, $F \sim F(q, N-p-q-1)$ and under the alternative, F has noncentral F distribution with the same degrees of freedom and a noncentrality parameter that we discuss shortly. Power will be equal to $P(F > f_{1-\alpha,q,N-p-q-1})$, where $F \sim F(q, N-p-q-1, \Lambda)$, calculated as $1 - \mathcal{F}_{q,N-p-q-1,\Lambda}(f_{1-\alpha,q,N-p-q-1})$.

Noncentrality parameter via multiple correlation coefficient

We discuss two ways of expressing the noncentrality parameter, one using multiple correlation coefficients and the other using a partial correlation coefficient. The multiple correlation coefficients approach can be used for a test set T of any size. The partial correlation coefficient approach can be used when T is a single predictor. The two approaches are mathematically equivalent when T is a single predictor.

Using the multiple correlation coefficients approach, the noncentrality parameter is

$$\Lambda = N \frac{\rho^2_{Y|TC} - \rho^2_{Y|C}}{1 - \rho^2_{Y|TC}}. \tag{10.22}$$

Using this parameterization requires specifying two out of three quantities, $\rho^2_{Y|TC}$, $\rho^2_{Y|C}$ and the difference $\rho^2_{Y|TC} - \rho^2_{Y|C}$. By specifying any two, we can solve for the third.

Example 10.10. We are planning a study that will test whether a set of two "test" predictors is significant in a multiple linear regression model with three control covariates. We expect the reduced model (control predictors only) will have $\rho^2_{Y|C} = 0.25$ and the full model (control + test predictors) will have $\rho^2_{Y|TC} = 0.35$. What is the power to conclude that at least one of the two predictors explains important variation in Y after controlling for the 3 covariates when $N = 60$, at $\alpha = 0.05$?

```
library(powertools)
mlrF.partial(N = 60, p = 3, q = 2, Rsq.red = 0.25, Rsq.full = 0.35,
    power = NULL)
[1] 0.7571183
```

Power is about 0.76.

Noncentrality parameter via partial correlation coefficient

The other parameterization of the noncentrality parameter uses a partial correlation coefficient. This approach can be used when the "test" set of predictors is a single predictor. We will call this test predictor X.

Multiple linear regression

A **partial correlation coefficient** measures the degree of linear association between two variables after controlling for some other variables. The partial correlation between Y and X controlling for a set of variables C, which we denote as $r_{YX|C}$, is the "controlled" version of the Pearson correlation coefficient, r_{YX}. We can get the partial correlation between Y and X controlling for C by: regressing Y on C and getting the residuals; regressing X on C and getting the residuals; the correlation between these two sets of residuals is the partial correlation between Y and X controlling for C. Using $e_{i,Y|C}$ and $e_{i,X|C}$ to denote these residuals for individual i, the sample partial correlation coefficient is

$$r_{YX|C} = \frac{\widehat{Cov}(e_{i,X|C}, e_{i,Y|C})}{\sqrt{\widehat{Var}(e_{i,X|C})\widehat{Var}(e_{i,Y|C})}} = \frac{\sum_{i=1}^{N} e_{i,X|C}\, e_{i,Y|C}}{\sqrt{\sum_{i=1}^{N} e_{i,X|C}^2 \sum_{i=1}^{N} e_{i,Y|C}^2}}.$$

We denote the population partial correlation between Y and X controlling for C as $\rho_{YX|C}$. Note that this is not the same as a multiple correlation coefficient; the squared multiple correlation coefficient $\rho_{Y|XC}^2$ is the population parameter version of the R^2 obtained when regressing Y on X and C. Using the partial correlation coefficient approach to test for the significance of a predictor X after controlling for a set of variables C, the noncentrality parameter is

$$\Lambda = N \frac{\rho_{YX|C}^2}{1 - \rho_{YX|C}^2}. \tag{10.23}$$

Power can be calculated as $1 - \mathcal{F}_{1,N-p-2,\Lambda}(f_{1-\alpha,1,N-p-2})$. Here, p is the number of predictors in the "reduced" model that does not include X. $N-p-2$ is the error degrees of freedom for the full model. In the notation of (10.21), the denominator degrees of freedom are $N-p-q-1$, where $q=1$.

Using this parameterization of the noncentrality parameter entails specifying only a single quantity, the square of the partial correlation coefficient. This can be more convenient than the multiple correlation coefficient approach, which involves specifying more quantities.

Example 10.11. Suppose we plan to test whether the level of an immune marker is associated with a fatigue score, after controlling for four potential confounders. What is the power to detect a partial correlation of $\rho_{YT|C} = 0.2$, given $N = 150$ and $\alpha = 0.05$?

```
library(powertools)
mlrF.partial(N = 150, p = 4, pc = 0.2, power = NULL)
[1] 0.6996332
```

Power is about 0.70.

10.3.8 Effect size for partial F tests

Based on Cohen [36], the effect size for a partial F test is

$$f^2 = \frac{\rho_{YT|C}^2}{1 - \rho_{YT|C}^2}.$$

Thus we have $\Lambda = Nf^2$. As discussed in Section 10.3.2, Cohen defined small, medium and large effect sizes as $f^2 = 0.02, 0.15$ and 0.35, respectively. These are equivalent to partial correlations of about $0.14, 0.36$ and 0.51.

Example 10.12. In Example 10.11, we specified a partial correlation of $\rho_{YT|C} = 0.2$. This corresponds to an f^2 effect size of

```
0.2^2 / (1 - 0.2^2)
[1]   0.04166667
```

which is relatively "small" by the rule of thumb.

11
Generalized linear regression

11.1 Power for generalized linear models

Linear regression models were discussed in Chapter 10. A linear regression model relates the mean of an outcome variable Y to a set of predictor variables $X_1, \ldots, X_p$ as $E(Y|X_1, \ldots, X_p) = \beta_0 + \beta_1 X_1 + \ldots + \beta_p X_p$. A generalized linear model (GLM) is a generalization of linear regression that relates the mean outcome to a set of predictors using a link function g,

$$g(E(Y|X_1, \ldots, X_p)) = \beta_0 + \beta_1 X_1 + \ldots + \beta_p X_p.$$

Linear regression is a GLM with an identity link function. Other commonly used GLMs include the logistic regression model, which is used for binary outcomes, $Y = 0$ or 1, and uses a logit link function,

$$\log\left(\frac{P(Y=1|X_1,\ldots,X_p)}{1 - P(Y=1|X_1,\ldots,X_p)}\right) = \beta_0 + \beta_1 X_1 + \ldots + \beta_p X_p$$

and the Poisson regression model, which is used for outcome variables that are counts, $Y = 0, 1, 2, \ldots$ and uses a log link function,

$$\log(E(Y|X_1, \ldots, X_p)) = \beta_0 + \beta_1 X_1 + \ldots + \beta_p X_p.$$

The presence of a nonlinear link function makes the derivation of power formulas more challenging. A general framework for power was presented by Demidenko [51, 52]. We discuss the general framework in this section and discuss logistic and Poisson regression specifically in subsequent sections.

For a GLM with a single predictor, $g(E(Y|X_1)) = \beta_0 + \beta_1 X_1$, the estimated regression coefficients $\hat{\beta}_0$ and $\hat{\beta}_1$ and their asymptotic variance-covariance matrix can be obtained using the method of maximum likelihood. Inference usually focuses on β_1. The hypothesis $H_0: \beta_1 = \beta_1^{(0)}$ can be tested using a Wald test statistic, which takes the form

$$Z = \frac{\hat{\beta}_1 - \beta_1^{(0)}}{\sqrt{\widehat{Var}(\hat{\beta}_1)}}.$$

DOI: 10.1201/9780429488788-11

The variance of $\hat{\beta}_1$ takes the form V/N, where N is the total sample size; more on V in a moment. Z has a standard normal distribution asymptotically when H_0 is true. Under the alternative that $\beta_1 = \beta_1^{(A)}$, for a two-sided test at level α, power can be approximated using

$$\Phi\left(\frac{\beta_1^{(A)} - \beta_1^{(0)}}{\sqrt{V/N}} + z_{\alpha/2}\right) \tag{11.1}$$

and the total sample size required for power of $1 - \beta$ is approximately

$$N \geq \frac{(z_{1-\alpha/2} + z_{1-\beta})^2 V}{\left(\beta_1^{(A)} - \beta_1^{(0)}\right)^2}. \tag{11.2}$$

What remains is to find an expression for V. Let $\boldsymbol{\beta} = (\beta_0, \beta_1)'$ represent the column vector of parameters and let $\hat{\boldsymbol{\beta}} = (\hat{\beta}_0, \hat{\beta}_1)'$ be the column vector of maximum likelihood estimates. The estimates have a multivariate normal distribution asymptotically with

$$\sqrt{N}\left(\hat{\boldsymbol{\beta}} - \boldsymbol{\beta}\right) \xrightarrow{d} \mathcal{N}(\mathbf{0}, \boldsymbol{I}^{-1})$$

where $\boldsymbol{I}$ is the expected Fisher information matrix, which has the form

$$\boldsymbol{I} = -E\begin{bmatrix} \frac{\partial^2 l(\beta_0,\beta_1)}{\partial \beta_0^2} & \frac{\partial^2 l(\beta_0,\beta_1)}{\partial \beta_0 \beta_1} \\ \frac{\partial^2 l(\beta_0,\beta_1)}{\partial \beta_0 \beta_1} & \frac{\partial^2 l(\beta_0,\beta_1)}{\partial \beta_1^2} \end{bmatrix} = \begin{bmatrix} I_{00} & I_{01} \\ I_{01} & I_{11} \end{bmatrix} \tag{11.3}$$

where $l(\beta_0, \beta_1)$ is the log-likelihood function and the expectation is taken with respect to X. The variance of $\hat{\beta}_1$ is gotten as the second diagonal element of the inverse of (11.3) and has the form

$$Var(\hat{\beta}_1) = \frac{1}{N} \frac{I_{00}}{I_{00}I_{11} - I_{01}^2}\bigg|_{(\hat{\beta}_0, \hat{\beta}_1)} = \frac{V}{N} \tag{11.4}$$

where $V = \frac{I_{00}}{I_{00}I_{11} - I_{01}^2}\big|_{(\hat{\beta}_0, \hat{\beta}_1)}$. Thus to get V, we need to take expectations of the second-order partial derivatives of the log-likelihood function with respect to the distribution of the predictor X. As a result, V depends on the distribution of X and it does not have a closed form except in special cases. This dependence on the distribution of X is what makes sample size and power calculations for GLMs more complex than they are for linear regression.

> ▶ Power for generalized linear regression models depends on the distribution of the predictors, which limits the cases in which we can derive closed form expressions for power.

11.2 Logistic regression

For the reasons explained in Section 11.1, closed form power formulas for logistic regression are available for a limited set of situations. We discuss models with a single predictor and with a set of multivariate normal predictors. For the cumulative logit (proportional odds) model, see Section 8.4.

11.2.1 One predictor

Logistic regression with one predictor models the conditional probability of a binary outcome, $Y = 1$ or 0, given the value of a predictor X as

$$P(Y = 1|X) = \frac{\exp(\beta_0 + \beta_1 X)}{1 + \exp(\beta_0 + \beta_1 X)}.$$

We can rewrite this relationship as the simple logistic regression model,

$$\log\left(\frac{P(Y = 1|X)}{1 - P(Y = 1|X)}\right) = \beta_0 + \beta_1 X. \tag{11.5}$$

β_0 is the log odds of $Y = 1$ when $X = 0$. Interest usually focuses on β_1, which is the expected change in the log odds of $Y = 1$ associated with a one unit increase in X. Interpretation usually focuses on the odds ratio (OR), which is

$$\text{OR} = \exp(\beta_1) = \frac{\text{odds}(Y = 1|X = c+1)}{\text{odds}(Y = 1|X = c)} = \frac{\frac{P(Y=1|X=c+1)}{P(Y=0|X=c+1)}}{\frac{P(Y=1|X=c)}{P(Y=0|X=c)}}.$$

The odds ratio is interpreted as the multiplicative change in the odds of $Y = 1$ associated with a one unit increase in X. β_1 is the log of the odds ratio.

As explained in Section 11.1, $Var(\hat{\beta}_1)$ has the general form V/N, and one of the steps in obtaining V is to take the expectations of the second-order partial derivatives of the log-likelihood function with respect to the distribution of the predictor. For a simple logistic regression model, these partial derivatives take the form

$$\begin{bmatrix} \frac{e^{\beta_0+\beta_1 x}}{(1+e^{\beta_0+\beta_1 x})^2} & \frac{xe^{\beta_0+\beta_1 x}}{(1+e^{\beta_0+\beta_1 x})^2} \\ \frac{xe^{\beta_0+\beta_1 x}}{(1+e^{\beta_0+\beta_1 x})^2} & \frac{x^2 e^{\beta_0+\beta_1 x}}{(1+e^{\beta_0+\beta_1 x})^2} \end{bmatrix}. \tag{11.6}$$

The expression for V is relatively simple only in the case of a binary predictor. Suppose that the predictor X in model (11.5) is binary and takes values 1 and 0 with probability π_x and $1 - \pi_x$, respectively. In a randomized trial where $X = 1$ if assigned to treatment and 0 if assigned to control, π_x denotes the probability of being assigned to treatment. We can find that for a binary X,

$$V = \frac{1}{(1-\pi_x)p_0(1-p_0)} + \frac{1}{\pi_x p_1(1-p_1)} \tag{11.7}$$

where $p_0 = P(Y=1|X=0)$ and $p_1 = P(Y=1|X=1)$. This expression for V can be used in equations (11.1) and (11.2) to estimate power and sample size. Needed inputs for a calculation are π_x and the values of p_1 and p_0 under the alternative.

Note that for a binary predictor, the odds ratio can be expressed as $\frac{p_1/(1-p_1)}{p_0/(1-p_0)}$. If we are given values for the odds ratio and p_1, we can solve for p_0. Similarly, if we are given the odds ratio and p_0, we can solve for p_1. This is illustrated in the following example.

Example 11.1. A study proposes to examine the association between smoking and Type 2 diabetes using data that approximates a random sample from the population. The investigators plan to fit a simple logistic regression model with diabetes as the outcome Y and ever smoked as the predictor ($X=1$ if ever smoked and 0 otherwise). The prevalence of ever-smoked in the population is expected to be 0.3, and the probability that an individual who has never smoked will have diabetes is assumed to be 0.1. What sample size is needed to have at least 80% power to reject $H_0: \beta_1 = 0$ when the true odds ratio is 3, at two-sided α of 0.05?

The wp.logistic function from the WebPower package can be used to perform the calculation. Zhang and Yuan [242] is a book on the WebPower package, which has a variety of functions. Calculations can also be performed online at http://webpower.psychstat.org. The function has the following syntax:

```
library(WebPower)
wp.logistic(n, p0, p1, alpha, power,
    alternative = c("two.sided", "less", "greater"),
    family = c("Bernoulli", exponential", "lognormal",
    "normal", "Poisson", "uniform"), parameter = NULL)
```

where p0 is $P(Y=1|X=0)$ and p1 is $P(Y=1|X=1)$ under the alternative. The input family is the distribution of the predictor; for a binary covariate as in this example, specify Bernoulli. The input parameter is the parameter(s) for the predictor's distribution; for Bernoulli, this parameter is $P(X=1)$.

To use the function, we need to specify p_0 and p_1, but in the example, we are given the odds ratio (OR = 3) and $p_0 = 0.1$. We can find p_1 as:

```
or <- 3
p0 <- 0.1
K <- or * (p0 / (1 - p0))
p1 <- K / (1 + K)  ;  p1
[1] 0.25
```

Thus an OR of 3 and p_0 of 0.1 imply that $p_1 = 0.25$. We are now ready to use the function:

```
wp.logistic(n = NULL, p0 = 0.1, p1 = 0.25, alpha = 0.05, power = 0.8,
   alternative = "two.sided", family = "Bernoulli", parameter = 0.3)
```

Power for logistic regression

```
    p0   p1      beta0    beta1        n alpha power
   0.1 0.25 -2.197225 1.098612 218.8331  0.05   0.8
```

URL: http://psychstat.org/logistic

The calculation suggests that we need a sample size of about 220.

Similar calculations can be performed using an online calculator provided at https://www.dartmouth.edu/~eugened/power-samplesize.php as a companion to the papers by Demidenko [51, 52]. This online calculator computes power, sample size or minimum detectable odds ratio. It also supports power and sample size calculations for logistic regression models with two binary predictors, with or without an interaction.

For other distributions of X, taking the expectations in equation (11.6) with respect to the distribution of X requires integration, which is performed in functions such as wp.logistic in the WebPower package. We illustrate with an example of a normally distributed covariate:

Example 11.2. Researchers are interested in the association between math scores in the first year of college and subsequent graduation. Math scores are standardized and are assumed to follow a standard normal distribution. For the standard normal distribution, one unit of X corresponds to one standard deviation. It is expected that students with standardized test scores of 0 and 1 have probabilities of graduating of 0.6 and 0.7, respectively. What is the sample size needed to detect an effect of test score on graduation with 90% power? Assume a two-sided α of 0.05.

Note that simple logistic regression models assume that the odds ratio associated with a one-unit increase in X is the same everywhere on the distribution of X. Here, the assumed odds ratio associated with a one-unit increase in X can be calculated as follows:

```
p1 <- 0.7
p0 <- 0.6
or <- (p1 / (1 - p1)) / (p0 / (1 - p0))  ; or
[1] 1.555556
```

Thus we are assuming that a one standard deviation increase in test score is associated with an increase in the odds of graduation of about 1.6, everywhere on the distribution of test scores.

We can perform the sample size calculation with wp.logistic as follows. For family = "normal", parameter should be specified as a vector of the mean and standard deviation of the normal distribution of the predictor.

```
library(WebPower)
wp.logistic(n = NULL, p0 = 0.6, p1 = 0.7, alpha = 0.05, power = 0.9,
    alternative = "two.sided", family = "normal", parameter = c(0, 1))

Power for logistic regression

    p0  p1    beta0     beta1          n alpha power
    0.6 0.7 0.4054651 0.4418328 254.7801  0.05   0.9
```

This suggests that we need at least 255 students.

The wp.logistic function in the WebPower package also performs calculations for the cases of predictor distributions that are exponential, lognormal, Poisson and uniform.

11.2.2 Multivariate normal predictors

The multiple logistic regression model with p predictor variables is

$$log\left(\frac{P(Y=1|X_1,\ldots,X_p)}{1-P(Y=1|X_1,\ldots,X_p)}\right) = \beta_0 + \beta_1 X_1 + \ldots + \beta_p X_p. \qquad (11.8)$$

Often, the hypothesis of interest involves the effect of one variable after controlling for other variables in the model, that is, a test of $H_0: \beta_1 = 0$ when the model includes $X_2, \ldots, X_p$, and we will focus on this setting.

As discussed in Section 11.1, power for logistic regression depends on the distribution of the predictors. For multiple logistic regression, some research has been done for the case that $X_1, \ldots, X_p$ have a multivariate normal distribution. Denote the variance of the maximum likelihood estimator of β_1 from a model with only X_1 as a predictor as $Var_1(\hat{\beta}_1)$ and from a model with p total covariates as $Var_p(\hat{\beta}_1)$. Then (see Whittemore [229])

$$Var_p(\hat{\beta}_1) \approx \left(\frac{1}{1 - \rho^2_{X_1|X_2 X_3 \ldots X_p}}\right) Var_1(\hat{\beta}_1)$$

where $\rho^2_{X_1|X_2 X_3 \ldots X_p}$ is the squared population multiple correlation coefficient relating X_1 to $X_2, \ldots, X_p$. As discussed in Section 10.3.1, $\rho^2_{X_1|X_2 X_3 \ldots X_p}$ is the population analogue of the sample multiple correlation coefficient, $R^2_{X_1|X_2 X_3 \ldots X_p}$, which is the R^2 obtained when X_1 is regressed on $X_2, \ldots, X_p$. Since $0 \leq \rho^2_{X_1|X_2 X_3 \ldots X_p} \leq 1$, dividing by $1 - \rho^2_{X_1|X_2 X_3 \ldots X_p}$ will inflate the

Logistic regression

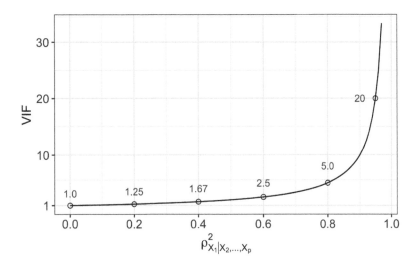

FIGURE 11.1: Variance inflation factor (VIF) as a function of $\rho^2_{X_1|X_2X_3...X_p}$, which is the population analogue of $R^2_{X_1|X_2X_3...X_p}$, the R^2 obtained when X_1 is regressed on $X_2, \ldots, X_p$.

variance. We can consider $1/(1 - \rho^2_{X_1|X_2X_3...X_p})$ to be a type of variance inflation factor (VIF).

Given that the required sample size N is directly proportional to the variance of the estimator (see equation (11.2)), it has been suggested by Hsieh et al. [102] that the sample size requirement for the multiple logistic regression model be obtained by multiplying the N required for a simple logistic regression by the VIF,

$$\frac{1}{1 - \rho^2_{X_1|X_2X_3...X_k}}. \tag{11.9}$$

Figure 11.1 shows how the VIF varies as a function of $\rho^2_{X_1|X_2X_3...X_p}$. The relationship suggests that, for example, when $\rho^2_{X_1|X_2X_3...X_p} = 0.2$, the sample size should be inflated by 25% to maintain power.

Hsieh et al. [102] report that this VIF approach works well for both multivariate normal and binary covariates. The VIF approach has been widely used regardless of the nature of the covariates; however, the accuracy of this approach in other contexts has not been well studied.

Example 11.3. In Example 11.2, we calculated that the sample size required to detect an effect of math test score (a normally distributed predictor) on the outcome of college graduation with 90% power and two-sided α of 0.05

was about 255. Suppose that we plan to adjust for four normally distributed covariates. We expect that the linear association of X_1 with $X_2, \ldots X_5$ will be in the "medium" range, corresponding to $\rho^2_{X_1|X_2\ldots X_5} = 0.13$ (see Section 10.3.2). The variance inflation factor is

```
rhosq <- 0.13
vif <- 1 / (1 - 0.13)  ; vif
[1]   1.149425
```

This suggests inflating the sample size by about 15%, which gives:

```
255 * vif
[1] 293.1034
```

Given the uncertainties and assumptions involved in this calculation, we may wish to round this value up to 300 or higher.

11.3 Poisson regression

Poisson regression is commonly used to model count data. Count data represent the number of occurrences of an event, for example, the number of species on a plot of land or the number of asthma exacerbations experienced by a patient, and can take only non-negative integer values. The Poisson regression model assumes that a count outcome variable Y has a Poisson distribution,

$$P(Y = y) = \frac{\lambda^y \exp(-\lambda)}{y!}, \quad y = 0, 1, 2, \ldots$$

where the mean of Y, $\lambda = E(Y)$, is related to values of covariates as

$$\log(\lambda) = \beta_0 + \beta_1 X_1 + \ldots + \beta_p X_p.$$

Similar to the situation with logistic regression, power calculations are more complicated for Poisson regression than they are for linear regression. Analytic approaches have been developed only for the case of a single covariate. When there is a single covariate X, the mean count is modeled as $\lambda = e^{\beta_0} e^{\beta_1 X}$; e^{β_0} is interpreted as the mean count when $X = 0$ and e^{β_1} is interpreted as the multiplicative factor by which the mean count is changed due to a one-unit increase in X.

Usually we are interested in hypothesis tests regarding β_1. The general approach to power for GLMs such as Poisson regression models is described in Section 11.1. The main result is that we need an expression for $Var(\hat{\beta}_1)$, which has the form V/N, where N is the sample size and V is a function of the

Poisson regression

elements of I, the expected Fisher information matrix. For Poisson regression with one predictor, I takes the form [242]

$$I = \begin{bmatrix} I_{00} & I_{01} \\ I_{01} & I_{11} \end{bmatrix} = -E \begin{bmatrix} e^{\hat{\beta}_0 + \hat{\beta}_1 x} & x e^{\hat{\beta}_0 + \hat{\beta}_1 x} \\ x e^{\hat{\beta}_0 + \hat{\beta}_1 x} & x^2 e^{\hat{\beta}_0 + \hat{\beta}_1 x} \end{bmatrix} \quad (11.10)$$

where the expectation is taken with respect to the distribution of X. The estimated variance of $\hat{\beta}_1$ is $\frac{1}{N} \frac{I_{00}}{I_{00} I_{11} - I_{01}^2}|_{(\hat{\beta}_0, \hat{\beta}_1)}$. If the distribution of X is known, computation of the expectations can be accomplished using integration. The wp.poisson function in the WebPower package implements this approach for a variety of distributions of X; see Zhang and Yuan [242] for further documentation. The calculations can also be performed online at http://psychstat.org/poisson. We provide an example.

Example 11.4. In a clinical trial, patients with asthma will be randomized to two conditions and compared on the number of asthma exacerbations over a 5-month follow up period. In the control condition, the mean number of exacerbations is expected to be 10. In the treatment condition, the mean number is expected to be 8. Patients will be randomized 2:1 to treatment and control. What is the sample size required for 80% power, two-sided α of 0.05?

We can use the wp.poisson function from the WebPower package to conduct the calculation. The syntax is

```
library(WebPower)
wp.poisson(n, exp0, exp1, alpha, power, alternative,
   family = c("Bernoulli", "exponential", "lognormal", "normal",
   "Poisson", "uniform"), parameter)
```

where exp0 is $\exp(\beta_0)$, the mean count when $X = 0$, exp1 is $\exp(\beta_1)$, the relative (multiplicative) change in the event rate due to a one-unit increase in X and parameter is the parameter(s) of the predictor distribution. In our example, exp0 is 10, exp1 is 8/10 and the predictor is Bernoulli with $P(X = 1) = 2/3$. We compute sample size as follows:

```
wp.poisson(n = NULL, exp0 = 10, exp1 = 8/10, alpha = 0.05, power = 0.8,
   alternative = "two.sided", family = "Bernoulli", parameter = 2/3)

Power for Poisson regression

        n power alpha exp0 exp1    beta0        beta1
 76.84446   0.8  0.05   10  0.8 2.302585   -0.2231436

URL: http://psychstat.org/poisson
```

Rounding up to the next multiple of 3, this suggests that we need 78 patients, with 26 in the control group and 52 in the treatment group.

11.4 Additional resources

The pwrss package also has functions for power and sample size for testing a single coefficient in logistic regression (pwrss.z.logistic) and Poisson regression (pwrss.z.poisreg).

The Poisson distribution has the constraint that the value of the mean, λ, is also the value of the variance. The negative binomial distribution is often chosen over the Poisson model for count data that are overdispersed, that is, when the variance exceeds the mean. Some resources for power and sample size for outcomes with a negative binomial distribution include the NBDesign package, for which Zhu et al. [244] is the main reference and the function n_glm in the skewsamp package; see Cundill et al. [47].

As we have discussed, the situations in which power for a GLM can be directly computed are limited. In general, when analytic expressions for power are not available, an alternative is to use simulation to compute power. Power by simulation was discussed in Section 2.10. The simglm package is designed to simulate regression models, including both linear regression and generalized linear mixed models with up to three levels of nesting. Power simulations allow for the specification of missing data, unbalanced designs and different random error distributions.Vignettes and examples are available at https://github.com/lebebr01/simglm.

12
Crossover studies

12.1 Introduction

Most of the study designs considered thus far have been **parallel group designs**. In a parallel group design, participants are randomized to receive one condition; for example, they may be randomized to Treatment T or Treatment R (T stands for "test" and R stands for "reference"). For some studies, it can be advantageous to use a **crossover design**. In a crossover design, participants are randomized to receive a **sequence** of conditions, that is, an ordering of treatment conditions, over multiple time periods. For example, they may be randomized to receive T in the first period followed by R in the second period, or R followed by T. Figure 12.1 provides an example contrasting a parallel and a crossover design.

In a parallel design, responses to different treatments are measured on different participants. In a crossover trial, the response of a participant to Treatment T can be contrasted with the same participant's response to Treatment R. This removes between-patient variation from the contrast between treatments and makes crossover trials potentially more efficient than parallel group trials with the same number of subjects.

Figure 12.1(B) illustrates a classic 2×2 crossover design, also called an AB/BA or TR/RT design. In this design, participants are randomized to either TR or RT. In this chapter, we will consider 2×2 designs as well as 2×2 designs with replications. In designs involving replications, subjects repeat the same treatment sequence. For example, a 2×2 crossover design with two replications randomizes subjects to either TRTR or RTRT and a 2×2 crossover design with three replications randomizes subjects to either TRTRTR or RTRTRT. We will label such trials as $(2\times2)2$ and $(2\times2)3$, with the last number indicating the number of replications. A wide variety of other crossover designs are possible, involving higher numbers of sequences, periods and treatments.

Crossover designs often include a **washout period** between treatment periods, of sufficient duration to allow subjects to return to their baseline status. Washout periods help ensure that the effects of a treatment do not carry over to subsequent periods. If treatment effects do carry over to subsequent periods, this is called a **carryover effect** or **residual effect**. Crossover designs can also have **period effects**, which occur when patients do systematically better or worse in later periods because their health status or some other

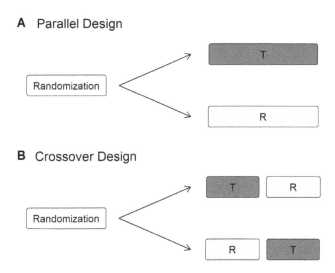

FIGURE 12.1: Comparison of parallel and crossover designs with Treatments T and R.

factor has changed over time, independent of treatment, or **sequence effects**, in which sequences themselves are associated with systematically higher or lower outcomes.

Crossover studies have certain advantages over parallel group studies. As previously mentioned, because each subject serves as their own control, in theory, crossover designs are more statistically efficient, and therefore require fewer subjects than do parallel designs. Additionally, patient enrollment into the study may be easier because each patient is guaranteed to receive all treatments, rather than only one treatment (and possibly only the reference treatment), as in a parallel design.

Disadvantages of crossover designs include increased complexity and longer study duration compared to a parallel group design. Longer duration increases the risk of period effects and patient dropout. If carryover, period and/or sequence effects occur, this can make it difficult to obtain an unbiased estimate of the treatment effect. A crossover design is not appropriate when a treatment can alter a subject permanently. Hence, crossover designs should not be used to compare treatments that are intended to provide a cure.

Crossover designs are commonly used in bioavailability and bioequivalence pharmacology trials to study the pharmacokinetics of a compound in the human body. For additional information on the design and analysis of such trials, see, for example, Chow and Liu [32]. There are many nuances and considerations involved in the design and analysis of crossover trials that are beyond the scope of this book. Readers are encouraged to consult more general references such as Jones and Kenward [109] or Senn [201] for a more thorough handling of issues in crossover trials.

In this chapter, we discuss the 2 × 2 crossover design and the $(2 \times 2)r$ crossover design, which is a 2 × 2 design with $r > 1$ replications. We consider designs that compare means under different treatments. Some of the material here is adapted from Chow et al. [33] and Senn [201].

12.2 2 × 2 crossover design

12.2.1 Model

In this section, we consider the 2 × 2 crossover design in Figure 12.1(B). We label the two treatments as the test (T) and reference (R) treatments. Subjects will be randomized to TR or RT. We assume that n subjects are randomized to each sequence, for a total of $2n$ subjects.

Let Y_{ijk} be the response of the ith subject, $i = 1, \ldots, n$, in the jth sequence, $j = 1, 2$, under the kth treatment, $k = T$ or R. A model for the responses is

$$Y_{ijk} = \mu_k + \gamma_{jk} + s_{ik} + \epsilon_{ijk}$$

where μ_k is the mean for treatment k, γ_{jk} is a fixed effect for the jth sequence under treatment k, s_{ik} is a random effect for subject i under treatment k and ϵ_{ijk} is a random error term. The parameter γ_{jk} allows the effect of a treatment to differ between sequences. Other parametrizations of the fixed effects are possible.

For power and sample size calculations, the focus is on the random terms. The random effects (s_{iT}, s_{iR}) allow each subject's mean under treatment k to vary from the population mean μ_k and are assumed to be bivariate normal with mean 0 and covariance matrix

$$\Sigma = \begin{bmatrix} \sigma_{BT}^2 & \rho\sigma_{BT}\sigma_{BR} \\ \rho\sigma_{BT}\sigma_{BR} & \sigma_{BR}^2 \end{bmatrix}.$$

The variances σ_{BT}^2 and σ_{BR}^2 pertain to variability between subjects, and therefore are subscripted with B. ρ is the correlation between an individual's responses under the two different treatments.

The error terms ϵ_{ijT} and ϵ_{ijR} allow for a subject's response to vary from their subject-specific mean response under treatment k, $\mu_k + s_{ik}$, and are assumed to be independent normal random variables with mean 0 and variances that can differ between treatments, σ_{WT}^2 and σ_{WR}^2. The subscript W indicates that these are within-subject variances.

To estimate the difference in means between treatments, $\mu_T - \mu_R$, we estimate for each subject the difference d_{ij} between their responses under treatments T and R,

$$d_{ij} = Y_{ijT} - Y_{ijR}.$$

Although d_{ij} has both i and j subscripts, each subject i is randomized to only one sequence j, and so for each subject, there is a single d_{ij}. Then $\mu_T - \mu_R$ can be estimated as the average over the $2n$ subjects,

$$\bar{d}_{..} = \frac{1}{2n} \sum_{j=1}^{2} \sum_{i=1}^{n} d_{ij}$$

Because the $2n$ subjects are independent, $Var(\bar{d}_{..})$ is equal to $Var(d_{ij})/(2n)$. Under the model assumptions, $Var(d_{ij})$, which we denote as σ_d^2, can be found to be

$$\begin{aligned}\sigma_d^2 &= Var(Y_{ijT}) + Var(Y_{ijR}) - 2Cov(Y_{ijT}, Y_{ijR}) \\ &= \sigma_{BT}^2 + \sigma_{WT}^2 + \sigma_{BR}^2 + \sigma_{WR}^2 - 2\rho\sigma_{BT}\sigma_{BR} \\ &= (\sigma_{BT}^2 + \sigma_{BR}^2 - 2\rho\sigma_{BT}\sigma_{BR}) + (\sigma_{WT}^2 + \sigma_{WR}^2)\end{aligned} \quad (12.1)$$

where in the last line we group the between- and within-subject variance components for clarity. If the simplifying assumption is made that the variances do not differ by treatment, so $\sigma_{BT}^2 = \sigma_{BR}^2 = \sigma_B^2$ and $\sigma_{WT}^2 = \sigma_{WR}^2 = \sigma_W^2$, equation (12.1) simplifies to

$$\sigma_d^2 = 2\left[(1-\rho)\sigma_B^2 + \sigma_W^2\right] \quad (12.2)$$

and we have that the variance of the estimator of the treatment effect is

$$Var(\bar{d}_{..}) = \frac{(1-\rho)\sigma_B^2 + \sigma_W^2}{n}. \quad (12.3)$$

From the data, an estimate of $Var(d_{ij})$ can be obtained as

$$\widehat{Var}(d_{ij}) = \hat{\sigma}_d^2 = \frac{1}{2(n-1)} \sum_{j=1}^{2} \sum_{i=1}^{n} (d_{ij} - \bar{d}_{..})^2$$

and $\widehat{Var}(\bar{d}_{..}) = \hat{\sigma}_d^2/(2n)$ Note that while we can estimate σ_d^2 in a standard 2×2 crossover design, we cannot estimate all of the variance components in equation (12.1) separately with this design. For more information on estimating variance components in crossover trials, see Chow and Liu [32].

12.2.2 Power and sample size

Tests with the null hypotheses $H_0: \mu_T - \mu_R = \Delta_0$, $H_0: \mu_T - \mu_R \leq \Delta_0$ or $H_0: \mu_T - \mu_R \geq \Delta_0$ (these null hypotheses will cover nonequality, noninferiority and superiority by a margin, discussed further in a moment) can be conducted using the test statistic

$$T = \frac{\bar{d}_{..} - \Delta_0}{\sqrt{\widehat{Var}(\bar{d}_{..})}} = \frac{\bar{d}_{..} - \Delta_0}{\hat{\sigma}_d/\sqrt{2n}}.$$

When the null hypothesis is true, T has a central t distribution with $2n-2$ degrees of freedom. Under an alternative that the true difference in means is Δ_A, T has a noncentral t distribution with noncentrality parameter

$$\lambda = \frac{\sqrt{2n}(\Delta_A - \Delta_0)}{\sigma_d}. \tag{12.4}$$

where σ_d^2 is given by equation (12.1) or (12.2). The power for a test at level α can be calculated as

$$\text{Power (lower-tail test)} = \mathcal{T}_{2n-2,\lambda}(t_{\alpha,2n-2}) \tag{12.5}$$
$$\text{Power (upper-tail test)} = 1 - \mathcal{T}_{2n-2,\lambda}(t_{1-\alpha,2n-2})$$
$$\text{Power (two-sided test)} = 1 - \mathcal{F}_{1,2n-2,\Lambda}(f_{1-\alpha,1,2n-2}).$$

where $\Lambda = \lambda^2$.

When sample sizes are large (a common rule of thumb is $n \geq 30$), for a test of equality/nonequality, a normal approximation for the sample size required for power of $1 - \beta$ when using a two-sided test at level α as

$$n \geq \frac{(z_{1-\alpha/2} + z_{1-\beta})^2 \sigma_d^2}{2(\Delta_A - \Delta_0)^2} \tag{12.6}$$

where n is the number of subjects in each sequence, for a total of $2n$ subjects (equal allocation to sequences is assumed). For a one-sided tests at level α, replace $\alpha/2$ with α.

Tests of noninferiority and superiority by a margin. For a noninferiority trial with noninferiority margin $m > 0$, the term $\Delta_A - \Delta_0$ is replaced by $\Delta_A + m$ in the noncentrality parameter (12.4) and in the sample size equation (12.6). For superiority by a margin $m > 0$, $\Delta_A - \Delta_0$ is replaced by $\Delta_A - m$. We are assuming in both cases that $\Delta_A \geq 0$. See Chapter 4 for more discussion of noninferiority and superiority by a margin.

Tests of equivalence. Crossover designs are commonly used for bioequivalence studies. Power and sample size for equivalence tests, including the two one-sided test (TOST) procedure, are discussed in Section 4.6. The hypotheses are $H_0: |\mu_T - \mu_R| \geq m$ versus $H_A: |\mu_T - \mu_R| < m$. As discussed in Section 4.6, a conservative estimate of power (actual power may be higher) can be obtained as

$$\text{Power (TOST)} \geq 1 - 2\mathcal{T}_{2n-2,\lambda}(t_{1-\alpha,2n-2})$$

where the noncentrality parameter λ is

$$\lambda = \frac{\sqrt{2n}(m - |\Delta_A|)}{\sigma_d}.$$

For large samples, sample size can be estimated using a normal approximation as

$$n \geq \frac{(z_{1-\alpha} + z_{1-\beta/2})^2 \sigma_d^2}{2(m - |\Delta_A|)^2}$$

where n is the number of subjects allocated to each sequence, for a total of $2n$ subjects.

Example 12.1. Suppose a 2×2 crossover trial is planned to test $H_0 : \mu_T = \mu_R$. There will be equal allocation to the two sequences. The expected means for test and reference treatments are 9 and 8 respectively. The standard deviations are assumed to be $\sigma_{BT} = \sigma_{BR} = 4$ and $\sigma_{WT} = \sigma_{WR} = 1$, with $\rho = 0.5$ for the correlation between two measurements on the same subject. Desired power is 80% for a two-sided test with $\alpha = 0.05$. Note that we generally expect that the variance between two observations from different subjects (σ_B^2) will be greater than the variance between two observations from the same subject (σ_W^2).

The crsize function in the designsize package supports power and sample size calculations for crossover trials and uses the noncentral t for computations. It supports tests of equality/non-equality, noninferiority, superiority by a margin and equivalence, specified using the type option. m indicates the number of replicates, with m = 1 for a standard 2×2 crossover trial (note that we use r to denote number of replications). k is the ratio of sample sizes in the two sequences. r1 and r2 specify the proportion of periods each subject spends in Treatments 1 and 2, which are 0.5 and 0.5 for a standard 2×2 crossover trial. beta is type II error.

```
library(designsize)
crsize(type = "equal", m = 1, k = 1, mur = 8, mut = 9,
       sigbr = 4, sigbt = 4, rho = 0.5, sigwr = 1, sigwt = 1,
       alpha = 0.05, beta = 0.20, r1 = 0.5, r2 = 0.5)

"Sample size determination under Crossover Design"
           Factor-1 Factor-2 Total
Sequence-1      36       36    72
Sequence-2      36       36    72
Total           72       72   144
```

This indicates that we need 72 subjects in each sequence, for a total of 144 subjects.

What factors affect power? Factors that affect power can be determined by examining the noncentrality parameter, given in equation (12.4). As expected, power increases as the number of subjects n in each sequence increases. The denominator of the noncentrality parameter is

$$\sigma_d = \sqrt{\sigma_{BT}^2 + \sigma_{BR}^2 - 2\rho\sigma_{BT}\sigma_{BR} + (\sigma_{WT}^2 + \sigma_{WR}^2)}$$
$$= \sqrt{2\left[(1-\rho)\sigma_B^2 + \sigma_W^2\right]}$$

when variances do not differ between treatment conditions. Power decreases as σ_d increases. This variance term involves the between-subject variances, the within-subject variances, and the correlation between the two measurements on the same subject ρ. Higher values of any of the variances will decrease power while higher correlation will increase power.

12.3 $(2 \times 2)r$ crossover design

12.3.1 Model

The classic 2×2 crossover design considered in Section 12.2 has several disadvantages. The sequence, period and carryover effects are confounded with each other (another term is "aliased") and cannot be estimated separately. This is because the 2×2 design can support estimating four fixed effect parameters, one for each sequence-period, whereas disentangling the treatment, sequence, period and carryover effects requires estimating additional fixed effects. Additionally, the within- and between-subject variances for each treatment cannot be estimated independently. These limitations can be addressed by using a $(2 \times 2)r$ crossover design with $r \geq 2$ replicates.

Table 12.1 displays a 2×2 crossover design with 2 replications, which we denote as $(2 \times 2)2$. Subjects are randomized to two sequences, TRTR or RTRT. The full sequences are constructed by repeating each 2-period sequence. The design can be further extended by adding more replications; for example, a 2×2 design with 3 replications, denoted $(2 \times 2)3$, randomizes subjects to either TRTRTR or RTRTRT.

Let Y_{ijkl} be the lth replicate or response, $l = 1, \ldots, r$, of the ith subject, $i = 1, \ldots, n$, in the jth sequence, $j = 1, 2$, under the kth treatment, $k = T$ or R. A model for the responses is

$$Y_{ijkl} = \mu_k + \gamma_{jk} + s_{ik} + \epsilon_{ijkl}$$

where μ_k is the mean for treatment k, γ_{jk} is a fixed effect for the jth sequence under treatment k, s_{ik} is a random effect for subject i under treatment k and ϵ_{ijkl} is an error term. The random effects (s_{iT}, s_{iR}) are assumed to be

TABLE 12.1: $(2 \times 2)r$ crossover design with $r = 2$ replicates.

Replication	1		2	
Period	1	2	3	4
Sequence 1	T	R	T	R
Sequence 2	R	T	R	T

bivariate normal with mean 0 and covariance matrix

$$\Sigma = \begin{bmatrix} \sigma_{BT}^2 & \rho\sigma_{BT}\sigma_{BR} \\ \rho\sigma_{BT}\sigma_{BR} & \sigma_{BR}^2 \end{bmatrix}$$

and the error terms ϵ_{ijTl} and ϵ_{ijRl} are assumed to be independent normal random variables with mean 0 and variances that can differ between treatments, σ_{WT}^2 and σ_{WR}^2. See Section 12.2 for more explanation of these variance components.

To estimate the difference in means between treatments, $\mu_T - \mu_R$, we estimate for each subject their mean response under each treatment, which involves averaging over the replications,

$$\bar{Y}_{ijT\cdot} = \frac{1}{r}\sum_{l=1}^{r} Y_{ijTl} \quad \text{and} \quad \bar{Y}_{ijR\cdot} = \frac{1}{r}\sum_{l=1}^{r} Y_{ijRl},$$

and then we obtain the difference,

$$d_{ij} = \bar{Y}_{ijT\cdot} - \bar{Y}_{ijR\cdot}.$$

The variance of d_{ij} can be found to be

$$Var(d_{ij}) = \sigma_d^2 = \sigma_{BT}^2 + \sigma_{BR}^2 - 2\rho\sigma_{BT}\sigma_{BR} + \frac{1}{r}(\sigma_{WT}^2 + \sigma_{WR}^2). \quad (12.7)$$

Note that this variance formula reduces to that in equation (12.1) for a standard 2×2 crossover design when setting $r = 1$. When $\sigma_{BT}^2 = \sigma_{BR}^2 = \sigma_B^2$ and $\sigma_{WT}^2 = \sigma_{WR}^2 = \sigma_W^2$, we have

$$\sigma_d^2 = 2\left[(1-\rho)\sigma_B^2 + \frac{\sigma_W^2}{r}\right]$$

By comparing this equation to equation (12.2), we can see that having replications reduces the impact of within-subject variance.

By averaging over all $2n$ values of d_{ij}, we can obtain an estimate of the difference in means $\mu_T - \mu_R$ as

$$\bar{d}_{\cdot\cdot} = \frac{1}{2n}\sum_{j=1}^{2}\sum_{i=1}^{n} d_{ij},$$

which has variance $Var(\bar{d}_{..}) = \sigma_d^2/(2n)$. An estimate of σ_d^2 can be obtained as

$$\hat{\sigma}_d^2 = \frac{1}{2(n-1)} \sum_{j=1}^{2} \sum_{i=1}^{n} (d_{ij} - \bar{d}_{.j})^2$$

where $\bar{d}_{.j}$ is the average value of d_{ij} for sequence j,

$$\bar{d}_{.j} = \frac{1}{n} \sum_{i=1}^{n} d_{ij}$$

12.3.2 Power and sample size

Tests of the hypotheses $H_0\colon \mu_T - \mu_R = \Delta_0$, $H_0\colon \mu_T - \mu_R \leq \Delta_0$ or $H_0\colon \mu_T - \mu_R \geq \Delta_0$ can be conducted using the test statistic

$$T = \frac{\bar{d}_{..} - \Delta_0}{\sqrt{\widehat{Var}(\bar{d}_{..})}} = \frac{\bar{d}_{..} - \Delta_0}{\hat{\sigma}_d/\sqrt{2n}}.$$

When the null hypothesis is true, T has a central t distribution with $2n - 2$ degrees of freedom. Under an alternative that the true difference in means is Δ_A, T has a noncentral t distribution with noncentrality parameter

$$\lambda = \frac{\sqrt{2n}(\Delta_A - \Delta_0)}{\sigma_d}.$$

The power for a test at level α can be calculated as

$$\text{Power (lower-tail test)} = \mathcal{T}_{2n-2,\lambda}(t_{\alpha, 2n-2}) \qquad (12.8)$$
$$\text{Power (upper-tail test)} = 1 - \mathcal{T}_{2n-2,\lambda}(t_{1-\alpha, 2n-2})$$
$$\text{Power (two-sided test)} = 1 - \mathcal{F}_{1, 2n-2, \Lambda}(f_{1-\alpha, 1, 2n-2}).$$

where $\Lambda = \lambda^2$.

When sample sizes are large, we can estimate the required sample size using the same formula as given for the 2×2 crossover trial in equation (12.6). However, the variance σ_d^2 will consider the number of replications r and is computed as in equation (12.7). For tests of noninferiority, superiority by a margin, or equivalence, the modifications to the formulas for power and sample size are the same as described for the standard 2×2 crossover trial in Section 12.2.

What factors affect power? The denominator of the noncentrality parameter is

$$\sigma_d = \sqrt{\sigma_{BT}^2 + \sigma_{BR}^2 - 2\rho\sigma_{BT}\sigma_{BR} + \frac{1}{r}(\sigma_{WT}^2 + \sigma_{WR}^2)}$$
$$= \sqrt{2\left[(1-\rho)\sigma_B^2 + \frac{\sigma_W^2}{r}\right]}$$

when variances do not differ between treatment conditions. As r increases, the influence of the within-subject variances decreases. This can increase power, but the impact can be modest because σ_B^2 is usually the larger variance component. Other advantages of having replicates in a crossover design include that period, sequence and crossover effects can potentially be estimated, and the variance components σ_{BT}^2, σ_{BR}^2, σ_{WT}^2 and σ_{WR}^2 can be estimated.

Example 12.2. We repeat Example 12.1 but with $r = 2$ replicates. We use the crsize function from the designsize package, which performs calculations using the noncentral t distribution:

```
library(designsize)
# m is the number of replications
crsize(type = "equal", m = 2, k = 1, mur = 8, mut = 9,
       sigbr = 4, sigbt = 4, rho = 0.5, sigwr = 1, sigwt = 1,
       alpha = 0.05, beta = 0.20, r1 = 0.5, r2 = 0.5)

"Sample size determination under Crossover Design"
           Factor-1 Factor-2 Total
Sequence-1    34       34     68
Sequence-2    34       34     68
Total         68       68    136
```

This indicates that we need 68 subjects per sequence. This is a small reduction in sample size compared to the 2 × 2 crossover design with $r = 1$ and is due to reduction in the impact of within-subject variance. The greater advantages of having replications are the ability to independently estimate treatment, sequence, period and carryover effects as well as the within- and between-subject variances.

12.4 Efficiency of crossover designs

In Section 3.3, we discussed how two different study designs can be compared by examining their relative efficiency. Suppose that A and B are two different study designs that could be used to estimate a parameter θ. The relative efficiency of the estimators from the two designs, $\hat{\theta}_A$ and $\hat{\theta}_B$, is

$$\text{RE}(\hat{\theta}_A, \hat{\theta}_B) = \frac{Var(\hat{\theta}_B)}{Var(\hat{\theta}_A)}.$$

We compare the efficiency of a crossover design to that of a parallel group design from two perspectives. First, we compare designs with the same number

Efficiency of crossover designs

of subjects. Denote the standard 2 × 2 crossover design as Design A and the parallel group design as Design B. Suppose that n subjects are allocated to each arm. The parameter to be estimated is the difference in means between treatments, $\theta = \mu_T - \mu_R$. For simplicity, we assume that $\sigma_{BT}^2 = \sigma_{BR}^2 = \sigma_B^2$ and $\sigma_{WT}^2 = \sigma_{WR}^2 = \sigma_W^2$. For the crossover design (A),

$$Var(\hat{\theta}_A) = \frac{(1-\rho)\sigma_B^2 + \sigma_W^2}{n}.$$

see equation (12.3). For the parallel group design (B),

$$Var(\hat{\theta}_B) = Var(\bar{Y}_T - \bar{Y}_R) = \frac{\sigma_T^2 + \sigma_R^2}{n} = \frac{2\sigma_Y^2}{n}$$

where we assume equal variances across treatment arms, $\sigma_T^2 = \sigma_R^2 = \sigma_Y^2$. The variance σ_Y^2 is the total variance of an observation, which includes both the between-subject and within-subject variance (although we cannot apportion the total variance between these two sources when we have only one observation per subject), so that $\sigma_Y^2 = \sigma_B^2 + \sigma_W^2$. Thus we have

$$Var(\hat{\theta}_B) = \frac{2(\sigma_B^2 + \sigma_W^2)}{n}.$$

The relative efficiency is the ratio of the variances,

$$\frac{Var(\hat{\theta}_B)}{Var(\hat{\theta}_A)} = \frac{2(\sigma_B^2 + \sigma_W^2)}{(\sigma_B^2 + \sigma_W^2) - \rho\sigma_B^2} \quad (12.9)$$

where we have re-expressed $Var(\hat{\theta}_A)$ to make the ratio easier to interpret. Since we expect ρ to be positive, the numerator will be at least twice as large as the denominator. This means that a crossover design is expected to be at least twice as efficient as a parallel design and require fewer than half as many subjects to achieve the same power.

Example 12.3. In Example 12.1, for a 2×2 crossover trial, the assumed variance parameters were $\sigma_B = 4$, $\sigma_W = 1$ and $\rho = 0.5$. The relative efficiency of a crossover design relative to a parallel group design, assuming equal allocation to each arm, can be calculated as

```
sigmaB <- 4
sigmaW <- 1
rho <- 0.5
varA <- sigmaB^2 + sigmaW^2 - rho * sigmaB^2
varB <- 2 * (sigmaB^2 + sigmaW^2)
re_AB <- varB / varA
re_AB
[1] 3.777778
```

The relative efficiency is about 3.8. Since $1/3.7778 = 0.26$, this implies that the crossover trial would require only about 26% as many subjects as the parallel group trial to achieve the same level of power, assuming that we do not have issues such as carryover effects or attrition.

Another way to compare efficiency is to compare the two designs when the number of subjects and the number of observations per subject is equal. We compare an TR/RT crossover design to a TT/RR design, in which each subject receives the same treatment twice and is measured for the outcome twice. Denote this design as Design C. Assuming n subjects in each arm, this design will have variance

$$Var(\hat{\theta}_C) = \frac{2\sigma_B^2 + \sigma_W^2}{n}.$$

Compared to the parallel design, the impact of the within-subject variance is reduced. The ratio of the variances is

$$\frac{Var(\hat{\theta}_C)}{Var(\hat{\theta}_A)} = \frac{2\sigma_B^2 + \sigma_W^2}{(1-\rho)\sigma_B^2 + \sigma_W^2}.$$

Example 12.4. We continue the previous example with the same parameter values. The relative efficiency of Design A compared to Design C is

```
varC <- 2 * sigmaB^2 + sigmaW^2
re_AC <- varC / varA
re_AC
[1] 3.666667
```

The crossover design is still highly efficient compared to the design without crossover. Having replicates within subjects reduced the impact of the within-subject variance, but did nothing to reduce the impact of between-subject variance, which tends to be the larger component of total variance.

12.5 Additional resources

Crossover studies can be quite complex and it is necessary to develop a detailed analysis plan when designing one. Such a plan could involve testing for carryover, period and/or sequence effects and specifying the course of action

Additional resources 215

if such effects are found, and assessing inter- and intra-subject variabilities. Investigators should consult authoritative texts such as Chow and Liu [32] when designing such trials.

The `PowerTOST` package supports sample size and power calculations for many different crossover designs. It focuses on bioequivalence studies and the defaults assume that the data are lognormal, although it can be used for normal data. The `crsize` function in the `designsize` package supports a range of crossover designs involving two sequences and two treatments, including replications.

We have focused on sample size and power for crossover designs for comparing means. Sample size and power for crossover designs for proportions are discussed in Chow et al. [33].

13
Multisite trials

13.1 Introduction

Many studies collect data from participants who are naturally grouped in some manner. They may be grouped by organization or site – for example, by school, worksite, clinic or community – or they may be grouped by having the same health care provider or other change agent. Two types of randomized study designs involving grouped participants can be distinguished. In a **multisite** or **multicenter trial**, subjects are randomized to conditions within each group; each group has some participants assigned to the intervention condition and some assigned to the control condition. In a **cluster or group randomized trial**, randomization occurs at the level of the group; each group is randomized to a condition, and all of the participants in a particular group are assigned to received the same condition.

Data from multisite and cluster randomized trials have a hierarchical or multilevel data structure, with participants nested within groups. Due to the multilevel structure of the data, such trials involve correlated data and can be more complex to design and analyze than trials with independent observations. In this chapter, we first discuss multilevel data structures in general, and then discuss power and sample size for multisite trials in particular. Cluster randomized trials are discussed in Chapters 14 and 15.

13.2 Multilevel data structure

Data from multisite trials and cluster randomized trials are examples of hierarchical or multilevel data. In multilevel data, observations are nested within higher order sampling units. For example, the observations may be of students nested within schools, patients nested within primary care providers, or measurement occasions nested within individuals. These are examples of hierarchical data with two levels. Further levels of nesting can occur; for example, we may have students nested within classrooms that are nested within schools. We will label the bottom level as Level 1, the next higher level as

Level 2, etc. Thus students at Level 1 may be nested within classrooms at Level 2 that are nested within schools at Level 3.

Data from a multisite or cluster randomized trial can be considered to have arisen from a **multistage sampling** design [207]. In a single stage sampling design, Level 1 units are sampled directly in one step. Simple random sampling is an example of single stage sampling. In two-stage sampling, we first sample Level 2 units and then sample Level 1 units within the selected Level 2 units. For example, we may select clinics and then sample patients within clinics. Multisite trials and cluster randomized trials can be considered a type of multistage sampling called **cluster sampling**. In cluster sampling, the population of interest is regarded as grouped into clusters (for example, clinics, schools or villages), clusters are sampled, and then individuals are sampled from the selected clusters.

When we directly sample the units of interest, such as when selecting a simple random sample, the observations can generally be considered statistically independent. When we use two-stage cluster sampling, after selecting the Level 2 units, the selection of Level 1 units becomes restricted to those belonging to the selected Level 2 units. For example, after we have selected clinics, only patients at the selected clinics have a positive probability of being selected into the study sample; patients in clinics that were not sampled have zero probability of being in the sample.

A consequence of multistage sampling is that observations within the same higher-level sampling unit cannot be regarded as independent of other observations within the same unit; rather, they should be considered potentially correlated. Thus, after we have selected clinics, outcomes of patients within the same clinic are not statistically independent of each other, but rather are likely to be correlated to some degree. At an intuitive level, patients from the same clinic are likely to share certain characteristics (e.g., health behaviors, age, socioeconomic background) that make their outcomes more similar to each other than they are to outcomes of patients from different clinics.

Correlation of outcomes within higher-level sampling units is a key feature of multilevel data and needs to be accounted for as part of a study design and analysis. In this chapter and the following chapters on cluster randomized trials, we present multilevel models for data from such studies and consider how the multilevel data structure affects power and sample size requirements.

13.3 Considerations for multisite trials

In a multisite or multicenter trial, sites are selected for the study and then subjects are randomized to conditions within each site. There are potential advantages and limitations to using a multisite design. Advantages include the opportunity to increase recruitment by enrolling participants from more sites and having results that are more generalizable, because they are obtained from a wider range of settings. A potential limitation is the risk that the control group may be "contaminated" with unintended exposure to the intervention. The potential for contamination depends on the type of intervention. An intervention involving personal interaction (e.g., education, training) involves more risk of contamination than interventions involving medication or surgery, for example. Contamination tends to reduce the differences between the conditions and make the intervention effect harder to detect.

Another consideration for multisite trials is that the treatment effect could vary across the sites, with treatment having a greater effect at some sites than at others. A term for this phenomenon is **heterogeneity of the treatment effect**. This can impact power, as we discuss.

The power and sample size methods described here for multisite trials are based on the work of Raudenbush and Liu [184], Moerbeek and Teerenstra [158], Liu [142] and Spybrook [210]. We confine our attention to trials with two conditions, which we label as treatment or intervention and control. Liu [142] discusses multisite trials with three conditions.

We note that in a multisite trial design, site can be considered a blocking variable. **Blocking** is the arranging of experimental units in groups (blocks) that are similar to one another on one or more characteristics. Observations are then allocated to conditions within blocks [233]. Randomizing subjects to conditions within blocks helps to ensure that levels of the blocking variables are balanced across conditions. A multisite trial design is more than a blocked design, however; in a multisite design, the participants can be considered cluster sampled rather than individually sampled, which makes their outcomes correlated; the sample is obtained by first sampling clusters (sites) and then measuring individuals within sites.

13.4 Model for continuous outcomes

Suppose that study participants are recruited from a number of different sites and are randomized to two conditions within each site. A model for a continuous outcome Y_{ij} of participant i in site j is

$$Y_{ij} = \beta_{0j} + \beta_{1j} x_{ij} + \epsilon_{ij} \qquad (13.1)$$

where $\epsilon_{ij} \sim \mathcal{N}(0, \sigma_\epsilon^2)$. We code the treatment indicator x_{ij} as -0.5 for participants in the control condition and 0.5 for participants in the intervention condition. This is a type of effect coding [128]. The coefficient β_{1j} represents the treatment effect at site j. Note that β_{1j} is the change in the mean of Y associated with a one-unit increase in x_{ij}, namely, going from -0.5 to 0.5. Due to the effect coding of x_{ij}, β_{0j} represents the average of the means for

Model for continuous outcomes

the control and intervention conditions for site j. It is analogous to a "grand mean" (mean of the group means) in ANOVA (see Section 5.2).

We model β_{0j} and β_{1j} as the sum of an average component and a site-specific deviation:

$$\beta_{0j} = \gamma_{00} + u_{0j} \qquad (13.2)$$
$$\beta_{1j} = \gamma_{10} + u_{1j}$$

The parameter γ_{00} is the grand mean across sites (mean of the site-level means) and u_{0j} is a random effect representing the difference between site j's mean and the grand mean. The parameter γ_{10} represents the average treatment effect across sites and u_{1j} is a random effect representing the difference between site j's treatment effect and the average treatment effect. We assume the random effects are normally distributed, $u_{0j} \sim \mathcal{N}(0, \sigma_{u0}^2)$ and $u_{1j} \sim \mathcal{N}(0, \sigma_{u1}^2)$, and are independent of each other and of ϵ_{ij}. The variance σ_{u0}^2 quantifies how much mean outcomes vary from site to site conditional on treatment condition and σ_{u1}^2 quantifies how much the treatment effect varies from site to site.

Substituting the site-level coefficient models (13.2) into the participant-level outcome model (13.1), we obtain a single-equation model

$$Y_{ij} = (\gamma_{00} + u_{0j}) + (\gamma_{10} + u_{1j})x_{ij} + \epsilon_{ij}. \qquad (13.3)$$

Observations on participants from the same site share the same random effects u_{0j} and u_{1j}, which induces correlation among these observations. Thus observations from the same site are correlated and observations from different sites are considered independent. The term $u_{1j}x_{ij}$ represents an interaction between site and treatment condition, allowing the treatment effect to vary by site.

Figure 13.1 shows simulated multisite trial data. Panel (A) shows data from a trial with no interaction between treatment condition and site, i.e., the treatment effect is the same at all sites. Panel (B) shows data from a trial with such an interaction, i.e., the treatment effect varies from site to site. Each data set has 10 sites and there are 10 intervention and 10 control participants at each site. Conceptually, the average treatment effect γ_{10} is estimated by estimating the treatment effect within each site and then taking the average across the sites. Note that when a condition-by-site interaction is present, the difference between the intervention and control means within sites is more variable; in the illustration, some site-specific treatment effects are as high as 12.8 and some are even negative. This additional variability tends to reduce power.

Interest in a multisite trial usually focuses on the mean treatment effect γ_{10}, and power and sample size procedures focus on rejecting the null hypothesis $H_0: \gamma_{10} = \gamma_{(0)}$. The value of $\gamma_{(0)}$ is zero for a test of nonequality; tests of noninferiority and superiority by a margin can be conducted by setting $\gamma_{(0)} = m$ and conducting a one-sided test as discussed in Chapter 4. Power for

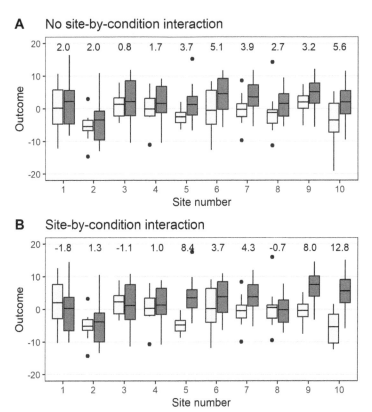

FIGURE 13.1: Data from a multisite trial (A) without and (B) with a site-by-condition interaction. Color represents condition (dark grey is intervention, light grey is control). Each boxplot summarizes data from 10 subjects. Intervention and control means within site are indicated by black lines within each box. Site level treatment effects β_{1j} are provided above the boxplots. When a site-by-condition interaction is present, the site level treatment effects are more variable.

testing hypotheses about γ_{10} are discussed in Section 13.6. It may also be of interest to test for the presence of heterogeneity of the treatment effect. Such tests involve the variance of the treatment effect, σ_{u1}^2; power and sample size procedures for such tests are discussed in Section 13.7.

Before discussing hypothesis testing and power and sample size procedures, we discuss the correlated data structure of a multisite trial and how it can be characterized using intraclass correlation coefficients. This is important for understanding and computing power.

13.5 Intraclass correlation coefficient

In multilevel models, variation in an outcome variable arises due to variation at two levels, variation of the mean outcome across sites and variation in outcomes of participants within the same site. Intraclass correlation coefficients (ICCs) are used to quantify how this variation is apportioned between levels.

To define the ICCs for multisite trial data, we start by finding the total variance of the outcome for individual i at site j, denoted σ_Y^2, as

$$Var(Y_{ij}) = Var(\gamma_{00} + u_{0j} + \gamma_{10}x_{ij} + u_{1j}x_{ij} + \epsilon_{ij}) \quad (13.4)$$
$$= Var(u_{0j} + u_{1j}x_{ij} + \epsilon_{ij})$$
$$= \sigma_{u0}^2 + \frac{1}{4}\sigma_{u1}^2 + \sigma_\epsilon^2.$$

Thus the total variance σ_Y^2 is the sum of the variance of the site-level means, $\sigma_{u0}^2 + \frac{1}{4}\sigma_{u1}^2$, and the variance of observations within sites, σ_ϵ^2. The variance of the site-level means has two components: σ_{u0}^2 arises from the random site effect and $\frac{1}{4}\sigma_{u1}^2$ arises from the random site-by-condition interaction. The factor of $\frac{1}{4}$ comes from squaring x_{ij}, which takes value -0.5 or 0.5. The ICC is defined as the proportion of the total variance that is due to variance at the site level,

$$\rho = \frac{\sigma_{u0}^2 + \frac{1}{4}\sigma_{u1}^2}{\sigma_{u0}^2 + \frac{1}{4}\sigma_{u1}^2 + \sigma_\epsilon^2}. \quad (13.5)$$

It can be shown that the ICC is also the correlation between two observations from the same site and in the same condition. ICC values vary between 0 and 1, with larger values indicating higher correlation of outcomes within site.

The ICC can be split into two parts, $\rho = \rho_0 + \rho_1$, where ρ_0 is the proportion of the variance that is due to the random site effect and ρ_1 is the proportion due to the random site-by-treatment interaction,

$$\rho = \rho_0 + \rho_1 = \frac{\sigma_{u0}^2}{\sigma_{u0}^2 + \frac{1}{4}\sigma_{u1}^2 + \sigma_\epsilon^2} + \frac{\frac{1}{4}\sigma_{u1}^2}{\sigma_{u0}^2 + \frac{1}{4}\sigma_{u1}^2 + \sigma_\epsilon^2}. \quad (13.6)$$

Example 13.1. For Figure 13.1, data were simulated from a model in which $\sigma_\epsilon^2 = 36, \sigma_{u0}^2 = 4$ and $\sigma_{u1}^2 = 0$ or 8. When there is no site-by-condition interaction ($\sigma_{u1}^2 = 0$), the total variance of an observation is $Var(Y_{ij}) = 4 + 36 = 40$ and $\rho = \rho_0 = 4/40 = 0.1$. When there is a site-by-condition interaction ($\sigma_{u1}^2 = 8$), $Var(Y_{ij}) = 42$ and the ICCs are $\rho_0 = 0.095$ and $\rho_1 = 0.048$, with $\rho = \rho_0 + \rho_1 = 0.143$.

Power formulas for multisite trials will generally involve either ICC values or values for the variance components, as we will see in the following sections.

13.6 Power for test of average treatment effect

In this section, we develop an expression for power for testing the null hypothesis that the average treatment effect is equal to a specified value, $H_0: \gamma_{10} = \gamma_{(0)}$. As the first step, we derive an estimate of the average treatment effect $\hat{\gamma}_{10}$ and its standard error, based on Raudenbush and Liu [184].

Suppose that there are J total sites and m participants at each site, and that they are assigned 1:1 to intervention and control conditions within each site. Unequal allocation and unequal numbers of participants per site are discussed in Sections 13.6.1 and 13.6.5. We estimate the treatment effect at each site and then average across sites to get the estimated average treatment effect $\hat{\gamma}_{10}$. In a balanced design with $m/2$ participants in each condition at each site, we can estimate the treatment effect at site j as the difference in the sample means for the treatment and control participants at the site, denoted as $\bar{Y}_{jT}$ and $\bar{Y}_{jC}$:

$$\hat{\beta}_{1j} = \bar{Y}_{jT} - \bar{Y}_{jC} = \frac{1}{m/2} \sum_{i=1}^{m/2} Y_{ijT} - \frac{1}{m/2} \sum_{i=m/2+1}^{m} Y_{ijC}$$

The average treatment effect is the mean of the site-specific treatment effects,

$$\hat{\gamma}_{10} = \frac{1}{J} \sum_{j=1}^{J} \hat{\beta}_{1j}. \tag{13.7}$$

Due to independence across sites, $Var(\hat{\gamma}_{10}) = \frac{1}{J} Var(\hat{\beta}_{1j})$, where $Var(\hat{\beta}_{1j}) = \frac{4\sigma_\epsilon^2}{m} + \sigma_{u1}^2$. This is the sum of the variance of the treatment effect within a site and the variance of the treatment effect across sites. Thus we can find that

$$Var(\hat{\gamma}_{10}) = \frac{\frac{4\sigma_\epsilon^2}{m} + \sigma_{u1}^2}{J} = \frac{4(\sigma_\epsilon^2 + \frac{1}{4}m\sigma_{u1}^2)}{mJ}. \tag{13.8}$$

The test statistic for testing $H_0: \gamma_{10} = \gamma_{(0)}$ is

$$T = \frac{\hat{\gamma}_{10} - \gamma_{(0)}}{\sqrt{Var(\hat{\gamma}_{10})}}. \tag{13.9}$$

When H_0 is true, T is distributed as $t(J-1)$. When some alternative $\gamma_{10} = \gamma_{(A)}$ is true, T has a noncentral t distribution, $T \sim t(J-1, \lambda)$, where the noncentrality parameter has the form

$$\lambda = \frac{\gamma_{(A)} - \gamma_{(0)}}{\sqrt{Var(\hat{\gamma}_{10})}} = \frac{\gamma_{(A)} - \gamma_{(0)}}{\sqrt{\frac{4\sigma_\epsilon^2/m + \sigma_{u1}^2}{J}}}. \tag{13.10}$$

There are several other ways to express λ, which we discuss shortly.

Power for test of average treatment effect

What factors affect power? As discussed in earlier chapters, power increases as the magnitude of the noncentrality parameter increases. As either of the variance components σ_ϵ^2 or σ_{u1}^2 increases, λ decreases and power is lower. As the sample size per site, m, or the number of sites, J, increases, power will increase. However, J is more influential than m; J affects the entire noncentrality parameter whereas m only affects the contribution of σ_ϵ^2.

Standardized effect size. The treatment effect in (13.10) is on the scale of the outcome variable. We can derive a standardized version of the treatment effect as follows. In Chapter 3, we defined the standardized effect size d as the difference between the intervention and control means in units of standard deviation of the outcome variable. For multisite trials, the total variance of Y, σ_Y^2, is given in equation (13.4). The standardized effect size can be defined as

$$d = \frac{\gamma_{(A)} - \gamma_{(0)}}{\sigma_Y} = \frac{\gamma_{(A)} - \gamma_{(0)}}{\sqrt{\sigma_{u0}^2 + \frac{1}{4}\sigma_{u1}^2 + \sigma_\epsilon^2}}. \quad (13.11)$$

Using d and the definitions of the ICCs in Section 13.5, we can express the noncentrality parameter as

$$\lambda = \frac{d}{\sqrt{\frac{4[1-\rho_0+(m-1)\rho_1]}{mJ}}}. \quad (13.12)$$

It is sometimes easier to specify the values of d and the ICCs than to specify the values of the variance components σ_{u1}^2 and σ_ϵ^2.

What factors affect power? *(continued)* Examination of expression (13.12) for λ indicates that the effects of the two ICCs on power are different. ρ_0 quantifies the proportion of the total variance of Y that is attributable to variation in site-level means, conditional on treatment condition, and as it increases, power increases. ρ_1 quantifies the proportion of the total variance of Y that is attributable to variation in the treatment effect across sites, and as it increases, power is reduced. The impact of ρ_1 tends to be larger than that of ρ_0 because it is multiplied by $m-1$. We can also infer that for a fixed total number of participants, $N = mJ$, combinations of m and J with larger values of m (i.e., more participants per site) will result in lower power.

Another approach to standardizing the treatment effect is to divide $\gamma_{(A)} - \gamma_{(0)}$ by the within-site standard deviation σ_ϵ rather than σ_Y. We denote this version of the standardized treatment effect as $d_\epsilon = (\gamma_{(A)} - \gamma_{(0)})/\sigma_\epsilon$; see, for example, Spybrook et al. [210]. With this approach, the noncentrality parameter becomes

$$\lambda = \frac{d_\epsilon}{\sqrt{\frac{\frac{4}{m}+VR}{J}}} \quad (13.13)$$

where $VR = \sigma_{u1}^2/\sigma_\epsilon^2$ is the variance ratio. This version of λ requires specification of only the variance ratio rather than both σ_{u1}^2 and σ_ϵ^2. In general, we expect that the within-site variance of individuals will be considerably larger than the variance between site means, with reasonable VRs in the range of 0.05–0.25. Because σ_ϵ^2 will tend to comprise a large percentage of the total variance σ_Y^2, d_ϵ will tend to be only slightly larger than d.

What factors affect power? *(continued)* Expression (13.13) adds the insight that power depends on the variance ratio. When VR is higher, λ is lower and power is reduced. VR is higher when there is more heterogeneity of the treatment effect across sites.

Power for average treatment effect. Power can be calculated as follows using any of the expressions (13.10), (13.12) or (13.13) for λ:

$$\text{Power (lower-tail test)} = P[T \leq t_{\alpha,J-1} \mid T \sim t(J-1,\lambda)] \quad (13.14)$$
$$= \mathcal{T}_{J-1,\lambda}(t_{\alpha,J-1})$$
$$\text{Power (upper-tail test)} = P[T \geq t_{1-\alpha,J-1} \mid T \sim t(J-1,\lambda)]$$
$$= 1 - \mathcal{T}_{J-1,\lambda}(t_{1-\alpha,J-1})$$
$$\text{Power (two-sided test)} = P[T^2 \geq f_{1-\alpha,1,J-1} \mid T^2 \sim F(1,J-1,\Lambda)]$$
$$= 1 - \mathcal{F}_{1,J-1,\Lambda}(f_{1-\alpha,1,J-1})$$

where $\Lambda = \lambda^2$. For a lower-tailed test, we expect $\lambda < 0$ and for an upper-tailed test, we expect $\lambda > 0$. Note that the degrees of freedom for the t and F distributions depend on the number of sites J.

Example 13.2. In Example 13.1, with simulated data displayed in Figure 13.1, there are $J = 10$ sites and $m = 20$ individuals per site with equal allocation, and the value of γ_{10} is 3. Suppose we wish to test $H_0: \gamma_{10} = 0$ with two-sided $\alpha = 0.05$. For the no-interaction and site-by-condition interaction scenarios, we have the following parameters:

	No interaction	Interaction
σ_ϵ^2	36	36
σ_{u0}^2	4	4
σ_{u1}^2	0	8
σ_Y^2	40	48
ρ_0	0.1	0.095
ρ_1	0	0.048
ρ	0.1	0.143
d	0.47	0.43
d_ϵ	0.50	0.50
VR	0	0.22
λ	3.536	2.493

The `multisite.cont` function computes power based on noncentrality parameter (13.12). For the no-interaction scenario, power can be computed as:

Power for test of average treatment effect 225

```
library(powertools)
multisite.cont(m = 20, J = 10, delta = 3, sd = sqrt(40), icc0 = 0.1,
   icc1 = 0, power = NULL)
[1] 0.8810671
```

Power is about 0.88. For the scenario with a site-by-condition interaction, power can be calculated as:

```
multisite.cont(m = 20, J = 10, delta = 3, sd = sqrt(48), icc0 = 0.095,
   icc1 = 0.048, power = NULL)
[1] 0.5268002
```

The power is considerably lower. This illustrates that the presence of a site-by-condition interaction can greatly reduce power. Note that in this scenario, the variance ratio $VR = \sigma_{u1}^2/\sigma_\epsilon^2$ is 0.22, which is large (see page 224) and indicates a high level of variability of the treatment effect from site to site.

13.6.1 Unequal allocation

Suppose that participants are allocated to treatment and control conditions within site such that $n_T/n_C = r$. Let $c = (1+r)^2/r$. Then $Var(\hat{\beta}_{1j}) = c\sigma_\epsilon^2/m + \sigma_{u1}^2$ and the noncentrality parameter can be expressed as

$$\lambda = \frac{\gamma_{(A)} - \gamma_{(0)}}{\sqrt{\frac{\frac{c\sigma_\epsilon^2}{m}+\sigma_{u1}^2}{J}}} = \frac{d}{\sqrt{\frac{c[1-\rho_0+(\frac{4m}{c}-1)\rho_1]}{mJ}}} = \frac{d_\epsilon}{\sqrt{\frac{c+mVR}{mJ}}}. \quad (13.15)$$

These versions of λ can be used in the power formulas (13.14).

Example 13.3. Suppose that for the trial in Example 13.2 we wish to allocate to intervention and control at each site with a 3:2 ratio. We use the condition-by-site interaction scenario. The power can be computed as follows:

```
multisite.cont(m = 20, alloc.ratio = 1.5, J = 10, delta = 0.43,
   sd = 1, icc0 = 0.095, icc1 = 0.048, power = NULL)
[1] 0.513528
```

Power is slightly lower than the power under equal allocation. Recall that for a two-sample comparison of means with equal variance, unequal allocation reduces power; see Section 3.2.4. We are assuming equal variance for treatment and control participants in these calculations and the same result applies.

13.6.2 Specifying ICC values

How can we select reasonable values for ρ_0 and ρ_1? Unfortunately, it can be difficult to find ICC values from multisite trials in the literature. If data from a pilot study or other prior studies are available, information on likely ICC values might be gleaned from them. Some reports suggest that ρ_0 values in the range of 0–0.15 are reasonable [223]. Since larger values of ρ_0 tend to increase power, it is important not to overestimate the value of ρ_0 used in a calculation to avoid overestimating power.

Raudenbush and Liu [184] propose 0.05, 0.10, and 0.15 as small, medium, and large ρ_1. This is based on reasoning about the dispersion of the site-specific standardized effect sizes that are implied by these values. An ICC of 0.05 implies that the standardized effect sizes across sites have a standard deviation of $\sqrt{0.05} \approx 0.22$. If site-specific effect sizes are normally distributed, we can expect about 95% of them to lie within ± 2 standard deviations of the mean effect size, and the range of site-specific standardized effect sizes (maximum minus minimum) should be about 4 SDs, in this case, about 0.88. Similarly, an ICC of 0.10 implies a standard deviation of $\sqrt{0.10} \approx 0.32$ and a range of about 1.26; and an ICC of 0.15 implies a standard deviation of $\sqrt{0.15} \approx 0.40$ and a range of about 1.6, which would reflect a great deal of variability in the effect sizes across sites. In general, values of ρ_1 that are "small" by these rules of thumb are probably reasonable to expect for most studies.

Example 13.4. In the site-by-condition interaction scenario of Example 13.1, ρ_1 is 0.048. This value implies that the range of site-specific standardized effect sizes (maximum minus minimum) is about $\sqrt{0.048} \times 4 \approx 0.88$. If we expected the mean standardized effect size to be 0.4, most of the site-specific standardized effect sizes would be expected to be within the interval $(-0.04, 0.84)$.

13.6.3 Design effect for multisite trial

For a multisite trial with equal allocation, the variance of the treatment effect estimator is, according to equation (13.8),

$$Var(\hat{\gamma}_{10}) = \frac{4(\sigma_\epsilon^2 + \frac{1}{4}m\sigma_{u1}^2)}{mJ}. \tag{13.16}$$

If the mJ observations were independent, the variance of the treatment effect estimator would be $4\sigma_Y^2/(mJ)$. The ratio of the variances is

$$\text{DE}_{\text{MS}} = \frac{\sigma_\epsilon^2 + \frac{1}{4}m\sigma_{u1}^2}{\sigma_Y^2} = 1 - \rho_0 + (m-1)\rho_1. \tag{13.17}$$

This is called the **design effect for a multisite trial**; it is the multiplicative factor by which the variance of the estimated treatment effect is changed due to the multisite design. Note that this design effect appears in formula (13.12) for the noncentrality parameter. For unequal allocation, the design effect is $1 - \rho_0 + (4m/c - 1)\rho_1$, where $c = (1+r)^2/r$ and $r = n_T/n_C$.

$\text{DE}_{\text{MS}} > 1$ implies that the multisite design is less efficient than a randomized trial with independent subjects and will require more total subjects for the same power. $\text{DE}_{\text{MS}} < 1$ implies that the multisite design is more efficient and will require fewer total subjects for the same power. Whether DE_{MS} is greater than or less than 1 depends on the relative values of ρ_0 and ρ_1. The DE_{MS} will exceed 1 if $(m-1)\rho_1 > \rho_0$ and be less than 1 if $(m-1)\rho_1 < \rho_0$ [158]. Thus a multisite trial has the potential to be more or less efficient than a randomized trial with the same number of independent subjects.

13.6.4 Sample size using normal approximation

If $\rho_0 = \rho_1 = 0$ or $m = 1$, $\text{DE}_{\text{MS}} = 1$ and the study design is equivalent to a two independent sample comparison of means, for which we could use a two-sample t test. Let N_{indep} denote the sample size for a two-sample t test derived using a normal approximation. Then the total sample size required for a multisite trial can be approximated as

$$N_{\text{MS}} \geq N_{\text{indep}} \text{DE}_{\text{MS}} \qquad (13.18)$$

where N_{MS} is the total number of participants, mJ. For example, using a two-sample t test with equal variances and equal allocation to calculate N_{indep}, the normal approximation sample size formula is

$$N_{\text{MS}} \geq N_{\text{indep}} \text{DE}_{\text{MS}} = \frac{4(z_{1-\alpha/2} + z_{1-\beta})^2}{d^2}[1 - \rho_0 + (m-1)\rho_1]. \qquad (13.19)$$

N_{MS} should be rounded up to the next whole number that is a multiple of m. As noted elsewhere, a normal approximation-based sample size calculation can underestimate the sample size required. The accuracy of the approximation increases as the degrees of freedom for the T statistic increase.

Often, when the outcome is continuous, the outcome variable will also be measured on the participants at baseline, and the analysis will adjusted for the baseline measurement. This typically increases power, as discussed in Section 13.6.6.

Example 13.5. We conduct a sample size calculation for a multisite trial using the design effect approach and using the more precise calculation. We assume a two-sided test at $\alpha = 0.05$, 80% power, 10 participants per site and equal allocation. We expect $d = 0.5$, $\rho_0 = 0$ and $\rho_1 = 0.05$. How many sites do we need? Using the design effect approach,

```
N_indep <- 4 * (qnorm(p = 0.975) + qnorm(p = 0.8))^2 / 0.5^2 ; N_indep
[1] 125.5821
DE_ms <- 1 - 0 + (10 - 1) * 0.05  ;  DE_ms
[1] 1.45
# use round_any function to round up to next multiple of 10:
library(plyr)
N_ms <- round_any(N_indep * DE_ms, 10, ceiling) ; N_ms
[1] 190
```

The design effect is 1.45, implying a need to inflate the sample size by 45%. After rounding up to the next multiple of 10, we estimate N_{MS} of 190. With $m = 10$, this equates to 19 sites. We get the more precise calculation provided by `multisite.cont` for comparison:

```
library(powertools)
multisite.cont(m = 10, J = NULL, delta = 0.5, sd = 1, icc0 = 0,
    icc1 = 0.05, power = 0.8)
[1] 20.21409
```

The more precise calculation suggests that we need 21 sites to have at least 80% power. The normal approximation result was similar but underestimated the number of sites required.

13.6.5 Unequal number of participants per site

Thus far we have assumed that the number of participants per site is equal. In practice, the number of participants often varies from site to site, which can increase the variance of the treatment effect estimator, resulting in a loss of efficiency and power [9]. We can quantify this loss of power by examining the relative efficiency (RE) of a multisite trial with unequal site sizes compared to one with equal sizes, when each has the same total sample size N.

Recall from Section 3.3 that the relative efficiency of Design A to Design B for estimating a parameter θ is the ratio of the variances, $\text{RE}(\hat{\theta}_A, \hat{\theta}_B) = Var(\hat{\theta}_B)/Var(\hat{\theta}_A)$, and that the RE also gives the ratio of the sample sizes required to achieve the same power under the two designs, $\text{RE}(\hat{\theta}_A, \hat{\theta}_B) = N_B/N_A$, when $Var(\hat{\theta}) \propto 1/N$, which is often the case. Denote the mean and standard deviation of site sizes as $\tilde{m}$ and $\tilde{s}$ so that $\text{CV} = \tilde{s}/\tilde{m}$ is the coefficient of variation of site size. Define $\rho_1^* = \frac{1}{4}\sigma_{u1}^2/(\frac{1}{4}\sigma_{u1}^2 + \sigma_\epsilon^2)$ and $K = \tilde{m}\rho_1^*/(1 + (\tilde{m} - 1)\rho_1^*)$. According to van Breukelen et al. [220], the relative efficiency is approximately

$$\text{RE}(\hat{\gamma}_{10}^{\text{uneq}}, \hat{\gamma}_{10}^{\text{eq}}) \approx 1 - \text{CV}^2 K(1 - K)$$

where $\hat{\gamma}_{10}^{\text{uneq}}$ and $\hat{\gamma}_{10}^{\text{eq}}$ are the variances of the treatment effect estimators under unequal and equal site sizes. The RE will be less than 1 unless $\tilde{s} = 0$ (i.e., no variation in site size). Note that ρ_1^* will generally be slightly larger than $\rho_1 = \frac{1}{4}\sigma_{u1}^2/(\sigma_{u0}^2 + \frac{1}{4}\sigma_{u1}^2 + \sigma_\epsilon^2)$. For practical purposes, one can set $\rho_1^* = \rho_1$.

To adjust a power calculation for the loss of power due to unequal site sizes, $Var(\hat{\gamma}_{01})$ in the noncentrality parameter should be divided by the RE. The `multisite.cont` function incorporates this functionality. For more discussion of the impact of varying cluster sizes, including alternative approximations of the RE, see [192, 220, 221].

Example 13.6. In Example 13.2, we had 20 subjects per site. Suppose that the number of subjects per site is expected to vary from 8 to 80 with a mean of 20. We can approximate the standard deviation of cluster size using the range rule (see page 181) as $(\max - \min)/4 = (80 - 8)/4 = 18$. We calculate power as follows:

```
library(powertools)
multisite.cont(m = 20, m.sd = 18, J = 10, delta = 3, sd = sqrt(48),
    icc0 = 0.095, icc1 = 0.048, power = NULL)
[1] 0.4411947
```

The power assuming equal site sizes was about 0.53. Thus power has been reduced due to varying site sizes.

13.6.6 Adjusting for an individual-level covariate

As discussed in Section 5.4, adjusting for a covariate can potentially reduce residual variance and thus increase the precision of the estimated treatment effect. When we add a person-level covariate v_{ij} to model (13.3), the model becomes

$$Y_{ij} = (\gamma_{00} + u_{0j}) + (\gamma_{10} + u_{1j})x_{ij} + \gamma_{20}v_{ij} + \tilde{\epsilon}_{ij} \qquad (13.20)$$

where γ_{20} is the regression coefficient associated with the covariate v_{ij}. When a covariate is added, the residual error may change; thus the error term is denoted as $\tilde{\epsilon}_{ij}$ in this model and we denote the new error variance as $\tilde{\sigma}_\epsilon^2$. If the proportion of the outcome variance that is explained by the covariate is $\rho_{Y|V}^2$, the error variance will be reduced by a factor of $1 - \rho_{Y|V}^2$:

$$\tilde{\sigma}_\epsilon^2 = (1 - \rho_{Y|V}^2)\sigma_\epsilon^2;$$

see Schochet [196]. Power can be calculated by using $\tilde{\sigma}_\epsilon^2$ rather than σ_ϵ^2 in the noncentrality parameter formula (13.10) or (13.13); see Spybrook et al. [210]. Note that the estimated treatment effect will now be adjusted for the covariate.

The degrees of freedom for the test of the covariate will have degrees of freedom that depends on the number of subjects; however, the degrees of freedom for the test of the treatment effect will be minimally affected.

Example 13.7. Continuing Example 13.6, suppose we plan to adjust for a baseline covariate. The covariate is expected to have correlation of about 0.4 with the outcome variable. In the case of a single covariate, the proportion of the variance of the outcome variable that is explained by the covariate is $0.4^2 = 0.16$ (see Section 5.4). This is inputted as the Rsq value:

```
library(powertools)
multisite.cont(m = 20, m.sd = 18, J = 10, delta = 3, sd = sqrt(48),
    icc0 = 0.095, icc1 = 0.048, Rsq = 0.16, power = NULL)
[1] 0.5062721
```

Power has increased due to adjustment for the covariate.

13.7 Power for test of heterogeneity of treatment effect

A key feature of multisite trials is that the treatment effect can vary from site to site. This treatment effect heterogeneity is quantified by the variance of the site-level treatment effects, σ_{u1}^2. A test for treatment effect heterogeneity tests $H_0: \sigma_{u1}^2 = 0$ versus $H_A: \sigma_{u1}^2 > 0$. We discuss power for this test in this section, based on Raudenbush and Liu [184] and Liu [142].

Having adequate power for testing the average treatment effect is usually the main concern of a multisite study, and testing for heterogeneity may be a secondary objective. Thus while we may want to compute power for a treatment effect heterogeneity test, power for this test usually does not drive the decision about sample size.

Recall that, at a conceptual level, the average treatment effect in a multisite trial is estimated by obtaining the estimated treatment effect at each site, $\hat{\beta}_{1j}$ for $j = 1, \ldots, J$, and then obtaining the average of these site-specific effects as $\hat{\gamma}_{01} = \frac{1}{J} \sum_{j=1}^{J} \hat{\beta}_{1j}$; see Section 13.6. (In reality, this simple approach only works with perfectly balanced data.) Consider the conditional variance of $\hat{\beta}_{1j}$ given β_{1j}; this is the variance of the treatment effect estimator at a single site j. The conditional variance is $Var(\hat{\beta}_{1j}|\beta_{1j}) = 4\sigma_\epsilon^2/m$. We can contrast the conditional variance with the unconditional variance $Var(\hat{\beta}_{1j})$, which is the overall variance of $\hat{\beta}_{1j}$ across all sites, which is $Var(\hat{\beta}_{1j}) = 4\sigma_\epsilon^2/m + \sigma_{u1}^2$ (see Section 13.6). The term σ_{u1}^2 accounts for the variance of the treatment effect across sites. We can estimate these variances from the data as (see [184])

$$\widehat{Var}(\hat{\beta}_{1j}|\beta_{1j}) = \frac{4\hat{\sigma}_\epsilon^2}{m}$$

$$\widehat{Var}(\hat{\beta}_{1j}) = \frac{1}{J-1}\sum_{j=1}^{J}(\hat{\beta}_{1j} - \hat{\gamma}_{10})^2 = \frac{4\hat{\sigma}_\epsilon^2}{m} + \hat{\sigma}_{u1}^2$$

where

$$\hat{\sigma}_\epsilon^2 = \frac{1}{J(m-2)}\sum_{j=1}^{J}\sum_{i=1}^{m}[Y_{ij} - (\hat{\beta}_{0j} + \hat{\beta}_{1j}x_{ij})]^2.$$

A test of $H_0: \sigma_{u1}^2 = 0$ versus $H_A: \sigma_{u1}^2 > 0$ can be conducted using the test statistic

$$W = \frac{\widehat{Var}(\hat{\beta}_{1j})}{\widehat{Var}(\hat{\beta}_{1j}|\beta_{1j})} = \frac{4\hat{\sigma}_\epsilon^2/m + \hat{\sigma}_{u1}^2}{4\hat{\sigma}_\epsilon^2/m}. \tag{13.21}$$

It can be shown that

$$E(4\hat{\sigma}_\epsilon^2/m + \hat{\sigma}_{u1}^2) = 4\sigma_\epsilon^2/m + \sigma_{u1}^2$$
$$E(4\hat{\sigma}_\epsilon^2/m) = 4\sigma_\epsilon^2/m$$

and that

$$\frac{4\hat{\sigma}_\epsilon^2/m + \hat{\sigma}_{u1}^2}{4\sigma_\epsilon^2/m + \sigma_{u1}^2} \sim \chi^2(J-1) \quad \text{and} \quad \frac{4\hat{\sigma}_\epsilon^2/m}{4\sigma_\epsilon^2/m} \sim \chi^2(J(m-2)),$$

and the two random variables are independent. Defining

$$\omega = \frac{4\sigma_\epsilon^2/m + \sigma_{u1}^2}{4\sigma_\epsilon^2/m},$$

W/ω has a central F distribution with $J-1$ and $J(m-2)$ degrees of freedom [184]. When $H_0: \sigma_{u1}^2 = 0$ is true, $\omega = 1$ and $W \sim F(J-1, J(m-2))$. The null hypothesis is rejected at level α if $W > f_{1-\alpha, J-1, J(m-2)}$. When ω equals some alternative value $\omega_A > 1$, W/ω_A also has a central F distribution with the same degrees of freedom. Power can be computed as

$$P(W > f_*) = P\left(\frac{W}{\omega_A} > \frac{1}{\omega_A}f_*\right) = P\left(F > \frac{1}{\omega_A}f_*\right) \tag{13.22}$$

$$= 1 - \mathcal{F}_{J-1, J(m-2)}\left(\frac{1}{\omega_A}f_*\right)$$

where $f_* = f_{1-\alpha, J-1, J(m-2)}$.

What factors affect power? Power for the test of treatment effect heterogeneity is determined by the value of ω_A as well as the sample sizes at the two levels, m and J, which appear in the degrees of freedom of the F statistic. There are several ways that ω can be expressed. We have

$$\omega = \frac{4\sigma_\epsilon^2/m + \sigma_{u1}^2}{4\sigma_\epsilon^2/m} = \frac{4\sigma_\epsilon^2 + m\sigma_{u1}^2}{4\sigma_\epsilon^2} = 1 + \frac{m\sigma_{u1}^2}{4\sigma_\epsilon^2} = 1 + \frac{m}{4}VR$$

where $VR = \sigma_{u1}^2/\sigma_\epsilon^2$; see Section 13.6. Thus ω_A can be specified using m and VR. More subjects per site or larger VR increases ω_A and the power of the test. The number of sites J affects power through the degrees of freedom of the F distribution. Raudenbush and Liu [184] provide more discussion.

Note that higher values of VR increase the power to detect heterogeneity of the treatment effect but decrease the power for a test of the average treatment effect. Usually, adequate power for testing the average treatment effect is the main concern of a study, and testing for heterogeneity of the treatment effect is a secondary concern.

Example 13.8. A multisite trial will have 30 sites and 10 subjects per site, with equal allocation to two conditions. If the true values of σ_{u1}^2 and σ_ϵ^2 are 8 and 36, what is the power to detect treatment effect heterogeneity?

```
library(powertools)
multisite.hte(m = 10, J = 30, VR = 8 / 36, v = TRUE)

Power for test of heterogeneity of treatment effect in multisite trials

     m1, m2 = 5, 5
          J = 30
         VR = 0.2222222
      alpha = 0.05
      power = 0.5087035

NOTE: m1, m2 are the number of subjects within site in condition 1,
    condition 2 (total of m1 + m2 per site)
```

The power is about 51%. Note that the variance ratio is 0.22, which is considered to be relatively large (see page 224). Power to detect heterogeneity will often be low, but this is usually not the primary objective.

13.8 Binary outcomes

We discuss power for binary outcomes in multisite trials based largely on Moerbeek et al. [161] and Moerbeek and Teerenstra [158]. For a binary outcome

Binary outcomes

$Y_{ij} = 0, 1$ in a multisite trial, one can use the multilevel logistic regression model

$$\log\left(\frac{P(Y_{ij} = 1 | x_{ij}, u_{0j}, u_{1j})}{1 - P(Y_{ij} = 1 | x_{ij}, u_{0j}, u_{1j})}\right) = (\gamma_{00} + u_{0j}) + (\gamma_{10} + u_{1j})x_{ij}$$

where $x_{ij} = 0.5$ if individual i at site j is in the intervention condition and $x_{ij} = -0.5$ if in the control condition, and u_{0j} and u_{1j} are normally distributed random effects with $u_{0j} \sim \mathcal{N}(0, \sigma_{u0}^2)$ and $u_{1j} \sim \mathcal{N}(0, \sigma_{u1}^2)$, assumed to be independent of each other. For expected outcome proportions p_T and p_C in the treatment and control conditions, γ_{00} is the average of the log odds, $[\log(p_T/(1-p_T)) + \log(p_C/(1-p_C))]/2$, and γ_{10} is the log odds ratio (OR), $\log\left[\frac{p_T/(1-p_T)}{p_C/(1-p_C)}\right]$. The random effect u_{0j} allows the average of the log odds to differ across sites; we can think of it as allowing the baseline probability of the outcome to differ across sites. The random effect u_{1j} allows the log odds ratio to vary across sites.

The log odds ratio γ_{10} is the parameter of interest for estimating the treatment effect. The variance of $\hat{\gamma}_{10}$ can be estimated as [161]

$$Var(\hat{\gamma}_{10}) \approx 1.2 \times \frac{4(\sigma_\epsilon^2 + \frac{1}{4}m\sigma_{u1}^2)}{mJ} \tag{13.23}$$

where σ_ϵ^2 is a subject-level variance component, which can be calculated as

$$\sigma_\epsilon^2 = \frac{1}{4}\left[\frac{1}{(1-\pi_T)p_C(1-p_C)} + \frac{1}{\pi_T p_T(1-p_T)}\right] \tag{13.24}$$

where π_T is the proportion of participants randomized to the treatment condition. Expression (13.23) for the variance is equivalent to that for continuous outcomes in equation (13.8), with substitution of the expression for σ_ϵ^2 and multiplication by a factor of 1.2 to improve accuracy; see [161] for details.

Suppose we wish to test $H_0: \gamma_{10} = \gamma_{(0)}$. Asymptotically, the test statistic

$$Z = \frac{\hat{\gamma}_{10} - \gamma_{(0)}}{\sqrt{\widehat{Var}(\hat{\gamma}_{10})}}$$

has a standard normal distribution when the null hypothesis is true. Power can be approximated as

$$\Phi\left(\frac{|\gamma_{(A)} - \gamma_{(0)}|}{\sqrt{1.2 \times \frac{4(\sigma_\epsilon^2 + \frac{1}{4}m\sigma_{u1}^2)}{mJ}}} - z_{1-\alpha}\right) \tag{13.25}$$

for a one-sided test. The required number of sites given site size m can be approximated as

$$J \geq \frac{(z_{1-\alpha} + z_{1-\beta})^2 \times 1.2 \times \left[4\left(\frac{\sigma_\epsilon^2}{m} + \frac{1}{4}\sigma_{u1}^2\right)\right]}{(\gamma_{(A)} - \gamma_{(0)})^2}. \tag{13.26}$$

For two-sided tests, substitute $\alpha/2$ for α.

Selecting plausible values of σ_{u1}^2. To use formula (13.25) or (13.26), a value for σ_{u1}^2 is needed. This parameter is the variance of the treatment effect across sites, with the treatment effect on the log odds scale. To arrive at a plausible estimate, we can reason as follows [158]. Because the treatment effects across sites are expected to be normally distributed with mean γ_{01} and variance σ_{u1}^2, we expect that about 95% of the sites will have treatment effects, on the log odds scale, that lie in the interval $(\gamma_{01} - 1.96\sigma_{u1}, \gamma_{01} + 1.96\sigma_{u1})$. To get the interval on the more familiar odds ratio scale, we exponentiate the endpoints and obtain $\left[e^{\gamma_{01} - 1.96\sigma_{u1}}, e^{\gamma_{01} + 1.96\sigma_{u1}}\right]$. This interval gives the plausible range of odds ratios across sites, with $e^{\gamma_{01} - 1.96\sigma_{u1}}$ being the lowest OR we expect to observe and $e^{\gamma_{01} + 1.96\sigma_{u1}}$ being the highest. By examining such intervals for a range of values of σ_{u1}, we can be guided to select a plausible value of σ_{u1}. This is illustrated in the following example.

Example 13.9. A multisite trial is planned in which the expected probability of the outcome is $p_C = 0.1$ in the control and $p_T = 0.2$ in the treatment condition. To select a plausible value of σ_{u1}, we consider a range of possible values and the 95% interval for site-level ORs that they imply. We can use the ms.varexplore function to facilitate:

```
library(powertools)
ms.varexplore(pc = 0.1, pt = 0.2)
```

OR: 2.25

sigma.u1	OR.lower	OR.upper
0.1	1.85	2.74
0.2	1.52	3.33
0.3	1.25	4.05
0.4	1.03	4.93
0.5	0.84	6.00
0.6	0.69	7.29
0.7	0.57	8.87
0.8	0.47	10.79
0.9	0.39	13.13
1.0	0.32	15.97

The output shows that when σ_{u1} is 0.5, the OR would be less than 1 for some sites, indicating worse outcomes under treatment than under the control condition at those sites, and some sites would have ORs as high as 6, indicating very strong treatment effects. $\sigma_{u1} = 0.4$ gives a more plausible range of ORs across sites; most sites are expected to show a benefit of treatment (OR> 1), but a few might show little or no benefit (OR $\approx$ 1).

Binary outcomes

Having selected a plausible value of σ_{u1}, we can calculate the required sample size. We assume a test of H_0: $\gamma_{01} = 0$ with two-sided $\alpha = 0.05$. There will be $m = 30$ participants per site with equal allocation to conditions. What is the required number of sites to achieve 90% power?

```
library(powertools)
multisite.bin(m = 30, J = NULL, pc = 0.1, pt = 0.2, sigma.u = 0.4,
    power = 0.9)
[1] 25.25981
```

Rounding up to the next whole number, we need 26 sites.

13.8.1 Design effect approach

Another approach to sample size calculation for a multisite trial with a binary outcome is to calculate the sample size required for a trial with independent observations and then inflate this value using a design effect. In Chapter 6, we discussed testing H_0: $p_1 - p_2 = \Delta_0$ versus H_A: $p_1 - p_2 \ne \Delta_0$ for two groups of independent subjects. When the expected outcome proportions are p_{1A} and p_{2A}, the required total sample size, using the normal approximation to the binomial distribution and assuming equal allocation, is

$$N \geq \frac{2(z_{1-\alpha/2} + z_{1-\beta})^2 [p_{1A}(1 - p_{1A}) + p_{2A}(1 - p_{2A})]}{(p_{1A} - p_{2A} - \Delta_0)^2}. \tag{13.27}$$

Using the design effect approach, we would multiply this N by a design effect for a multisite trial to arrive at the required sample size accounting for the multisite design.

A difficulty with this approach is obtaining a plausible estimate of the design effect in the context of a binary outcome. For continuous outcomes, the design effect for a multisite trial is $1 - \rho_0 + (m-1)\rho_1$ (Section 13.6.3). It is unclear whether this formula can be applied to a binary outcome and what values should be used for the ICCs. There are several different ways of defining an ICC for binary data [63]; most notably, there is a distinction between an ICC from a cluster-level proportions model and an ICC from a cluster-level log-odds model; we discuss this topic further in Section 14.3.2. There are also numerous methods proposed for estimating ICCs from binary data [237]. Furthermore, the data from such trials will generally be analyzed using a statistical method suitable for correlated data, such as a multilevel logistic regression model, and in general, the power analysis approach should be consistent with the planned analysis method. Thus this approach should only be used with caution.

13.9 Additional resources

The `PowerUpR` package is a comprehensive package for evaluating sample size and power for studies with multilevel data, including multisite and cluster randomized trials with up to four levels, for continuous outcomes [56, 143]. There is a companion ShinyApp available at https://www.causalevaluation.org/power-analysis.html and a reference manual [12].

The `WebPower` package has power and sample size functions for two-arm and three-arm multisite trials, `wp.mrt2arm` and `wp.mrt3arm`. These functions assume a continuous outcome and require as input the within-site error variance σ_ϵ^2 and the variance of the treatment effects σ_{u1}^2. Equal allocation is assumed.

14
Cluster randomized trials: parallel designs

14.1 Introduction

In a **cluster randomized trial**, also called a **group randomized trial**, pre-existing groups of individuals such as clinics, schools or communities are randomized to conditions, with all individuals in the same group receiving the same treatment. At follow-up, outcomes are measured at the individual level.

A cluster randomized design may be selected over an individually randomized design for several reasons. Cluster randomization can prevent "contamination", that is, the potential for the control group to be exposed to the intervention. The intervention may naturally be implemented at the group level, e.g., a clinic-wide change in procedures. Additionally, it may be less costly or logistically easier to implement the intervention at the cluster level.

Data from cluster randomized trials have a **hierarchical** or **multilevel data structure**, with participants nested within groups. As discussed in Section 13.2, such data can be considered to have arisen from a **multistage sampling** design [207], in which we first sample higher-level units (for example, clinics) and then sample lower-level units within the higher-level units (for example, patients within clinics). A consequence of multistage sampling is that observations within the same higher-level sampling unit cannot be regarded as independent of other observations within the same unit; rather, they are potentially correlated. The correlated data structure created by randomization at the cluster level can have a substantial impact on power and sample size requirements and it is important to account for the cluster randomized design when powering a study.

A design related to a cluster randomized design is the **individually randomized group treatment** trial (IRGTT). In an IRGTT, participants are randomized to study conditions individually but receive some or all of their assigned condition in a group setting with other participants or through an intervention provider shared with other participants. Most commonly, participants assigned to the intervention condition are clustered into groups whereas control participants are not, although in some studies, control participants may also be grouped after randomization to receive the control condition. This design is also called a **partially clustered design** when it entails clustering in one condition but not in the other.

DOI: 10.1201/9780429488788-14

In this chapter, we discuss power and sample size for cluster randomized trials and IRGTTs with **parallel designs**. In a parallel design, units are randomized to one condition with no crossover to a different condition during the trial. A parallel cluster randomized design can be contrasted with designs that involve clusters transitioning to different conditions during the study, with repeated assessments of the outcome variable under different conditions. These designs include cluster randomized crossover trials and stepped wedge trials. We refer to such studies as longitudinal cluster randomized trials. We include parallel cluster randomized trials with a baseline measurement of the outcome variable in this category. We discuss power and sample size for such trials in Chapter 15.

There are many books and articles on designing cluster randomized trials [25, 58, 83, 158, 164, 191]. The National Institutes of Health has a website with design considerations and sample size calculators for cluster randomized trials, individually randomized group treatment trials and stepped wedge trials at https://researchmethodsresources.nih.gov/. We provide additional resources for specific designs in this chapter and the next.

We discuss power and sample size for continuous outcomes in Section 14.2 and binary outcomes in Section 14.3. Additional resources for parallel cluster randomized trials are provided in Section 14.4. Individually randomized group treatment trials are discussed in Section 14.5. We briefly discuss extensions to designs with three or more levels of data and split-plot designs, which have randomization to different treatment factors at different levels, in Section 14.6.

14.2 Continuous outcomes

14.2.1 Model

A basic model for a continuous outcome of individual i in cluster j, denoted Y_{ij}, is

$$Y_{ij} = \mu_j + \epsilon_{ij}, \tag{14.1}$$

where μ_j is the mean for cluster j and $\epsilon_{ij} \sim \mathcal{N}(0, \sigma_\epsilon^2)$ is an error term. Thus each cluster has its own mean and individuals within the cluster have outcomes that vary around that mean. A basic model for the mean of cluster j is

$$\mu_j = \gamma_0 + u_j \tag{14.2}$$

where γ_0 denotes the population mean, assumed to be fixed, and $u_j \sim \mathcal{N}(0, \sigma_u^2)$ is a random effect representing the difference between cluster j's mean and the population mean. The random effect u_j captures the effects of variables that tend to make outcomes of individuals in cluster j systematically higher or lower than the outcomes of individuals in other clusters, e.g., the different

Continuous outcomes

health risk profiles of patients at different clinics. The random terms ϵ_{ij} and u_j are assumed to be mutually independent.

In a cluster randomized trial, the intervention is applied at the cluster level and has its effect on the cluster mean. Let w_j be a cluster-level covariate that takes value -0.5 if the cluster is assigned to the control condition and 0.5 if assigned to the intervention condition. Adding this covariate to the cluster mean model yields

$$\mu_j = \gamma_0 + \gamma_1 w_j + u_j \tag{14.3}$$

where γ_0 is the grand mean (mean of the means in the control and intervention conditions) and γ_1 is the difference in means between the two conditions. Note that w_j is subscripted only by j because treatment is assigned at the cluster level. By substituting (14.3) into (14.1), we obtain a single equation model,

$$Y_{ij} = \gamma_0 + \gamma_1 w_j + u_j + \epsilon_{ij}. \tag{14.4}$$

Figure 14.1 presents simulated data for two cluster randomized trials, each with 10 clusters (5 control and 5 intervention) and 20 observations per cluster. The model parameter values are $\gamma_0 = 0$, $\gamma_1 = 5$, $\sigma_\epsilon^2 = 36$ and either $\sigma_u^2 = 1$ (low variance of cluster means) or $\sigma_u^2 = 16$ (high variance of cluster means). Conceptually, estimating the treatment effect involves: estimating each cluster mean; estimating the mean for the treatment condition by averaging the cluster means for clusters assigned to treatment; estimating the mean for the control condition by averaging the cluster means for clusters assigned

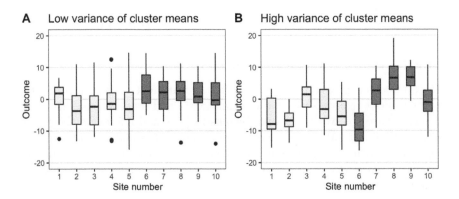

FIGURE 14.1: Boxplots of simulated data from two cluster randomized trials showing the impact of variation of the cluster-level means. In Panel (A), the variance of the cluster means is low; in Panel (B), the variance is higher. Color represents condition (light grey: control, dark grey: intervention). Means within each cluster are represented by the black lines in each box. The treatment effect γ_1 is 5 in both panels. Higher variance of the cluster-level means as in Panel (B) will result in higher variance of the estimated treatment effect.

to control; then taking the difference. Higher variance of the cluster means will increase the variance of the treatment effect estimator, making it more difficult to detect a treatment effect. Factors affecting power are discussed in more detail in Section 14.2.2.

Inspection of model (14.4) reveals that the total variance of an observation Y_{ij} is the sum of two variance components, one at the cluster level (σ_u^2) and the other at the individual level (σ_ϵ^2),

$$Var(Y_{ij}) = \sigma_Y^2 = \sigma_u^2 + \sigma_\epsilon^2. \tag{14.5}$$

Further, the covariance of two different observations from the same cluster, $Cov(Y_{ij}, Y_{i'j})$, $i \neq i'$, is equal to σ_u^2. Thus the correlation between two different observations from the same cluster is

$$Corr(Y_{ij}, Y_{i'j}) = \frac{\sigma_u^2}{\sigma_Y^2} = \frac{\sigma_u^2}{\sigma_u^2 + \sigma_\epsilon^2} = \rho. \tag{14.6}$$

This correlation is called the **intraclass correlation coefficient** (ICC) and denoted as ρ. In addition to being interpretable as a correlation coefficient, the ICC also quantifies the proportion of the total variance of the outcome that is attributable to variance of the cluster-level means. We can also see this by noting that $\sigma_u^2 = \rho \sigma_Y^2$. As discussed in the next section, the ICC is a key parameter influencing power in a cluster randomized trial. Note that because σ_u^2 and σ_ϵ^2 are non-negative, $0 \leq \rho \leq 1$.

Equation (14.6) implies that within a cluster, the correlation between any two observations is equal, namely, it is equal to the constant ρ. This is termed **exchangeable correlation structure**, also called **compound symmetry**.

14.2.2 Power for test of treatment effect

To develop an expression for power for tests regarding the treatment effect γ_1, we first derive expressions for the estimator $\hat{\gamma}_1$ and its variance. The derivations are based on Moerbeek and Teerenstra [158] and references therein. We assume that J total clusters are randomized with equal allocation to two conditions, with $J/2$ clusters in each condition, and that there are an equal number of participants m in each cluster. Denote the cluster means in each condition as

$$\bar{Y}_{.jT} = \frac{1}{m} \sum_{i=1}^{m} Y_{ijT} \quad \text{and} \quad \bar{Y}_{.jC} = \frac{1}{m} \sum_{i=1}^{m} Y_{ijC}$$

and denote the means of the cluster-level means in each condition as

$$\bar{Y}_{..T} = \frac{1}{J/2} \sum_{j=1}^{J/2} \bar{Y}_{.jT} \quad \text{and} \quad \bar{Y}_{..C} = \frac{1}{J/2} \sum_{j=J/2+1}^{J} \bar{Y}_{.jC}$$

Continuous outcomes

An unbiased estimate of γ_1 can be obtained as the difference of these means,

$$\hat{\gamma}_1 = \bar{Y}_{..T} - \bar{Y}_{..C}$$

The next step is to find $Var(\hat{\gamma}_1)$. Because clusters are assumed to be independent, we have that

$$Var(\hat{\gamma}_1) = Var(\bar{Y}_{..T}) + Var(\bar{Y}_{..C}) = \frac{4}{J}Var(\bar{Y}_{.j}) \qquad (14.7)$$

where $Var(\bar{Y}_{.j})$ is the variance of a cluster-level mean, which in model (14.4) is assumed to be the same in each condition, $Var(\bar{Y}_{.jT}) = Var(\bar{Y}_{.jC}) = Var(\bar{Y}_{.j})$. Using rules for the variance of the sum of correlated random variables, $Var(\bar{Y}_{.j})$ can be found to be

$$Var(\bar{Y}_{.j}) = \frac{1}{m}\left[Var(Y_{ij}) + (m-1)Cov(Y_{ij}, Y_{i'j})\right] = \frac{\sigma_Y^2}{m}\left[1 + (m-1)\rho\right]. \qquad (14.8)$$

Putting together (14.7) and (14.8), we obtain

$$Var(\hat{\gamma}_1) = \frac{4\sigma_Y^2}{mJ}\left[1 + (m-1)\rho\right]. \qquad (14.9)$$

Using (14.5) and (14.6), we can also express this variance as

$$Var(\hat{\gamma}_1) = \frac{4}{mJ}\left(\sigma_\epsilon^2 + m\sigma_u^2\right). \qquad (14.10)$$

A test of $H_0 : \gamma_1 = \gamma_{(0)}$ in model (14.4) can be conducted using the test statistic

$$T = \frac{\hat{\gamma}_1 - \gamma_{(0)}}{\sqrt{\widehat{Var}(\hat{\gamma}_1)}}. \qquad (14.11)$$

When the null hypothesis is true, $T \sim t(J-2)$. Under an alternative $\gamma_1 = \gamma_{(A)}$, T has a noncentral t distribution with noncentrality parameter

$$\lambda = \frac{\gamma_{(A)} - \gamma_{(0)}}{\sqrt{Var(\hat{\gamma}_1)}}. \qquad (14.12)$$

Power can be calculated as follows:

$$\begin{aligned}\text{Power (lower-tail test)} &= P[T \leq t_{\alpha, J-2} \mid T \sim t(J-2, \lambda)] \qquad (14.13)\\ &= \mathcal{T}_{J-2,\lambda}(t_{\alpha, J-2})\\ \text{Power (upper-tail test)} &= P[T \geq t_{1-\alpha, J-2} \mid T \sim t(J-2, \lambda)]\\ &= 1 - \mathcal{T}_{J-2,\lambda}(t_{1-\alpha, J-2})\\ \text{Power (two-sided test)} &= P[T^2 \geq f_{1-\alpha, 1, J-2} \mid T^2 \sim F(1, J-2, \Lambda)]\\ &= 1 - \mathcal{F}_{1, J-2, \Lambda}(f_{1-\alpha, 1, J-2})\end{aligned}$$

where $\Lambda = \lambda^2$. For a lower-tailed test, we expect λ to be negative and for an upper-tailed test, we expect λ to be positive. Note that the degrees of freedom for the t and F distributions depend on the number of clusters J. In general, for balanced data (clusters of equal size), the degrees of freedom are $J - q - 1$, where q is the number of cluster-level covariates, including the covariate indicating treatment assignment.

What factors affect power? Power increases as the magnitude of the noncentrality parameter λ increases; thus power increases as the magnitude of the true treatment effect $\gamma_{(A)}$ or the difference $\gamma_{(A)} - \gamma_{(0)}$ increases, and decreases as $Var(\hat{\gamma}_1)$ increases. The variance can be expressed in a number of different ways, each of which gives insights into what factors affect power for a parallel cluster randomized trial. From the expression

$$Var(\hat{\gamma}_1) = \frac{4\sigma_Y^2}{mJ}[1 + (m-1)\rho] \qquad (14.14)$$

it is clear that the variance will increase and thus power will decrease as the total variance of an observation or the ICC increases, and the variance will decrease as the number of clusters J increases. Expressing the variance as

$$Var(\hat{\gamma}_1) = 4\left(\frac{\sigma_\epsilon^2}{mJ} + \frac{\sigma_u^2}{J}\right) \qquad (14.15)$$

helps to differentiate the impacts of number of clusters and cluster size. As total number of clusters J increases, the contributions of both components of the variance decrease. However, increasing cluster size m only reduces the first component; it has no effect on the influence of the variance of the cluster means. Thus at some point, increasing the number of individuals per cluster will have little impact on power. In general, power will be driven more by number of clusters than by cluster size.

> ▶ In a cluster randomized trial, power is generally influenced more by the number of clusters than by the size of the clusters.

Using standardized effect sizes. As previously discussed (Section 2.4), it can be useful to express a treatment effect as a standardized effect size. Here, the standardized effect size is $d = (\gamma_{(A)} - \gamma_{(0)})/\sigma_Y$, with $\gamma_{(A)}/\sigma_Y$ when $\gamma_{(0)} = 0$. The noncentrality parameter can then be expressed as

$$\lambda = \frac{d}{\sqrt{\frac{4[1+(m-1)\rho]}{mJ}}}. \qquad (14.16)$$

This expression involves only d, ρ and the sample sizes at the two levels, which can be convenient for calculations.

Continuous outcomes   243

Example 14.1. Suppose we are planning a parallel cluster randomized trial that will involve a total of 16 clusters with 30 participants per cluster. Clusters will be allocated equally to two conditions. If the expected standardized effect size is $d = 0.4$, what is the power for an upper-tailed, one-sided test at level 0.025? The ICC is assumed to be 0.05.

The function crt.parallel.cont allows one to specify different ICCs in each arm (see Section 14.2.7). In this example, they are both equal to 0.05. J1 is the number of clusters in arm 1; by default, equal allocation to two arms is assumed. Unequal allocation is discussed in Section 14.2.8.

```
library(powertools)
crt.parallel.cont(m = 30, J1 = 8, delta = 0.4, icc1 = 0.05, icc2 = 0.05,
   alpha = 0.025, sides = 1, power = NULL)
[1] 0.7401059
```

Power is about 74%.

14.2.3   Design effect and sample size using normal approximation

As discussed in Section 14.2.2, in a cluster randomized trial with $J/2$ clusters of size m in each condition, the variance of the treatment effect estimator, which is the mean difference in outcomes between conditions, is

$$\frac{4\sigma_Y^2}{mJ}\left[1 + (m-1)\rho\right]. \tag{14.17}$$

For an individually randomized trial with the same number of subjects, that is, $mJ/2$ in each condition, this variance would be $4\sigma_Y^2/(mJ)$. The ratio of the variances, for a parallel cluster randomized trial to that for an individually randomized trial, is

$$1 + (m-1)\rho \tag{14.18}$$

and is called the **design effect** for a cluster randomized trial. We will denote it as DE_{CRT}. DE_{CRT} is the multiplicative factor by which the variance of the estimated treatment effect is increased due to clustering. When $\rho > 0$, DE_{CRT} will be greater than one; hence another term for the design effect is the "variance inflation factor" (not to be confused with other meanings of the term variance inflation factor, such as in multiple linear regression; see Section 11.2.2). The design effect reduces to 1 when we have clusters of size 1 or when $\rho = 0$, i.e., independent observations. For a cluster randomized trial, we usually expect $\text{DE}_{\text{CRT}} > 1$.

TABLE 14.1: Values of $DE_{CRT} = 1 + (m-1)\rho$ for selected values of cluster size m and intraclass correlation coefficient ρ.

ρ	m					
	10	20	50	100	200	500
0.001	1.009	1.019	1.049	1.099	1.199	1.499
0.002	1.018	1.038	1.098	1.198	1.398	1.998
0.005	1.045	1.095	1.245	1.495	1.995	3.495
0.010	1.090	1.190	1.490	1.990	2.990	5.990
0.020	1.180	1.380	1.980	2.980	4.980	10.980
0.050	1.450	1.950	3.450	5.950	10.950	25.950
0.100	1.900	2.900	5.900	10.900	20.900	50.900

The design effect also gives an approximate multiplicative factor by which the sample size needs to be increased due to clustering in order to achieve the same power. Let N_{indep} denote the sample size for a parallel trial with independent subjects. Then the total sample size required for a comparable parallel cluster randomized trial, N_{CRT}, can be approximated as

$$N_{\text{CRT}} \approx N_{\text{indep}} DE_{\text{CRT}} \qquad (14.19)$$

where N_{CRT} is the total number of participants, mJ. For example, using a normal approximation for a two-sample t test with equal variances and equal allocation to calculate N_{indep}, we obtain

$$N_{\text{CRT}} \geq N_{\text{indep}} DE_{\text{CRT}} = \frac{4(z_{1-\alpha/2} + z_{1-\beta})^2}{d^2}[1 + (m-1)\rho]. \qquad (14.20)$$

N_{CRT} should be rounded up to the next whole number that is a multiple of $2m$, to allow for equal allocation of clusters to the two arms.

Table 14.1 displays values of DE_{CRT} for selected values of cluster size and ICC. Even a small ρ can lead to high design effects if clusters are large. For example, an ICC of 0.02 and cluster size of 10 leads to DE_{CRT} of 1.18, while the same ICC and a cluster size of 200 leads to DE_{CRT} of 4.98, which is about five times the variance, and five times as many subjects, compared to independent observations.

The approximation may underestimate the sample size required for the cluster randomized trial due to the mismatch in the degrees of freedom, which tend to be much lower for a cluster randomized trial compared to an individually randomized trial. The next example illustrates the design effect approach to sample size calculation for a cluster randomized trial and compares it to the more accurate calculation.

Continuous outcomes

Example 14.2. We conduct a sample size calculation for a parallel cluster randomized trial using the design effect approach and using the more precise calculation. We assume a two-sided test at $\alpha = 0.05$, 80% power, 20 participants per site and equal allocation. We expect $d = 0.4$ and $\rho = 0.05$. How many sites do we need? Using the design effect approach,

```
N_indep <- 4 * (qnorm(p = 0.975) + qnorm(p = 0.8))^2 / 0.4^2 ; N_indep
[1] 196.222
DE_crt <- 1 + (20 - 1) * 0.05  ;  DE_crt
[1] 1.95
# use round_any function to round up to next multiple of 40:
library(plyr)
N_crt <- round_any(N_indep * DE_crt, 40, ceiling)  ;  N_crt
[1] 400
```

The design effect is 1.95, indicating a need to double the sample size due to the clustered design. After rounding up to the next multiple of $2m = 40$, we estimate that we need N_{CRT} of 400. With $m = 20$, this equates to 20 clusters, with 10 in each arm.

We get the more precise calculation provided by `crt.parallel.cont`, which uses power formulas (14.13), for comparison:

```
library(powertools)
crt.parallel.cont(m = 20, J1 = NULL, delta = 0.4, icc1 = 0.05,
   icc2 = 0.05, power = 0.8)
[1] 10.61766
```

Rounding up to a whole number of clusters in each arm, the more accurate calculation indicates that we need 11 clusters per arm to achieve at least 80% power. The normal approximation result was similar but underestimated the number of clusters required.

14.2.4 Cluster size for a fixed number of clusters

In some studies, we may have a fixed number of clusters available but have flexibility as to the number of participants to enroll per cluster. In this setting, we want to find m to achieve the desired level of power for a given J. An approximate closed-form formula for m can be obtained by setting N_{CRT} equal to mJ in sample size formula (14.20) and solving for m, yielding [87]

$$m = \lceil \frac{1-\rho}{J/N_{\text{indep}} - \rho} \rceil \qquad (14.21)$$

where $N_{\text{indep}} = 4(z_{1-\alpha/2} + z_{1-\beta})^2/d^2$, the number of subjects required for a trial with no clustering (assuming equal allocation and equal variances), and the notation $\lceil x \rceil$ means to take the ceiling of x, i.e., next highest integer. A more precise solution can be obtained by numerically solving the power equation for m using software.

However, as discussed in Hemming et al. [87], it may not be possible to achieve the desired level of power with a fixed number of clusters simply by increasing cluster size. Recall (page 242) that the variance of the treatment effect estimator can be expressed as

$$Var(\hat{\gamma}_1) = 4\left(\frac{\sigma_\epsilon^2}{mJ} + \frac{\sigma_u^2}{J}\right).$$

Increasing m only reduces the first component. Taking the limit as $m \to \infty$, the lower bound on the variance is $4\sigma_u^2/J = 4\rho\sigma_Y^2/J$. Since the variance for a trial with independent subjects is $4\sigma_Y^2/N_{\text{indep}}$, this leads to the condition $J > \rho N_{\text{indep}}$ as a feasibility check. If this inequality does not hold, then desired power cannot be achieved, even with very large clusters.

If the number of available clusters cannot be increased, investigators might choose to determine the smallest effect size that can be detected with the available power, for example, or consider modifications to the trial design to increase power.

Example 14.3. Suppose that 12 hospitals are available to participate in a study and we wish to know how many patients to sample from each hospital to achieve 80% power with a two-sided test at $\alpha = 0.05$. We wish to detect a standardized effect size of $d = 0.35$ and assume $\rho = 0.05$. When we run the crt.parallel.cont function, it gives an error message:

```
library(powertools)
crt.parallel.cont(m = NULL, J1 = 6, delta = 0.35, icc1 = 0.05,
   icc2 = 0.05, power = 0.8)
Error in crt.parallel.cont(m = NULL, J1 = 6, delta = 0.35,
   : desired power unable to be achieved with given specifications
```

Checking the feasibility condition, we first find N_{indep}, which we can do using:

```
ttest.2samp(n1 = NULL, delta = 0.35, sd1 = 1, power = 0.8, sides = 2)
[1] 129.1121
```

The output indicates that we need at least 129 in each group or a total of at least $N_{\text{indep}} = 258$. We find $\rho N_{\text{indep}} = 0.05 \times 258 = 12.9$ which exceeds $J = 12$, so the feasibility check fails. In this scenario, we cannot achieve 80% power with only 12 clusters simply by increasing the number of patients per clinic.

Continuous outcomes

> ► Cluster randomized trials with a limited number of clusters have limited power. It may not be possible to achieve desired power with a small number of clusters simply by increasing cluster size.

14.2.5 Specifying ICC values

Specifying the magnitude of the ICC for a planned cluster randomized trial can be challenging. ICC values depend on the outcome and the setting. If data from a previous study or pilot study are available, this can be used to specify a plausible value for the expected ICC. Literature is also available on ICC values for various contexts. For example, ICCs in the range of 0–0.10 were reported in a review of primary care trials [1, 61]. ICCs tend to be small for large geographically defined clusters such as towns or counties, often < 0.01 or even < 0.001, and larger (often 0.01–0.05) for clusters composed of organizations such as schools or worksites. ICCs for tightly knit clusters such as families tend to be even larger, often > 0.2 [57, 165].

In general, it is advisable to perform a sensitivity analysis by calculating power or sample size for a range of plausible values of important parameters whose values are uncertain, including the ICC in a cluster randomized trial. An additional option is to conduct a sample size re-estimation. A sample size re-estimation in this case would involve planning for an interim analysis during the study in which the ICC is estimated from accumulated data and then recalculating the number of clusters required. Because such an interim analysis would not involve making a decision about study hypotheses, it does not inflate the Type I error rate. For further information, see [131, 181].

14.2.6 Varying cluster sizes

Thus far we have assumed that all clusters are the same size. In many studies, clusters have varying sizes. When cluster sizes vary, the variance of the treatment effect estimator is increased, and therefore efficiency and power are reduced [9, 62, 220]. The loss of efficiency can be quantified as the relative efficiency of a cluster randomized trial with unequal cluster sizes compared to one with equal sizes, given the same J and overall total N. Recall from Section 3.3 that the relative efficiency of Design A to Design B for estimating a parameter θ is the ratio of the variances, $\text{RE}(\hat{\theta}_A, \hat{\theta}_B) = Var(\hat{\theta}_B)/Var(\hat{\theta}_A)$.

Let $\tilde{m}$ and $\tilde{s}$ denote the mean and standard deviation of the distribution of cluster sizes. An approximation of the relative efficiency of unequal versus equal cluster sizes given the same J and total N is (see van Breukelen et al. [220]

$$1 - \text{CV}^2 K(1-K) \qquad (14.22)$$

where $\text{CV} = \tilde{s}/\tilde{m}$, the coefficient of variation of cluster sizes, and $K = \tilde{m}\rho/[1+(\tilde{m}-1)\rho]$. This relative efficiency formula was also discussed for multisite trials (see Section 13.6.5). The relative efficiency will be less than 1 unless $\tilde{s} = 0$, i.e., no variation in cluster size. In a power calculation, $Var(\hat{\gamma}_1)$ in the noncentrality parameter should be divided by the relative efficiency to account for the loss of efficiency.

Other authors [6, 123, 147] present other approaches for handling varying cluster sizes. For example, Eldridge et al. [62] suggest using as the design effect $1 + [(\text{CV}^2 + 1)\tilde{m} - 1]\rho$ rather than $1 + [m - 1]\rho$. If the clusters are known to have sizes $m_1, \ldots, m_J$ with mean cluster size $\tilde{m}$, the relative efficiency is

$$\left(\frac{\tilde{m} + \psi}{\tilde{m}}\right) \frac{1}{J} \sum_{j=1}^{J} \left(\frac{m_j}{m_j + \psi}\right)$$

where $\psi = (1 - \rho)/\rho$ [220].

Often investigators have a good idea of the expected mean cluster size but may not have a good prior estimate of the standard deviation of the cluster sizes. To estimate the standard deviation, one strategy is to use the **range rule**, which suggests that if a distribution is roughly normal, the standard deviation of a sample can be approximated as one-fourth of the range [219]. Thus $\tilde{s}$ can be estimated by making educated guesses for the minimum and maximum cluster sizes likely to be observed and computing $\tilde{s} \approx (\max - \min)/4$. This is illustrated in the following example.

Example 14.4. In Example 14.1, with 8 clusters allocated to each condition, all clusters of equal size 30, d of 0.4 and ICC of 0.05, we found that power for a one-sided test with α of 0.025 was 74%. Suppose that the cluster sizes are expected to vary from 6 to 70 with a mean of 30. We approximate the standard deviation of cluster sizes as $\tilde{s} = (70 - 6)/4 = 16$. The re.clustsize.cont function computes relative efficiency due to varying cluster sizes:

```
library(powertools)
re.clustsize.cont(m = 30, m.sd = 16, icc = 0.05)
[1] 0.9324726
```

The relative efficiency is about 93%, indicating that we can expect some loss of power. The crt.parallel.cont function accounts for this when a non-zero value is specified for the standard deviation of cluster sizes m.sd:

```
crt.parallel.cont(m = 30, m.sd = 16, J1 = 8, delta = 0.4,
   icc1 = 0.05, icc2 = 0.05, alpha = 0.025, sides = 1, power = NULL)
[1] 0.7104195
```

There is a modest drop in power to 71%.

The expected increase in the sample size needed to achieve the same power as a trial with equal cluster sizes is about $1/\text{RE} = 1.072$, i.e., the sample size needs to be increased by about 7%. Setting J1 = NULL and power = 0.8, the number of clusters needed per arm for 80% power increases from 9.08 to 9.65 when `m.sd` increases from 0 to 16. After rounding up to the next whole number, we find that 10 clusters in each arm is suggested under both scenarios.

How much efficiency loss can we expect in general? Candel et al. [26, 27] suggest that if the ratio of the largest to the smallest cluster size is less than 2, the impact on power is likely to be minimal and no adjustment is needed. Eldridge et al. [62] suggest that a CV of cluster sizes of less than 0.23 will have minimal impact. van Breukelen et al. [220] suggest that for distributions of cluster sizes likely to be encountered in practice, the loss of efficiency due to varying cluster sizes seldom exceeds 10%.

14.2.7 Unequal ICCs

Thus far we have assumed that the ICC is the same across study arms. In some studies, the ICC might differ across arms. For example, a group therapy intervention that involves interaction among cluster members may result in a higher ICC in the intervention arm. When we expect different ICCs in the two treatment arms, the variance of the treatment effect estimate is, assuming balanced data,

$$Var(\hat{\gamma}_1) = \frac{2\sigma_Y^2}{mJ}\left\{[1 + (m-1)\rho_1] + [1 + (m-1)\rho_2]\right\},$$

which simplifies to equation (14.17) when $\rho_1 = \rho_2$. This expression can be used in the noncentrality parameter formula to calculate power. Unequal values of ICCs can be specified in the `crt.parallel.cont` function.

Related to the topic of different ICCs in different treatment conditions is the individually randomized group treatment trial (IRGTT) design, discussed in Section 14.5. In IRGTT, clustering occurs in the treatment condition but not the control condition.

14.2.8 Unequal allocation

Thus far, we have assumed equal numbers of clusters in each arm. Sometimes there are logistical, scientific or cost reasons to allocate unequal numbers of clusters to conditions. Let J_1 and J_2 denote the numbers of clusters in arms 1 and 2, respectively. The variance of the treatment effect estimator becomes, also allowing for different ICCs in the two arms,

$$Var(\hat{\gamma}_1) = \frac{\sigma_Y^2}{m}\left[\frac{1 + (m-1)\rho_1}{J_1} + \frac{1 + (m-1)\rho_2}{J_2}\right].$$

Unequal allocation can be specified in the `crt.parallel.cont` function by specifying `J1` and `J.ratio`, specified as J_2/J_1.

14.2.9 Covariates

As discussed for ANCOVA (Section 5.4), regression adjustment for covariates in a randomized trial can reduce residual variance and thereby improve precision and power. In a single-level model, if we add a covariate X that is uncorrelated with other predictors in the model and whose correlation with the outcome Y is ρ_{XY}, the error variance is reduced by a factor $1 - \rho_{XY}^2$. We can express this relationship as

$$\sigma_{Y|X}^2 = \sigma_Y^2 (1 - \rho_{XY}^2)$$

with the subscripting of $\sigma_{Y|X}^2$ indicating that this is the conditional variance of Y given X.

In a cluster randomized trial, the model can include covariates at the individual level and/or the cluster level. The impacts of covariates at the two levels are different, as we discuss next.

14.2.9.1 Cluster-level covariates

A cluster-level covariate might be the specialty of a health care provider in a trial randomizing providers, or geographic location in a trial randomizing schools. The results here are based Moerbeek et al. [158, 160]. When a cluster-level covariate z_j is added, model (14.4) becomes

$$Y_{ij} = \tilde{\gamma}_0 + \tilde{\gamma}_1 w_j + \tilde{\gamma}_2 z_j + \tilde{u}_j + \tilde{\epsilon}_{ij}$$

where the tildes are used to indicate that the values of the regression coefficients and random terms may be different in this adjusted model. The variance components in the adjusted model could also be different; we denote them as $\tilde{\sigma}_u^2$ and $\tilde{\sigma}_\epsilon^2$.

How do $\tilde{\sigma}_u^2$ and $\tilde{\sigma}_\epsilon^2$ compare to σ_u^2 and σ_ϵ^2, the variance components in the model without covariate adjustment? Since a cluster-level covariate takes the same value for all members of a cluster, it cannot explain variation among individuals within a cluster. Therefore the within-cluster variance is unchanged and $\tilde{\sigma}_\epsilon^2 = \sigma_\epsilon^2$. For the cluster-level variance, we have

$$\tilde{\sigma}_u^2 = (1 - \rho_B^2)\sigma_u^2 \qquad (14.23)$$

where ρ_B is the between-cluster residual correlation between the outcome and the covariate [206]. ρ_B^2 is the percent of variance of the outcome that is explained by the cluster-level covariate [210]. When there is more than one cluster-level covariate, ρ_B^2 is the percent of variance of the outcome that is explained by the set of cluster-level covariates. The ICC becomes

$$\tilde{\rho} = \frac{\tilde{\sigma}_u^2}{\sigma_Y^2} = \frac{(1-\rho_B^2)\sigma_u^2}{\sigma_Y^2} = (1-\rho_B^2)\rho.$$

Continuous outcomes

The variance of the treatment effect estimator becomes

$$Var(\hat{\tilde{\gamma}}_1) = \frac{4(\sigma_\epsilon^2 + m\tilde{\sigma}_u^2)}{mJ} = \frac{4\sigma_Y^2 [1 + (m-1)\tilde{\rho}]}{mJ}$$
$$= \frac{4\sigma_Y^2 [1 + (m-1)(1-\rho_B^2)\rho]}{mJ}.$$

The quantity in square brackets is the design effect when a cluster-level covariate is included, and simplifies to the standard design effect when $\rho_B = 0$. Power can be calculated using this expression for $Var(\hat{\gamma}_1)$ in the noncentrality parameter.

Because $1 - \rho_B^2 \le 1$, we have $1 + (m-1)(1-\rho_B^2)\rho \le 1 + (m-1)\rho$; hence the design effect is reduced due to a cluster-level covariate. However, for each covariate, one additional degree of freedom is lost for the t distribution; the degrees of freedom are $J - q - 1$, where q is the number of cluster-level covariates, including the intervention assignment indicator. This impact could offset a potential power gain, especially if the number of clusters is limited.

Example 14.5. In Example 14.1, with 8 clusters allocated to each condition, all clusters of equal size 30, d of 0.4 and ICC of 0.05, we found that power for a one-sided test with α of 0.025 was 74%. Suppose we plan to adjust for a cluster-level covariate that we expect will explain about 10% of the total variance of the outcome. What is the impact on power?

```
library(powertools)
crt.parallel.cont(m = 30, J1 = 8, delta = 0.4, ncov = 1, RsqB = 0.1,
    icc1 = 0.05, icc2 = 0.05, alpha = 0.025, sides = 1, power = NULL)
[1] 0.7605778
```

The power has increased by about 2 percentage points.

14.2.9.2 Individual-level covariates

Now we consider individual-level covariates. Denote an individual-level covariate as c_{ij} and let $c_{.j}$ denote the mean of c_{ij} for cluster j. The recommended model for including an individual-level covariate is the following, which includes a within-cluster covariate $c_{ij} - c_{.j}$ and a cluster-level covariate $c_{.j}$ (see [156, 167]):

$$Y_{ij} = \tilde{\gamma}_0 + \tilde{\gamma}_1 w_j + \tilde{\gamma}_2 c_{.j} + \tilde{\gamma}_3 (c_{ij} - c_{.j}) + \tilde{u}_j + \tilde{\epsilon}_{ij}$$

The tildes are used to indicate that these parameters may differ from the corresponding parameters in the model without the covariate. The regressor $c_{ij} - c_{.j}$ represents how the covariate value varies within a cluster while $c_{.j}$ represents how the mean value of the covariate varies from cluster to cluster.

The effects of these two covariates on the outcome can be different. Omitting the between-cluster part of the covariate and only including c_{ij} in the model can increase the cluster-level variance component, which can decrease precision in estimating the treatment effect [156].

When adjusting for an individual-level covariate, both the within-cluster and between-cluster variances can be affected. The relationships between the adjusted and unadjusted variances are

$$\tilde{\sigma}_\epsilon^2 = \left(1 - \frac{m}{m-1}\rho_W^2\right)\sigma_\epsilon^2 \text{ and } \tilde{\sigma}_u^2 = \left(1 - \rho_B^2 + \frac{1}{m-1}\rho_W^2\right)\sigma_u^2$$

where ρ_W and ρ_B are the within-cluster and between-cluster residual correlations between the outcome Y_{ij} and the covariate c_{ij}; see [156, 207]. Somewhat different formulas have been presented by other authors [21, 183, 215]. The design effect is now

$$1 + [m(1 - \rho_B^2) - 1]\rho - \frac{m\rho_W^2(1 - 2\rho)}{m-1}.$$

This formula can be substituted for the standard design effect in formulas for power and sample size. ρ_B^2 is the percent of the variance of the outcome that is explained by variation in the cluster-level means $c_{\cdot j}$ and ρ_W^2 is the percent explained by variation of the covariate within cluster. When there are multiple covariates, ρ_B^2 and ρ_W^2 are the percent of variance explained by the full sets of covariates.

The regressor $c_{\cdot j}$ is a cluster-level covariate and impacts the degrees of freedom. Thus when using the recommended modeling approach, there will be one degree of freedom lost for each cluster- or individual-level covariate.

Example 14.6. In Example 14.5, suppose that we plan to additionally adjust for an individual-level covariate with $\rho_W = 0.5$. The cluster mean-centered regressor for this covariate will also be included, but we lack a good estimate of its impact on ρ_B^2, so we keep $\rho_B^2 = 0.1$. What is the impact on power?

```
library(powertools)
crt.parallel.cont(m = 30, J1 = 8, delta = 0.4, ncov = 2, RsqB = 0.1,
    RsqW = 0.5^2, icc1 = 0.05, icc2 = 0.05, alpha = 0.025, sides = 1,
    power = NULL)
[1] 0.7987004
```

The power is increased to about 80%.

▶ Power for a cluster randomized trial can potentially be increased by controlling for a cluster- or individual-level covariate that helps to explain

Binary outcomes

> variation in the outcome. However, adjusting for covariates also reduces the degrees of freedom, which can counteract the increase in power.

There are several different ways of approaching how adjustment for an individual-level covariate in a cluster randomized trial impacts power. Another approach, which is based on using a longitudinal model for repeated measures of the outcome variable at baseline and follow up in a cluster randomized design, is discussed in Section 15.3.

14.3 Binary outcomes

We discuss three approaches to power and sample size for parallel cluster randomized trials with a binary outcome. The first approach is based on a multilevel logistic regression model, which is a common modeling approach for clustered binary data. The second approach is based on applying a design effect to a sample size calculation for a two independent samples test of proportions. The third method is based on generalized estimating equations (GEE), which is another common method for analyzing correlated binary data.

In general, the sample size calculation method should correspond to the planned method of analysis. For parallel cluster randomized trials with a binary outcome, multilevel logistic regression and GEE are the two most commonly used methods of analysis [43, 44].

14.3.1 Multilevel logistic regression model approach

When a cluster randomized trial has a binary outcome, it is common to analyze the data using a logistic regression model with a random effect for cluster. For participant i in cluster j, we consider the model [158]

$$\log\left(\frac{P(Y_{ij} = 1 | x_j, u_j)}{1 - P(Y_{ij} = 1 | x_j, u_j)}\right) = \gamma_0 + \gamma_1 x_j + u_j$$

where x_j is the intervention condition indicator taking value -0.5 for control and 0.5 for intervention clusters and $u_j \sim \mathcal{N}(0, \sigma_u^2)$. For expected outcome proportions p_T and p_C in the treatment and control groups, γ_0 is the average of the log odds, $[\log(p_T/(1-p_T)) + \log(p_C/(1-p_C))]/2$, and γ_1 is the log odds ratio, $\log\left[\frac{p_T/(1-p_T)}{p_C/(1-p_C)}\right]$. The random effect for cluster, u_j, allows the probability of the outcome to depend on cluster, with the probability in cluster j equal to $P(Y_{ij} = 1 | x_j, u_j) = \exp(\gamma_0 + \gamma_1 x_j + u_j)/(1 + \exp(\gamma_0 + \gamma_1 x_j + u_j))$.

The log odds ratio γ_1 is the parameter of interest for estimating the treatment effect. If we allocated $J/2$ clusters to each condition, the variance of $\hat{\gamma}_1$

in this model is approximately

$$Var(\hat{\gamma}_1) = 1.2 \times \frac{4(\sigma_\epsilon^2 + m\sigma_u^2)}{mJ}$$

where m is cluster size, J is total number of clusters, and σ_ϵ^2 is the individual-level variance of the outcome [158]. The factor of 1.2 is due to use of second order penalized quasilikelihood (PQL) for estimation, which is recommended [161]. To test $H_0\colon \gamma_1 = \gamma_{(0)}$, we can use the test statistic

$$Z = \frac{\hat{\gamma}_1 - \gamma_{(0)}}{\sqrt{\widehat{Var}(\hat{\gamma}_{10})}}$$

which has a standard normal distribution asymptotically when H_0 is true. When the true log odds ratio is $\gamma_{(A)}$, power can be approximated as

$$\Phi\left(\frac{|\gamma_{(A)} - \gamma_{(0)}|}{\sqrt{Var(\hat{\gamma}_1)}} - z_{1-\alpha}\right) \quad (14.24)$$

for a one-sided test. For two-sided, substitute $\alpha/2$ for α. The required total number of clusters can be estimated as

$$J \geq 1.2 \times \frac{4(z_{1-\alpha/2} + z_{1-\beta})^2 \left(\dfrac{\sigma_\epsilon^2}{m} + \sigma_u^2\right)}{(\gamma_{(A)} - \gamma_{(0)})^2} \quad (14.25)$$

To use this approach, we need to specify values for $\gamma_{(A)}$, σ_ϵ^2 and σ_u^2. $\gamma_{(A)}$ and σ_ϵ^2 can be calculated from p_C and p_T:

$$\gamma_{(A)} = \log\left(\frac{p_T/(1-p_T)}{p_C/(1-p_C)}\right)$$

and

$$\sigma_\epsilon^2 \approx \frac{1}{2}\left[\frac{1}{p_C(1-p_C)} + \frac{1}{p_T(1-p_T)}\right].$$

σ_u^2 is the variance of the log odds across sites, given treatment condition. To arrive at a plausible estimate, we can reason in a manner similar to that in Section 13.8 for multisite trials. The log odds of the outcome for cluster j is $\gamma_0 + \gamma_1 x_j + u_j$. Because $u_j \sim \mathcal{N}(0, \sigma_u^2)$, we can expect that the log odds among clusters assigned to control could plausibly range within ± 1.96 standard deviations, that is, from $\gamma_0 - \frac{1}{2}\gamma_1 - 1.96\sigma_u$ to $\gamma_0 - \frac{1}{2}\gamma_1 + 1.96\sigma_u$. Transforming these log odds to probabilities, we expect that about 95% of the outcome probabilities across control clusters will be in the interval

$$\left[\frac{e^{\gamma_0 - \frac{1}{2}\gamma_1 - 1.96\sigma_u}}{1 + e^{\gamma_0 - \frac{1}{2}\gamma_1 - 1.96\sigma_u}}, \frac{e^{\gamma_0 - \frac{1}{2}\gamma_1 + 1.96\sigma_u}}{1 + e^{\gamma_0 - \frac{1}{2}\gamma_1 + 1.96\sigma_u}}\right].$$

Similarly, we expect that about 95% of the outcome probabilities across intervention clusters will be in the interval

$$\left[\frac{e^{\gamma_0+\frac{1}{2}\gamma_1-1.96\sigma_u}}{1+e^{\gamma_0+\frac{1}{2}\gamma_1-1.96\sigma_u}}, \frac{e^{\gamma_0+\frac{1}{2}\gamma_1+1.96\sigma_u}}{1+e^{\gamma_0+\frac{1}{2}\gamma_1+1.96\sigma_u}} \right].$$

By examining such intervals for a range of σ_u values, we can be guided to select a plausible value of σ_u. We illustrate in the following example.

Example 14.7. Researchers are planning to evaluate an intervention to reduce nicotine use among young people. The study will randomize schools to intervention and control conditions. The outcome variable is intention to use nicotine products (yes/no), assessed using a student survey. The researchers expect mean outcome proportions of 0.15 among students at intervention schools and 0.25 among students at control schools. If there will be 60 students per school, how many schools are needed for 80% power, with α of 0.05, two-sided, to test $H_0: \gamma_1 = 0$?

To help find plausible values for σ_u, we use the crt.varexplore function, which gives the 95% intervals for outcome proportions across clusters in the control and intervention conditions for a range of different σ_u values:

```
library(powertools)
crt.varexplore(pc = 0.25, pt = 0.15)

pc: 0.25 ; pt: 0.15
```

sigma.u	pc.lower	pc.upper	pt.lower	pt.upper
0.1	0.22	0.29	0.13	0.18
0.2	0.18	0.33	0.11	0.21
0.3	0.16	0.38	0.09	0.24
0.4	0.13	0.42	0.07	0.28
0.5	0.11	0.47	0.06	0.32
0.6	0.09	0.52	0.05	0.36
0.7	0.08	0.57	0.04	0.41
0.8	0.06	0.62	0.04	0.46
0.9	0.05	0.66	0.03	0.51
1.0	0.04	0.70	0.02	0.56

Based on this output, we might choose a σ_u in the range of 0.3–0.4, depending on what we think is a reasonable range of cluster-level outcome proportions for the setting. We calculate required number of clusters for $\sigma_u = 0.3$:

```
crt.parallel.bin(m = 60, J = NULL, pc = 0.25, pt = 0.15,
    sigma.u = 0.3, power = 0.8)
[1] 18.61033
```

Rounding up to the next even integer to account for equal allocation, we get $J = 20$ total schools, which corresponds to $20 \times 60 = 1200$ total students.

Accounting for varying cluster sizes. Candel and van Breukelen [27] provide a formula for the relative efficiency of unequal versus equal cluster sizes that can be used as an adjustment factor in power and sample size formulas when the outcome is binary. The relative efficiency depends on mean cluster size, the coefficient of variation of cluster sizes, the outcome proportions and σ_u^2; see [27] for details. The crt.parallel.bin function implements this method when a non-zero value is specified for m.sd. The impact of varying cluster sizes on power in cluster randomized trials with binary outcomes is also discussed in [5, 115]. It has been suggested that sampling 14% more clusters is sufficient to account for the efficiency loss due to varying cluster sizes in many cases [27].

14.3.2 Design effect approach for binary outcomes

In Section 14.2.3, we discussed a design effect approach to sample size calculation for a cluster randomized trial with a continuous outcome. This involved calculating the sample size required for a trial with independent outcomes and then inflating by a design effect of the form $1 + (m-1)\rho$.

An analogous approach for binary outcomes is to calculate the sample size required for a trial with a binary outcome that has independent observations and then inflate this value using a design effect. To test $H_0\colon p_1 - p_2 = \Delta_0$ versus $H_A\colon p_1 - p_2 \neq \Delta_0$ with independent observations, the required total sample size, using the normal approximation to the binomial distribution and assuming equal allocation, is

$$N_{\text{indep}} \geq \frac{2(z_{1-\alpha/2} + z_{1-\beta})^2 [p_1(1-p_1) + p_2(1-p_2)]}{(p_1 - p_2 - \Delta_0)^2}$$

where p_1 and p_2 are the expected outcome proportions in the two conditions; see Chapter 6. What should be used for the design effect?

One answer comes from viewing the data as arising from a **cluster-level proportions model**, which is a hierarchical model for clustered binary data that is an alternative to the mixed logistic model [38, 42, 55, 63, 135]. Consider a single population of clusters. Under the cluster-level proportions model, each observation i in cluster j, Y_{ij}, is Bernoulli with cluster-specific success probability p_j. The p_j are assumed to be random variables. Denote their mean and variance as $E(p_j) = p$ and $Var(p_j) = V$. Often, a beta distribution is assumed for the p_j, which leads to a beta-binomial model, but the main result does not depend on the particular distribution. Under this model, we have $E(Y_{ij}) = E(p_j) = p$ and $Var(Y_{ij}) = p(1-p)$. It can be shown that the covariance of two observations from the same cluster, $i \neq i'$, is $Cov(Y_{ij}, Y_{i'j}) =$

Binary outcomes

V [38]. Thus the correlation between two observations from the same cluster is

$$\rho = \frac{V}{p(1-p)}. \tag{14.26}$$

Let $\hat{p} = \frac{1}{mJ}\sum_{j=1}^{J}\sum_{i=1}^{m} Y_{ij}$ be the overall sample proportion across all observations, assuming J clusters of size m. We can find that this is an unbiased estimate of p and that the variance of $\hat{p}$ is

$$Var(\hat{p}) = \frac{p(1-p)}{mJ}\left[1 + (m-1)\rho\right].$$

Since for independent observations, $Var(\hat{p})$ would be $p(1-p)/mJ$, $1+(m-1)\rho$ can be considered the design effect under this model.

Now suppose that $J/2$ clusters are randomized to a treatment condition and $J/2$ to a control condition. Denote the success proportions in the two conditions as p_1 and p_2. We can estimate these proportions as $\hat{p}_k = \frac{1}{mJ/2}\sum_{j=1}^{J/2}\sum_{i=1}^{m} Y_{ijk}$ for $k = 1, 2$. The intervention effect can be estimated as the difference in sample proportions, $\hat{p}_1 - \hat{p}_2$, which has variance

$$Var(\hat{p}_1 - \hat{p}_2) = \frac{p_1(1-p_1)}{mJ/2}\mathrm{DE}_1 + \frac{p_2(1-p_2)}{mJ/2}\mathrm{DE}_2$$

where the design effects are $\mathrm{DE}_k = 1 + (m-1)\rho_k = 1 + (m-1)\frac{V_k}{p_k(1-p_k)}$, with V_k denoting the variance of the cluster-level proportions in condition k. This leads to a design effect-based sample size formula,

$$N_{\mathrm{CRT}} \geq \frac{2(z_{1-\alpha/2} + z_{1-\beta})^2[p_1(1-p_1)\mathrm{DE}_1 + p_2(1-p_2)\mathrm{DE}_2]}{(p_1 - p_2 - \Delta_0)^2}.$$

If we assume that $\rho_1 = \rho_2 = \rho$, then

$$N_{\mathrm{CRT}} \geq \frac{2(z_{1-\alpha/2} + z_{1-\beta})^2[p_1(1-p_1) + p_2(1-p_2)]\mathrm{DE}}{(p_1 - p_2 - \Delta_0)^2}.$$

Caveats. To use this approach, one must specify suitable values for ρ_1 and ρ_2. It can be difficult to find such values reported in the literature. Further, there are several different ways of defining an ICC for binary data and numerous different methods for estimating such ICCs [63, 237], which can create uncertainty about whether a particular reported value may be appropriate. One approach is to use the range rule to estimate V_1 and V_2, then use these estimates together with p_1 and p_2 to obtain estimates of ρ_1 and ρ_2. Note that due to the dependence of ρ here on the outcome proportion, it is unlikely that the design effects will be identical in two study conditions even if $V_1 = V_2$.

In the mixed logistic model, the between-cluster variance component σ_u^2 is on the log-odds scale and in the cluster-level proportions model, the between-cluster variance V is on the proportions scale. Thus these two quantities are not directly comparable and there is no closed-form relationship between them. An approximate relationship obtaining using a Taylor expansion is $\rho_h \approx \sigma_u^2 p(1-p)$ [63].

Another consideration is that the data from such trials will generally be analyzed using a common statistical method suitable for correlated data, such as a multilevel logistic regression model or generalized estimating equations and in general, the power analysis approach should be consistent with the planned analysis method. Beta-binomial models are not commonly used for randomized trials data analyses. All of these caveats should be kept in mind when using this approach.

Example 14.8. We repeat Example 14.7 using this approach. The expected outcome proportions are 0.15 and 0.25. Clusters are of size $m = 60$ students. How many schools are needed to achieve 80% power for a two-sided test of $H_0: p_T = p_C$ at $\alpha = 0.05$ for equal allocation?

First we calculate the sample size for independent observations:

```
library(powertools)
prop.2samp(n1 = NULL, p1 = 0.15, p2 = 0.25, alpha = 0.05, power = 0.8)
[1] 247.2397
```

This indicates a total of about 494 participants. Now we need estimates of the design effects. If we assume that cluster-level proportions will vary around the mean proportion for each condition by ±0.1, then $V_1 = V_2 = 0.05^2 = 0.0025$ and

```
p1 <- 0.15
p2 <- 0.25
V <- 0.05^2
# rhoh1:
V / (p1 * (1 - p1))
[1] 0.01960784
# rhoh2
V / (p2 * (1 - p2))
[1] 0.01333333
```

The values of the two design effects are relatively close; we will assume a value of 0.017 for both for simplicity. Now we inflate by the design effect:

```
de <- 1 + (60 - 1) * 0.017   ;   de
[1] 2.003
# total required N is:
N <- 494 * de   ;   N
[1] 989.482
library(plyr)
round_any(N, 120, ceiling)
[1] 1080
```

Rounding up to the next multiple of 120 (the number of students for two schools, one intervention and one control), this suggests that we need 1080 total student participants; this corresponds to 60 students at each of 18 schools.

14.3.3 Generalized estimating equations approach

The generalized estimating equations (GEE) approach [141, 241] is a popular method for analyzing correlated data, especially data with binary or other discrete outcomes, and has been used for many analyses of cluster randomized trials [83, 104, 164]. GEE requires only specification of the mean and covariance structure of the observations, not a full probability distribution. GEE yields population-average estimates of the effect of covariates using a "sandwich" variance estimator [103]. A major appeal of the GEE approach is that it is generally robust to misspecification of the covariance structure [144, 148].

Shih [203] presents sample size and power calculation methods that can be used for a cluster randomized trial with a binary outcome when the analysis method is GEE. The mean model uses a logit link

$$\log\left(\frac{P(Y=1|X)}{1-P(Y=1|X)}\right) = \beta_0 + \beta_1 X$$

where $X = 0, 1$ for the control and intervention conditions. The parameter β_1 is the log odds ratio, $\log\left(\frac{p_2/(1-p_2)}{p_1/(1-p_1)}\right)$, where p_1 and p_2 are the outcome proportions in the control and intervention conditions. It is assumed that the correlation structure is specified as exchangeable, i.e., all observations in a cluster are equally correlated, with $Corr(Y_{ij}, Y_{i'j}) = \rho$. This correlation coefficient is on the proportions scale and is essentially a Pearson correlation coefficient applied to binary observations. The required total number of clusters for testing $H_0: \beta_1 = 0$ when a fraction w are assigned to control and $1-w$ to intervention and clusters are of size m is calculated as

$$J = \frac{(z_{1-\alpha/2} + z_{1-\beta})^2 [1 + (m-1)\rho]}{m(\beta_1)^2} \left[\frac{1}{wp_1(1-p_1)} + \frac{1}{(1-w)p_2(1-p_2)}\right].$$

This formula corresponds to that for a simple logistic regression model with a single binary predictor, discussed in Section 11.2, with multiplication by the design effect $1 + (m-1)\rho$.

An important caveat for using the GEE method is that the sandwich estimator tends to underestimate the standard errors and thus can give an inflated type I error rate when the number of clusters is small. A minimum of 40 clusters has been suggested to avoid inflated type I errors [144, 148]; there are small sample corrections available, although they have been underutilized [104].

Example 14.9. We repeat Example 14.7 using the GEE approach. The specifications are $p_{TA} = 0.15$, $p_{CA} = 0.25$, clusters of 60 students, 80% power for a two-sided test of $H_0\colon p_T = p_C$ at $\alpha = 0.05$ with equal allocation.

First we use the wp.logistic function from the WebPower package to find the sample size assuming independent observations:

```
library(WebPower)
wp.logistic(n = NULL, p0 = 0.15, p1 = 0.25, alpha = 0.05, power = 0.8,
    alternative = "two.sided", family = "Bernoulli", parameter = 0.5)

Power for logistic regression

    p0   p1    beta0     beta1         n alpha power
  0.15 0.25 -1.734601 0.6359888 511.3719  0.05   0.8
```

Then we inflate by the design effect. We assume ρ of 0.017 as in Example 14.8 and thus the same design effect:

```
de <- 1 + (60 - 1) * 0.017 ;  de
[1] 2.003
# total required N is:
N <- 511.3719 * de ; N
[1]   1024.278
library(plyr)
round_any(N, 120, ceiling)
[1] 1080
```

Rounding up to the next multiple of 120, this suggests we need 1080 total participants, which corresponds to 60 students at each of 18 schools. This is the same sample size suggested by the cluster-level proportions design effect approach. Note that this is less than 40 clusters and type I error rates may be inflated unless a small sample bias correction is used in the analysis; see Huang et al [104] for more details and references.

14.4 Additional resources for parallel cluster randomized trials

There are several packages as well as several online tools for power calculation for parallel cluster randomized trials. Note that sometimes R packages are not posted on CRAN but can be accessed through authors' online resources or in the CRAN archives.

The WebPower package has a wide collection of tools for power analysis, including tools for cluster randomized trials. There is also a web application, available at https://webpower.psychstat.org, and a companion book, Zhang and Yuan [242].

The clusterPower package calculates power for parallel cluster randomized trials including multi-arm trials and some of the designs discussed in Chapter 15 using closed-form analytic solutions, and also estimates power using simulation. It handles normal, binary and count outcomes.

The CRTpowerdist package [175] focuses on attained power. Attained power is the power conditional on the realized allocation of units to study conditions and can differ from the pre-randomization expected power. For example, a two-arm trial that is expected to allocate 20 participants to each condition will attain less than the expected power if by chance it allocates 25 and 15 participants to the conditions. The package implements simulations and approximate analytic formulae and covers unequal cluster size, cross-sectional stepped wedge and parallel cluster randomized trials. Outcome types are continuous, binary and count. The analytic formula-based calculations are also implemented in a Shiny app.

The Research Methods Resources website of the National Institutes of Health includes sample size calculators for parallel cluster randomized trials, individually randomized group treatment trials and stepped wedge cluster randomized trials at https://researchmethodsresources.nih.gov/.

The Shiny CRT Calculator [91] is an app that is programmed in R and implemented using the R Shiny application. The app can be found at https://clusterrcts.shinyapps.io/rshinyapp. Source code and updates are located on GitHub at https://github.com/karlahemming/Cluster-RCT-Sample-Size-Calculator.

The PowerUpR package is a comprehensive package for evaluating sample size and power for studies with multilevel data, including multisite and cluster randomized trials with up to four levels, for continuous outcomes [56, 143]. There is a companion ShinyApp with a reference manual [12] available at https://www.causalevaluation.org/power-analysis.html. We discuss this further in Section 14.6.

14.5 Individually randomized group treatment trials

In the designs considered in this chapter thus far, the clusters or groups to which the study participants belong were in existence prior to randomization. In an individually randomized group treatment trial (IRGTT), individuals are randomized to study conditions and then organized into groups [179, 187]. The groups may be sets of individuals who receive their intervention together with other participants, such as a group-based exercise program, or the groups may be formed through the sharing of a common interventionist or facilitator, such as a therapist.

In some IRGTTs, grouping may occur in a similar manner in both study conditions. For example, study participants may be randomized to intervention and control conditions, and then participants in each condition are organized into meeting groups to receive a group-based intervention or a group-based control condition. When there is similar clustering in both conditions, the design can be handled as a parallel cluster randomized design. In other IRGTTs, only participants randomized to the intervention condition are organized into groups; participants assigned to the control condition are not subjected to any grouping. In this case, there is multilevel structure in the intervention condition and the outcomes of control participants can be regarded as independent. Some terms for this data structure are "partial nesting" or "partially clustered". We focus on this design in this section. Designs with differential clustering in the two conditions are discussed in Moerbeek and Teerenstra [158] as well as Hoover [101].

14.5.1 Continuous outcomes

14.5.1.1 Model

In this section, we present a model for an IRGTT with a continuous outcome based on [159, 158, 187]. To arrive at the full model, separate models are formulated for individuals in the control condition and in the intervention condition, then the two models are combined. In the control condition, the model for the outcome Y_i for individual i is

$$Y_i = \gamma_0 + r_i$$

where γ_0 is the mean outcome for control condition participants and $r_i \sim N(0, \sigma_r^2)$ is a random error term at the individual level. In the intervention condition, the model for the outcome Y_{ij} for participant i in group j is

$$Y_{ij} = \gamma_0 + \gamma_1 + u_j + \epsilon_{ij}$$

where γ_1 is the effect of the intervention, $u_j \sim N(0, \sigma_u^2)$ is a random error term at the group level, and $\epsilon_{ij} \sim N(0, \sigma_\epsilon^2)$ is a random error term at the individual level; these random effects are assumed to be independent. The model allows for correlation among individuals in the same group; the intraclass correlation is $\rho = \sigma_u^2 / (\sigma_u^2 + \sigma_\epsilon^2)$.

Defining an indicator variable I_{ij} equal to 1 if the individual is assigned to the intervention condition and 0 if assigned to control, the combined single-equation model is:

$$Y_{ij} = \gamma_0 + \gamma_1 I_{ij} + u_j I_{ij} + \epsilon_{ij} I_{ij} + r_i(1 - I_{ij}) \qquad (14.27)$$

with $r_i \sim N(0, \sigma_r^2)$, $u_j \sim N(0, \sigma_u^2)$ and $\epsilon_{ij} \sim N(0, \sigma_\epsilon^2)$, all mutually independent. Note that the total variance for individuals in the intervention condition,

$\sigma_u^2 + \sigma_\epsilon^2$, is not necessarily equal to the total variance σ_r^2 for individuals in the control condition; one condition could have higher total variance than the other.

14.5.1.2 Power for test of treatment effect

Suppose that we wish to test the null hypothesis $H_0: \gamma_1 = \gamma_{(0)}$. The treatment effect γ_1 can be estimated as

$$\hat{\gamma}_1 = \bar{Y}_{..T} - \bar{Y}_{.C}$$

where $\bar{Y}_{..T}$ is the mean for observations in the intervention condition and $\bar{Y}_{.C}$ is the mean for observations in the control condition. Let there be J groups each of size m in the intervention condition (we assume that the group sizes are constant), and let there be n total participants in the control condition. The variance of $Var(\hat{\gamma}_1)$ can be expressed as

$$Var(\hat{\gamma}_1) = \frac{m\sigma_u^2 + \sigma_\epsilon^2}{mJ} + \frac{\sigma_r^2}{n} = \sigma_r^2 \left(\frac{\Theta[1 + (m-1)\rho]}{mJ} + \frac{1}{n} \right) \quad (14.28)$$

where Θ is the ratio of the variances, $(\sigma_u^2 + \sigma_\epsilon^2)/\sigma_r^2$.

The null hypothesis $H_0: \gamma_1 = \gamma_{(0)}$ can be tested using the test statistic

$$T = \frac{\hat{\gamma}_1 - \gamma_{(0)}}{\sqrt{\widehat{Var}(\hat{\gamma}_1)}}$$

which has a central t distribution when H_0 is true. Hoover [101] suggests a Welch-Satterthwaite approximation for the degrees of freedom based on [53]. Defining the two terms in equation (14.28) as U_t and U_c, the approximation is

$$df \approx \frac{U_t^2 \left(\frac{J+1}{J-1} \right) + 2U_t U_c + U_c^2 \left(\frac{n+1}{n-1} \right)}{U_t^2 \left[\frac{J+1}{(J-1)^2} \right] + U_c^2 \left[\frac{n+1}{(n-1)^2} \right]}. \quad (14.29)$$

When the true treatment effect is $\gamma_{(A)}$, the test statistic has a noncentral t distribution with noncentrality parameter

$$\lambda = \frac{\gamma_{(A)} - \gamma_{(0)}}{\sqrt{Var(\hat{\gamma}_1)}} = \frac{\gamma_{(A)} - \gamma_{(0)}}{\sqrt{\frac{m\sigma_u^2 + \sigma_\epsilon^2}{mJ} + \frac{\sigma_r^2}{n}}} = \frac{\gamma_{(A)} - \gamma_{(0)}}{\sqrt{\sigma_r^2 \left(\frac{\Theta[1+(m-1)\rho]}{mJ} + \frac{1}{n} \right)}}. \quad (14.30)$$

When the treatment effect is standardized by the standard deviation of the outcome in the control condition, $d = \gamma_1/\sigma_r$, and $\gamma_{(0)} = 0$, the noncentrality parameter can be expressed as

$$\lambda = \frac{d}{\sqrt{\frac{\Theta[1+(m-1)\rho]}{mJ} + \frac{1}{n}}}. \quad (14.31)$$

Thus power can be calculated as

$$\text{Power (lower-tail test)} \approx P[T \le t_{\alpha,df} \mid T \sim t(df,\lambda)] \quad (14.32)$$
$$= \mathcal{T}_{df,\lambda}(t_{\alpha,df})$$
$$\text{Power (upper-tail test)} \approx P[T \ge t_{1-\alpha,df} \mid T \sim t(df,\lambda)]$$
$$= 1 - \mathcal{T}_{df,\lambda}(t_{1-\alpha,df})$$
$$\text{Power (two-sided test)} \approx P[T^2 \ge f_{1-\alpha,1,df} \mid T^2 \sim F(1,df,\Lambda)]$$
$$= 1 - \mathcal{F}_{1,df,\Lambda}(f_{1-\alpha,1,df})$$

where $\Lambda = \lambda^2$ and df are given in equation (14.29). For a lower-tailed test, we generally expect λ to be negative and for an upper-tailed test, we expect λ to be positive.

Example 14.10. Suppose that we plan an IRGTT that will randomize 200 individuals equally to an intervention condition and a control condition. Individuals randomized to the intervention condition will receive the intervention in groups of size 10. The standardized effect size is assumed to be $d = 0.4$ and the ratio of the total variances in the two conditions is assumed to be $\Theta = 1$. The ICC in the treatment condition is assumed to be 0.05. What is the power for a test of $H_0\colon \gamma_1 = 0$ with two-sided α of 0.05?

```
library(powertools)
irgtt.cont(m = 10, J = 10, n = 100, delta = 0.4, icc = 0.05, Theta = 1,
    power = NULL)
[1] 0.6518103
```

Power is about 0.65.

14.5.1.3 Sample size using normal approximation

If the test statistic for testing $H_0\colon \gamma_1 = 0$ had a normal distribution, we could calculate power for a two-sided test as

$$1 - \beta = \Phi\left(z_{\alpha/2} + |\lambda|\right) \quad (14.33)$$
$$= \Phi\left(z_{\alpha/2} + \frac{|d|}{\sqrt{\frac{\Theta[1+(m-1)\rho]}{mJ} + \frac{1}{n}}}\right)$$
$$z_{1-\beta} = z_{\alpha/2} + \frac{|d|}{\sqrt{\frac{\Theta[1+(m-1)\rho]}{mJ} + \frac{1}{n}}}$$
$$z_{1-\alpha/2} + z_{1-\beta} = \frac{|d|}{\sqrt{\frac{\Theta[1+(m-1)\rho]}{mJ} + \frac{1}{n}}}$$
$$\frac{\Theta[1+(m-1)\rho]}{mJ} + \frac{1}{n} = \frac{d^2}{(z_{1-\alpha/2} + z_{1-\beta})^2}.$$

Individually randomized group treatment trials 265

This formula can be solved for J, m or n. If we plan to allocate equal numbers of participants to the two conditions, then $mJ = n$ and the sample size required in each condition is

$$n = \frac{(z_{1-\alpha/2} + z_{1-\beta})^2(\Theta[1 + (m-1)\rho] + 1)}{d^2} \qquad (14.34)$$

for a total of $2n$ participants. Keep in mind that this approach will tend to underestimate the required sample sizes.

14.5.2 Binary outcomes

For binary outcomes in IRGTTs, we present an approach that uses the normal approximation to the binomial distribution with inflation by the design effect. This approach is expedient, but has some caveats. As discussed in Section 14.3.2, these include the difficulty of specifying suitable values for the ICCs when the outcomes are binary.

Suppose that the proportions with the outcome in the treatment and control conditions are expected to be p_T and p_C, respectively. As in Section 14.5.1.2, let J and m represent the number of groups and group size in the intervention condition, and let n represent the number of individual in the control condition, which does not entail any clustering. Suppose that we wish to test the hypothesis $H_0: p_T = p_C$. The intervention effect can be estimated as $\hat{p}_T - \hat{p}_C$, which will have variance approximately equal to

$$\frac{\hat{p}_T(1-\hat{p}_T)[1+(m-1)\rho]}{mJ} + \frac{\hat{p}_C(1-\hat{p}_C)}{n}.$$

The test statistic is

$$\frac{\hat{p}_T - \hat{p}_C}{\sqrt{\frac{\hat{p}_T(1-\hat{p}_T)[1+(m-1)\rho]}{mJ} + \frac{\hat{p}_C(1-\hat{p}_C)}{n}}}$$

and will have approximately a normal distribution. To find sample size to attain a desired level of power $1 - \beta$, we can set up and solve the equation

$$1 - \beta = \Phi\left(z_{\alpha/2} + \frac{p_T - p_C}{\sqrt{\frac{p_T(1-p_T)[1+(m-1)\rho]}{mJ} + \frac{p_C(1-p_C)}{n}}}\right),$$

arriving at

$$\frac{p_T(1-p_T)[1+(m-1)\rho]}{mJ} + \frac{p_C(1-p_C)}{n} = \frac{(p_T - p_C)^2}{(z_{1-\alpha/2} + z_{1-\beta})^2}.$$

This equation can be solved for J, m or n. If we plan to allocate equal numbers of participants to the two conditions, then $mJ = n$ and the sample size required in each condition is

$$n = \frac{(z_{1-\alpha/2} + z_{1-\beta})^2\{p_T(1-p_T)[1+(m-1)\rho] + p_C(1-p_C)\}}{(p_T - p_C)^2}$$

for a total of $2n$ participants.

Example 14.11. Suppose that in an IRGTT, the expected outcome proportions are $p_T = 0.6$ and $p_C = 0.8$. After individual randomization, intervention participants will be organized into groups of size 20 to receive intervention, while control condition participants will not be grouped. The ICC in the intervention condition is expected to be $\rho = 0.04$. What sample size is needed for 80% power, with two-sided α of 0.05?

If we plan to have equal allocation, then $n = mJ$, and we provide input to the function that is consistent with this relationship. A simple search finds the smallest J that achieves at least 80% power:

```
library(powertools)
irgtt.bin(m = 20, J = 6, n = 120, p1 = 0.8, p2 = 0.6, icc = 0.04,
    power = NULL)
[1] 0.8188213
```

This suggests that we need 6 groups, which entails 120 participants in each condition (total of 240). Keep in mind that the calculation uses a normal approximation and so may overestimate power.

14.5.3 Additional resources

The `clusterPower` package has functions for individually randomized group treatment trials. The functions use normal approximations and so will tend to overestimate power, especially when the number of clusters is small. Note that sometimes R packages are not posted on CRAN but can be accessed through authors' online resources or in the CRAN archives.

The Research Methods Resources website of the National Institutes of Health has guidance on research methods related to individually randomized group treatment trials as well as parallel cluster randomized trials and stepped wedge trials at https://researchmethodsresources.nih.gov. The website includes a sample size calculator.

14.6 Other multilevel trial designs

Standard multisite and cluster randomized trials have two levels, with individuals nested within sites/clusters. In some settings, such as educational settings, it is not uncommon to have studies that involve additional levels. For example, there may be students nested within classrooms nested within

Other multilevel trial designs

TABLE 14.2: Design options for trials with multilevel structure. CRT, cluster randomized trial; IRT, individually randomized trial; MS, multisite; MST, multisite trial.

	IRT	2-level MST	2-level CRT	3-level MST	3-level MS CRT	3-level CRT	4-level MS CRT
No. levels	1	2	2	3	3	3	4
Blocking level	–	2	–	2	3	–	4
Randomiz. level	1	1	2	1	2	3	3

schools (3 levels) or further nested within school districts (4 levels). Designs may have randomization at any of these levels.

Table 14.2 displays some design options for such trials. For all designs, we assume that outcomes are measured at the individual level. A standard individually randomized trial has one level, with randomization at that level. If there are two levels and randomization occurs at level 1, we have a standard multisite trial, as discussed in Chapter 13. In this case, there is blocking on site; randomization occurs within site. If there are two levels and randomization occurs at level 2, we have a standard cluster randomized trial.

When there are three levels, there are several different design options that depend on the level at which randomization occurs. Consider the case of students nested within classrooms nested within schools. If students are randomized within classrooms, then we have a 3-level multisite trial; if classrooms are randomized within schools, then we have a multisite cluster randomized trial; and if schools are the unit of randomization, then we have a cluster randomized trial.

Power and sample size calculations for such trials are extensions of the methods discussed in this book for multisite and cluster randomized trials. PowerUpR is a package for evaluating sample size and power for studies with multilevel data, including multisite and cluster randomized trials with up to four levels, for continuous outcomes [56, 143]. There is a companion ShinyApp with a reference manual [12] available at https://www.causalevaluation.org/power-analysis.html. This package also handles power for moderation and mediation analyses for many designs.

Another design option for multilevel trials is the **split-plot design** [50, 78, 121]. In a two-level split-plot design, there are two treatment factors, which we will call Factors A and B. First, sites are cluster-randomized to levels of Factor A, and then within sites, individuals are randomized to levels of Factor B. This is a type of factorial design (see Section 5.3) that results in individuals receiving all combinations of levels of Factors A and B. For example, the IQuaD trial randomized dental practices to provide either routine or personalized oral hygiene advice to all of their dental patients, and within each practice, patients were randomized to receive none, 6-monthly or 12-

monthly periodontal instrumentation procedures [34]. Sample size calculation procedures for 2×2 factorial split-plot designs have been developed by Tian et al. [216], who refer to this design as a hierarchical 2×2 factorial trial. The methods can be implemented in the H2x2Factorial package.

15
Cluster randomized trials: longitudinal designs

15.1 Introduction

Chapter 14 discussed parallel cluster randomized trials, in which each cluster is randomized to a condition and the outcome variable is measured at a single follow-up time point, after the treatment has been applied in the treatment condition and at a comparable time point in the control condition. This chapter covers cluster randomized trials with a longitudinal design, in which the outcome variable is measured at more than one time point. This includes parallel cluster randomized trials with a baseline measurement, cluster randomized crossover designs and stepped wedge designs.

We will call a cluster randomized trial with only a single measurement of the outcome variable, at follow up, a "simple" parallel design. Figure 15.1 compares simple parallel, parallel with a baseline measurement, crossover and stepped wedge cluster randomized trial designs. In a simple parallel cluster randomized trial (Panel (A)), each cluster is randomized to a condition and receives only that condition, and then the outcome is measured at follow-up. A **parallel cluster randomized trial with a baseline measurement** (Panel (B)) is similar, except that the outcome variable is also measured at baseline, before the treatment is applied to clusters assigned to the treatment condition and at a comparable time point in clusters assigned to the control condition. This is a common design, especially when the outcome variable is continuous. In a **cluster randomized crossover trial**, each cluster is randomized to a study arm that receives both the control condition and the treatment condition, but during different time periods. Panel (C) illustrates a 2×2 cluster randomized crossover design, in which clusters are randomized to receive either the control condition followed by the treatment condition or treatment followed by control. In a standard **stepped wedge cluster randomized trial**, clusters receive both the control and treatment condition, but transitions are only from control to treatment and different study arms transition to the treatment condition at different time periods. Panel (D) depicts a stepped wedge design in which all clusters start in the control condition and then a fixed number of clusters transition to the treatment condition at the start of

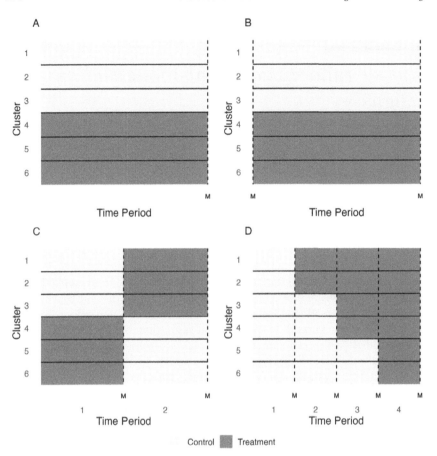

FIGURE 15.1: Schematic representation of different cluster randomized trial designs. Dashed lines labelled with "M" indicate times of measurement of the outcome variable. (A) Simple parallel cluster randomized trial, with three clusters allocated to the control condition and three clusters to the treatment condition; (B) Parallel cluster randomized trial with a baseline measurement; (C) Cluster randomized crossover design, with three clusters randomized to receive control then treatment and three clusters randomized to receive treatment then control; (D) Cluster randomized stepped wedge design, in which clusters are randomized to start the treatment at the beginning of different time periods. Two clusters are randomized to start treatment at Period 2, two are randomized to start at Period 3, and two are randomized to start at Period 4.

each time period. Other designs are possible, e.g., clusters may transition from control to treatment and then back to control.

Statistical models for each of these designs can be derived as special cases of a general model for a cluster randomized trial with longitudinal measurements. We discuss this general model in Section 15.2, with a focus on the correlation structure of the data and its parametrization, which are important for understanding and computing power. We discuss parallel cluster randomized trials with a baseline measurement in Section 15.3, cluster randomized crossover trials in Section 15.4, and stepped wedge trials in Section 15.5. We largely restrict attention to continuous outcomes, but provide resources for trials with binary and other types of outcomes.

15.2 Modeling framework for continuous outcomes

In this section, we describe a modeling framework for longitudinal cluster randomized trials. The framework will be applied to the various trial designs discussed in this chapter. Publications describing this modeling framework include Feldman and McKinlay [68] and Hooper et al. [100], with Li et al. [140] providing a particularly thorough synthesis of modeling options.

Among longitudinal cluster randomized trials, we can distinguish between cross-sectional designs and closed cohort designs. In a **cross-sectional design**, the measurements at different time points are taken on different individuals. In a **closed cohort design**, the same individuals are followed throughout the study, and thus the measurements at the different time points are taken on the same individuals. We discuss both types of designs.

15.2.1 Cross-sectional designs

Suppose that a study will involve a total of J clusters indexed by j and T time periods indexed by t. The clusters have been assigned to study arms indexed by k. In a cross-sectional design, different individuals are measured in each cluster at each time period. We assume an equal number m are measured in each cluster at each period and index individuals by i.

Exchangeable correlation. One model for the outcome of individual i in cluster j in study arm k at time t for a cross-sectional design is [107]

$$Y_{ijkt} = \mu_{kt} + c_j + s_{ijt} \qquad (15.1)$$

where μ_{kt} is a fixed effect and the other terms are random effects. The term μ_{kt} is the mean in study arm k at time t. This term will be parametrized further for specific study designs. In this section, the main focus is on the random effects and the correlation structure of the data. These are important in order to derive the variance of the estimator of the treatment effect and therefore the parameters that are needed for power calculations.

In model (15.1), c_j is a cluster-level random effect. This random effect is time-invariant; for any cluster j, it takes the same value at each time point. The term s_{ijt} is a subject-specific random effect; this term allows subjects within the same cluster and time period to vary in outcomes. The random effects are assumed to be normally distributed with mean zero and variances σ_c^2 and σ_{st}^2, respectively, and mutually independent. The total variance of an observation is $Var(Y_{ijkt}) = \sigma_Y^2 = \sigma_c^2 + \sigma_{st}^2$.

In model (15.1), the correlation between the outcomes of two different individuals in the same cluster in the same time period (the within-cluster, within-period ICC) is

$$\rho_w = Corr(Y_{ijkt}, Y_{i'jkt}) = \frac{\sigma_c^2}{\sigma_Y^2}.$$

This corresponds to the ICC in a simple parallel cluster randomized trial, which we denoted ρ in that context. Here, we add the subscript w to distinguish it from other ICCs that will be defined. In addition, in model (15.1), the correlation between the outcomes of two different individuals in the same cluster but different time periods (the within-cluster, between-period ICC), is also ρ_w: $Corr(Y_{ijkt}, Y_{i'jkt'}) = \sigma_c^2/\sigma_Y^2 = \rho_w$. This is termed **exchangeable** or **compound symmetry correlation structure**. Exchangeable correlation structure is illustrated in the top left panel of Figure 15.2. Each panel in this figure displays the correlation matrix for a vector of six observations taken from a single cluster over time. There are three time periods and in each period, two observations are collected from the cluster. The vector of observations is $(Y_{11}, Y_{21}, Y_{12}, Y_{22}, Y_{13}, Y_{23})$, where we only show the indices for individual i and period t, Y_{it}. For cross-sectional sampling, all observations are from different individuals. In an exchangeable structure, the correlation between any two individuals in the same cluster and same period is ρ_w, and the correlation between any two individuals in the same cluster and different periods is also ρ_w.

In model (15.1), a cluster-period mean takes the form

$$\bar{Y}_{\cdot jkt} = \frac{1}{m}\sum_{i=1}^{m} Y_{ijkt} = \frac{1}{m}\sum_{i=1}^{m}[\mu_{kt} + c_j + s_{ijt}]$$

$$= \mu_{kt} + c_j + \frac{1}{m}\sum_{i=1}^{m} s_{ijt}$$

and the variance of a cluster-period mean is

$$Var(\bar{Y}_{\cdot jkt}) = \sigma_c^2 + \frac{\sigma_{st}^2}{m} = \frac{\sigma_Y^2}{m}[1 + (m-1)\rho_w].$$

This is the same result that we found for the cluster-level mean in a simple parallel cluster randomized trial in equation (14.8). The covariance of two cluster-period means from the same cluster during different periods $t \neq t'$ is

$$Cov(\bar{Y}_{\cdot jkt}, \bar{Y}_{\cdot jkt'}) = Cov\left(c_j + \frac{\sum s_{ijt}}{m}, c_j + \frac{\sum s_{ijt'}}{m}\right)$$

$$= \sigma_c^2 = \sigma_Y^2 \rho_w$$

Modeling framework for continuous outcomes 273

	CROSS-SECTIONAL	CLOSED COHORT
	Exchangeable	Basic

$$\begin{pmatrix} 1 & \rho_w & \rho_w & \rho_w & \rho_w & \rho_w \\ \rho_w & 1 & \rho_w & \rho_w & \rho_w & \rho_w \\ \rho_w & \rho_w & 1 & \rho_w & \rho_w & \rho_w \\ \rho_w & \rho_w & \rho_w & 1 & \rho_w & \rho_w \\ \rho_w & \rho_w & \rho_w & \rho_w & 1 & \rho_w \\ \rho_w & \rho_w & \rho_w & \rho_w & \rho_w & 1 \end{pmatrix} \quad \begin{pmatrix} 1 & \rho_w & \rho_a & \rho_w & \rho_a & \rho_w \\ \rho_w & 1 & \rho_w & \rho_a & \rho_w & \rho_a \\ \rho_a & \rho_w & 1 & \rho_w & \rho_a & \rho_w \\ \rho_w & \rho_a & \rho_w & 1 & \rho_w & \rho_a \\ \rho_a & \rho_w & \rho_a & \rho_w & 1 & \rho_w \\ \rho_w & \rho_a & \rho_w & \rho_a & \rho_w & 1 \end{pmatrix}$$

	Nested exchangeable	Block exchangeable

$$\begin{pmatrix} 1 & \rho_w & \rho_b & \rho_b & \rho_b & \rho_b \\ \rho_w & 1 & \rho_b & \rho_b & \rho_b & \rho_b \\ \rho_b & \rho_b & 1 & \rho_w & \rho_b & \rho_b \\ \rho_b & \rho_b & \rho_w & 1 & \rho_b & \rho_b \\ \rho_b & \rho_b & \rho_b & \rho_b & 1 & \rho_w \\ \rho_b & \rho_b & \rho_b & \rho_b & \rho_w & 1 \end{pmatrix} \quad \begin{pmatrix} 1 & \rho_w & \rho_a & \rho_b & \rho_a & \rho_b \\ \rho_w & 1 & \rho_b & \rho_a & \rho_b & \rho_a \\ \rho_a & \rho_b & 1 & \rho_w & \rho_a & \rho_b \\ \rho_b & \rho_a & \rho_w & 1 & \rho_b & \rho_a \\ \rho_a & \rho_b & \rho_a & \rho_b & 1 & \rho_w \\ \rho_b & \rho_a & \rho_b & \rho_a & \rho_w & 1 \end{pmatrix}$$

	Exponential decay	Proportional decay

$$\begin{pmatrix} 1 & \rho_w & \rho_w\tau & \rho_w\tau & \rho_w\tau^2 & \rho_w\tau^2 \\ \rho_w & 1 & \rho_w\tau & \rho_w\tau & \rho_w\tau^2 & \rho_w\tau^2 \\ \rho_w\tau & \rho_w\tau & 1 & \rho_w & \rho_w\tau & \rho_w\tau \\ \rho_w\tau & \rho_w\tau & \rho_w & 1 & \rho_w\tau & \rho_w\tau \\ \rho_w\tau^2 & \rho_w\tau^2 & \rho_w\tau & \rho_w\tau & 1 & \rho_w \\ \rho_w\tau^2 & \rho_w\tau^2 & \rho_w\tau & \rho_w\tau & \rho_w & 1 \end{pmatrix} \quad \begin{pmatrix} 1 & \rho_w & \tau & \rho_w\tau & \tau^2 & \rho_w\tau^2 \\ \rho_w & 1 & \rho_w\tau & \tau & \rho_w\tau^2 & \tau^2 \\ \tau & \rho_w\tau & 1 & \rho_w & \tau & \rho_w\tau \\ \rho_w\tau & \tau & \rho_w & 1 & \rho_w\tau & \tau \\ \tau^2 & \rho_w\tau^2 & \tau & \rho_w\tau & 1 & \rho_w \\ \rho_w\tau^2 & \tau^2 & \rho_w\tau & \tau & \rho_w & 1 \end{pmatrix}$$

FIGURE 15.2: Illustration of different correlation structures for a longitudinal cluster randomized trial. Each panel displays the correlations among observations taken from a single cluster over time. There are 3 time periods and in each period, 2 observations are taken. Each panel is the correlation matrix for the vector of length 6 of the observations. Figure partly adapted from Li et al. [140].

and the correlation is

$$Corr\left(\bar{Y}_{\cdot jkt}, \bar{Y}_{\cdot jkt'}\right) = \frac{m\rho_w}{1 + (m-1)\rho_w}. \tag{15.2}$$

Nested exchangeable correlation. Exchangeable correlation may not be a realistic assumption in some studies. Rather, we may expect that the within-cluster, between-period ICC will be less than the within-cluster, within-period ICC. A model for the outcome of individual i in cluster j in study arm k at time t for a cross-sectional design that allows $\rho_b < \rho_w$ is [68, 100, 77]

$$Y_{ijkt} = \mu_{kt} + c_j + (ct)_{jt} + s_{ijt} \tag{15.3}$$

In this model, c_j is a time-invariant cluster-level random effect, taking the same value for all time periods, and $(ct)_{jt}$ is a time-varying or time-specific cluster-level random effect. The term $(ct)_{jt}$ allows the effect of being in cluster j to be different at different times; it is a cluster-by-time interaction term. The term s_{ijt} is a subject-specific random effect that allows subjects within the same cluster and time period to vary in outcomes. The random effects are assumed to be normally distributed with mean zero and variances σ_c^2, σ_{ct}^2 and σ_{st}^2, respectively, and mutually independent. The total variance of an observation is $Var(Y_{ijkt}) = \sigma_Y^2 = \sigma_c^2 + \sigma_{ct}^2 + \sigma_{st}^2$.

In this model, the correlation between the outcomes of two individuals in the same cluster and same time period is

$$\rho_w = Corr(Y_{ijkt}, Y_{i'jkt}) = \frac{\sigma_c^2 + \sigma_{ct}^2}{\sigma_Y^2}$$

and the correlation between the outcomes of two individuals in the same cluster but different time periods is

$$\rho_b = Corr(Y_{ijkt}, Y_{i'jkt'}) = \frac{\sigma_c^2}{\sigma_Y^2},$$

which constrains $\rho_b \leq \rho_w$. The random effects in model (15.3) induce a **nested exchangeable correlation structure**, also called **nested compound symmetry**, which is illustrated in the middle left panel of Figure 15.2.

Another useful parameter is the **cluster autocorrelation** (CAC), defined as

$$CAC = \frac{\sigma_c^2}{\sigma_c^2 + \sigma_{ct}^2} = \frac{\rho_b}{\rho_w}.$$

The CAC can be interpreted as the proportion of the cluster-level variance that is time-invariant [68]. CAC values close to 1 imply that a cluster's means tend to be very similar over time. We can describe the correlation structure in model (15.3) using (ρ_w, ρ_b) or (ρ_w, CAC).

In a model with nested exchangeable correlation structure, a cluster-period mean takes the form

$$\bar{Y}_{.jkt} = \mu_{kt} + c_j + (ct)_{jt} + \frac{1}{m}\sum_{i=1}^{m} s_{ijt}$$

and the variance of a cluster-period mean is

$$Var(\bar{Y}_{.jkt}) = \sigma_c^2 + \sigma_{ct}^2 + \frac{\sigma_{st}^2}{m} = \frac{\sigma_Y^2}{m}[1 + (m-1)\rho_w].$$

Modeling framework for continuous outcomes 275

The covariance of two cluster-period means from the same cluster during different periods $t \neq t'$ is

$$Cov\left(\bar{Y}_{\cdot jkt}, \bar{Y}_{\cdot jkt'}\right)$$
$$= Cov\left(c_j + (ct)_{jt} + \frac{\sum s_{ijt}}{m}, c_j + (ct)_{jt'} + \frac{\sum s_{ijt'}}{m}\right)$$
$$= \sigma_c^2 = \sigma_Y^2 \rho_w \text{CAC}$$

and the correlation is

$$Corr\left(\bar{Y}_{\cdot jkt}, \bar{Y}_{\cdot jkt'}\right) = \frac{m\rho_w \text{CAC}}{1 + (m-1)\rho_w}. \quad (15.4)$$

Exponential decay. The nested exchangeable correlation model has been extended to allow the between-period correlation to decay over time [117]. Such models are most relevant to designs with three or more periods such as stepped wedge trials, discussed in Section 15.5. The exponential decay model for cluster randomized longitudinal data with cross-sectional sampling of subjects can be expressed as

$$Y_{ijkt} = \mu_{kt} + \nu_{jt} + s_{ijt} \quad (15.5)$$

where s_{ijt} is a subject-specific random effect with variance σ_{st}^2 and each cluster j has a set of random effects over the time periods given by $\nu_j = (\nu_{j1}, \ldots, \nu_{jT})' \sim \mathcal{N}(0, \sigma_\nu^2 \mathbf{M})$, where a typical choice for $\mathbf{M}$ is an autoregressive structure, $\mathbf{M}(1, \tau)$, where τ is the decay rate. In such models, the decay in correlation is a function of the distance between time periods. In the autoregressive model, the total variance of an observation is $Var(Y_{ijkt}) = \sigma_\nu^2 + \sigma_{st}^2$ and the correlation between observations is

$$Corr(Y_{ijkt}, Y_{ijkt'}) = \begin{cases} \rho_w = \sigma_\nu^2/(\sigma_\nu^2 + \sigma_{st}^2), & \text{if } t = t' \\ \rho_{b,|t-t'|} = \sigma_\nu^2 \tau^{|t-t'|}/(\sigma_\nu^2 + \sigma_{st}^2), & \text{if } t \neq t' \end{cases} \quad (15.6)$$

The bottom left panel of Figure 15.2 provides an illustration of exponential decay (autoregressive) correlation structure.

15.2.2 Closed cohort designs

In a closed cohort model, the same individuals are measured in each cluster during each time period. Suppose that we have a total of J clusters indexed by j, each of which is assigned to a study arm indexed by k. Each cluster includes m individuals indexed by i, each of whom is measured at T time points indexed by t.

Basic cohort model. A basic model for the outcome of individual i in cluster j in study arm k at time t that allows for repeated measures on the same individuals is [13, 40]

$$Y_{ijkt} = \mu_{kt} + c_j + s_{ij} + (st)_{ijt} \quad (15.7)$$

where μ_{kt} is a fixed effect and the other terms are random effects. The term c_j is a time-invariant cluster-level random effect. The term s_{ij} is a time-invariant subject-specific random effect and $(st)_{ijt}$ is a random effect that reflects variation of an individual between different time points; the latter can be regarded as a subject-by-time interaction effect. The random effects are assumed to be normally distributed with mean zero and variances σ_c^2, σ_s^2 and σ_{st}^2 and mutually independent. The total variance of an observation is $Var(Y_{ijkt}) = \sigma_Y^2 = \sigma_c^2 + \sigma_s^2 + \sigma_{st}^2$.

In this model, the correlation between two observations from the same individual in different time periods is

$$Corr(Y_{ijkt}, Y_{ijkt'}) = \rho_a = (\sigma_c^2 + \sigma_s^2)/(\sigma_c^2 + \sigma_s^2 + \sigma_{st}^2)$$

and the correlation between two observations from different individuals, whether in the same period or different periods, is

$$Corr(Y_{ijkt}, Y_{i'jkt}) = Corr(Y_{ijkt}, Y_{i'jkt'}) = \rho_w = \sigma_c^2/(\sigma_c^2 + \sigma_s^2 + \sigma_{st}^2)$$

[138]. This correlation structure is illustrated in the top right panel of Figure 15.2. The same individual is measured in each period.

In a closed cohort design, we define the **subject autocorrelation** (SAC) as the proportion of the subject-level variance that is time-invariant [68]. In the basic cohort model, the SAC is

$$\text{SAC} = \frac{\sigma_s^2}{\sigma_s^2 + \sigma_{st}^2} = \frac{\rho_a - \rho_w}{1 - \rho_w}. \tag{15.8}$$

SAC values close to 1 imply that an individual's outcome values do not change much over time, after controlling for fixed effects. We can describe the correlation structure using (ρ_w, ρ_a) or (ρ_w, SAC).

In model (15.7), a cluster-period mean takes the form

$$\bar{Y}_{\cdot jkt} = \mu_{kt} + c_j + \frac{1}{m}\sum_{i=1}^{m} s_{ij} + \frac{1}{m}\sum_{i=1}^{m}(st)_{ijt}$$

and has variance

$$Var(\bar{Y}_{\cdot jkt}) = \sigma_c^2 + \frac{\sigma_s^2}{m} + \frac{\sigma_{st}^2}{m} = \frac{\sigma_Y^2}{m}[1 + (m-1)\rho_w].$$

The covariance of two cluster-period means from the same cluster during different periods $t \neq t'$ is

$$Cov\left(\bar{Y}_{\cdot jkt}, \bar{Y}_{\cdot jkt'}\right)$$
$$= Cov\left(c_j + \frac{\sum s_{ij}}{m} + \frac{\sum (st)_{ijt}}{m}, c_j + \frac{\sum s_{ij}}{m} + \frac{\sum (st)_{ijt'}}{m}\right)$$
$$= \sigma_c^2 + \frac{\sigma_s^2}{m} = \frac{\sigma_Y^2}{m}[\rho_a + (m-1)\rho_w]$$

Modeling framework for continuous outcomes 277

and the correlation is

$$Corr\left(\bar{Y}_{\cdot jkt}, \bar{Y}_{\cdot jkt'}\right) = \frac{\rho_a + (m-1)\rho_w}{1 + (m-1)\rho_w}. \tag{15.9}$$

Block exchangeable correlation. Model (15.7) assumes that the correlation between measurements collected from different individuals in the same cluster is the same regardless of whether the measurements are from the same period or different periods, which can be unrealistic. A model for the outcome of individual i in cluster j in study arm k at time t that relaxes this assumption is [68, 100, 77]

$$Y_{ijkt} = \mu_{kt} + c_j + (ct)_{jt} + s_{ij} + (st)_{ijt} \tag{15.10}$$

where μ_{kt} is a fixed effect and the other terms are random effects. This model includes random effects for both clusters and subjects, and for both, there are time-invariant and time-varying (time-specific) components. The terms c_j and $(ct)_{jt}$ are time-invariant and time-varying (time-specific) cluster-level random effects. The term s_{ij} is a time-invariant subject-specific random effect and $(st)_{ijt}$ is a random effect that reflects variation of an individual between different time points; the latter can be regarded as a subject-by-time interaction effect. The random effects are assumed to be normally distributed with mean zero and variances σ_c^2, σ_{ct}^2, σ_s^2 and σ_{st}^2 and are assumed to be mutually independent. The total variance of an observation is $Var(Y_{ijkt}) = \sigma_Y^2 = \sigma_c^2 + \sigma_{ct}^2 + \sigma_s^2 + \sigma_{st}^2$.

In this model, the correlation between the outcomes of two different individuals ($i \neq i'$) in the same cluster and same time period, i.e., the within-cluster, within-period ICC, is

$$\rho_w = Corr(Y_{ijkt}, Y_{i'jkt}) = \frac{\sigma_c^2 + \sigma_{ct}^2}{\sigma_Y^2}. \tag{15.11}$$

The within-cluster, between-period ICC, which is the correlation between the outcomes of two different individuals ($i \neq i'$) in the same cluster but different periods ($t \neq t'$), is

$$\rho_b = Corr(Y_{ijkt}, Y_{i'jkt'}) = \frac{\sigma_c^2}{\sigma_Y^2}.$$

Note that $\rho_b \leq \rho_w$. We can also define the within-cluster, within-subject correlation as the correlation between two measurements within the same subject at different times,

$$\rho_a = Corr(Y_{ijkt}, Y_{ijkt'}) = \frac{\sigma_c^2 + \sigma_s^2}{\sigma_Y^2}.$$

Note that $\rho_a \geq \rho_b$, that is, the correlation between two measurements on the same individual in different time periods will be stronger than the correlation between measurements of two different individuals in the same cluster but different time periods.

The random effects in model (15.10) induce a **block exchangeable correlation structure**, which is illustrated in the middle right panel of Figure 15.2. The correlation between different individuals in the same cluster and same period is ρ_w, the correlation between different individuals in the same cluster and different periods is ρ_b, and the correlation between different measurements on the same individual in different periods is ρ_a.

As for the cross-sectional design, we define the cluster autocorrelation as

$$\text{CAC} = \frac{\sigma_c^2}{\sigma_c^2 + \sigma_{ct}^2} = \frac{\rho_b}{\rho_w}. \tag{15.12}$$

The subject autocorrelation (SAC) in this model is

$$\text{SAC} = \frac{\sigma_s^2}{\sigma_s^2 + \sigma_{st}^2} = \frac{\rho_a - \rho_b}{1 - \rho_w}. \tag{15.13}$$

SAC values close to 1 imply that an individual's outcome values do not change much over time, after controlling for fixed effects. We can describe the correlation structure using (ρ_w, ρ_b, ρ_a) or $(\rho_w, \text{CAC}, \text{SAC})$.

In model (15.10), a cluster-period mean takes the form

$$\bar{Y}_{\cdot jkt} = \frac{1}{m}\sum_{i=1}^{m} Y_{ijkt} = \frac{1}{m}\sum_{i=1}^{m}\left[\mu_{kt} + c_j + (ct)_{jt} + s_{ij} + (st)_{ijt}\right]$$

$$= \mu_{kt} + c_j + (ct)_{jt} + \frac{1}{m}\sum_{i=1}^{m} s_{ij} + \frac{1}{m}\sum_{i=1}^{m}(st)_{ijt}$$

and the variance of a cluster-period mean is

$$Var(\bar{Y}_{\cdot jkt}) = \sigma_c^2 + \sigma_{ct}^2 + \frac{\sigma_s^2}{m} + \frac{\sigma_{st}^2}{m} = \frac{\sigma_Y^2}{m}[1 + (m-1)\rho_w].$$

The covariance of two cluster-period means from the same cluster during different periods $t \neq t'$ is

$$Cov\left(\bar{Y}_{\cdot jkt}, \bar{Y}_{\cdot jkt'}\right)$$
$$= Cov\left(c_j + (ct)_{jt} + \frac{\sum s_{ij}}{m} + \frac{\sum(st)_{ijt}}{m},\ c_j + (ct)_{jt'} + \frac{\sum s_{ij}}{m} + \frac{\sum(st)_{ijt'}}{m}\right)$$
$$= \sigma_c^2 + \frac{\sigma_s^2}{m} = \frac{\sigma_Y^2}{m}[\rho_a + (m-1)\rho_b] = \frac{\sigma_Y^2}{m}[m\rho_w\,\text{CAC} + (1-\rho_w)\text{SAC}]$$

and the correlation is

$$Corr\left(\bar{Y}_{\cdot jkt}, \bar{Y}_{\cdot jkt'}\right) = \frac{\rho_a + (m-1)\rho_b}{1 + (m-1)\rho_w} = \frac{m\rho_w\,\text{CAC} + (1-\rho_w)\text{SAC}}{1 + (m-1)\rho_w}. \tag{15.14}$$

Note that the basic cohort model has $\rho_b = \rho_w$ and the CAC is constrained to be 1.

Proportional exponential decay. The block exchangeable correlation model (15.10) has been extended to allow exponential decay of the between-period ICC and the within-individual ICC [137, 140]. This modeling option is most relevant to designs with three or more periods such as stepped wedge trials; see Section 15.5. We can formulate an exponential decay model for a closed cohort with the same form as the exponential decay model for cross-sectional sampling given in equation (15.5), with the further assumption of autoregressive structure for the residual errors,

$$\mathbf{s}_{ij} = (s_{ij1}, \ldots, s_{ijT})' \sim \mathcal{N}(0, \sigma_{st}^2 \, \mathbf{M}(1, \tau))$$

where τ is the decay rate shared with $\boldsymbol{\nu}_j$. This model is termed the **proportional decay model** because the same decay rate τ applies to both the within-individual ICC and the between-period ICC for different individuals. The within-cluster correlations between pairs of observations in this model are

$$Corr(Y_{ijt}, Y_{i'jt'}) = \begin{cases} \rho_w = \sigma_\nu^2/(\sigma_\nu^2 + \sigma_{st}^2) & \text{if } t = t', i \neq i' \\ \rho_{b,|t-t'|} = \rho_w \tau^{|t-t'|} & \text{if } t \neq t', i \neq i' \\ \rho_{a,|t-t'|} = \tau^{|t-t'|} & \text{if } i = i', t \neq t' \end{cases}$$

The bottom right panel of Figure 15.2 provides an illustration of proportional decay correlation structure.

15.2.3 Summary of models

Table 15.1 summarizes the models discussed in this section and their correlation parameters. An important factor in choosing between these models is the number of periods in the trial. Cross-sectional exchangeable is the standard choice for cluster randomized trials with one period, that is, just a follow up measurement of the outcome variable. For trials with two periods, nested exchangeable for cross-sectional sampling and block exchangeable for closed cohorts are common choices. For trials with three or more periods such as stepped wedge trials, those two modeling options can be considered along with models allowing for decay in correlation, with decay models generally providing a more realistic model for the data as the number of periods and the total length of the trial increases. Additional modeling options for stepped wedge trials are discussed in Section 15.5.

A general expression for the correlation between two cluster-period means from the same cluster during different time periods is

$$r = Corr\left(\bar{Y}_{\cdot jkt}, \bar{Y}_{\cdot jkt'}\right) = \frac{m\rho_w \, \text{CAC} + (1 - \rho_w)\text{SAC}}{1 + (m-1)\rho_w} \tag{15.15}$$

TABLE 15.1: Summary of models for longitudinal cluster randomized trials with a continuous outcome and their variance/correlation parameters. CAC, cluster autocorrelation; SAC, subject autocorrelation.

Design	Total variance σ_Y^2	Correlation parameters
Cross-sectional		
Exchangeable	$\sigma_c^2 + \sigma_{st}^2$	$\rho_w = \sigma_c^2/\sigma_Y^2$
Nested exchangeable	$\sigma_c^2 + \sigma_{ct}^2 + \sigma_{st}^2$	$\rho_w = (\sigma_c^2 + \sigma_{ct}^2)/\sigma_Y^2$
		$\rho_b = \sigma_c^2/\sigma_Y^2$
		CAC $= \rho_b/\rho_w$
Exponential decay	$\sigma_\nu^2 + \sigma_{st}^2$	$\rho_w = \sigma_\nu^2/\sigma_Y^2$
		$\rho_{b,|t-t'|} = \rho_w \tau^{|t-t'|}$
Closed cohort		
Basic	$\sigma_c^2 + \sigma_s^2 + \sigma_{st}^2$	$\rho_a = (\sigma_c^2 + \sigma_s^2)/\sigma_Y^2$
		$\rho_w = \sigma_c^2/\sigma_Y^2$
		SAC $= (\rho_a - \rho_w)/(1 - \rho_w)$
Block exchangeable	$\sigma_c^2 + \sigma_{ct}^2 + \sigma_s^2 + \sigma_{st}^2$	$\rho_w = (\sigma_c^2 + \sigma_{ct}^2)/\sigma_Y^2$
		$\rho_b = \sigma_c^2/\sigma_Y^2$
		$\rho_a = (\sigma_c^2 + \sigma_s^2)/\sigma_Y^2$
		CAC $= \rho_b/\rho_w$
		SAC $= (\rho_a - \rho_b)/(1 - \rho_w)$
Proportional decay	$\sigma_\nu^2 + \sigma_{st}^2$	$\rho_w = \sigma_\nu^2/\sigma_Y^2$
		$\rho_{b,|t-t'|} = \rho_w \tau^{|t-t'|}$
		$\rho_{a,|t-t'|} = \tau^{|t-t'|}$

where exchangeable correlation structure has CAC = 1 and SAC = 0, nested exchangeable has CAC in the interval $(0,1)$ and SAC = 0, basic cohort has CAC = 1 and SAC in the interval $(0,1)$, and block exchangeable has both CAC and SAC in the interval $(0,1)$.

Power and sample size calculations for longitudinal cluster randomized trials require estimates of the various ICCs and/or autocorrelations listed in Table 15.1. Ouyang et al. [177] present a tutorial on estimating ICCs for planning such trials.

15.3 Parallel cluster randomized trial with baseline measurement

In a parallel cluster randomized trial with a baseline measurement, the outcome variable is measured on participants at both baseline, prior to randomization, and at follow up. Study designs with a baseline measurement of the outcome variable are common, especially when the outcome variable is continuous. For example, a treatment trial for depression may collect a depressive symptoms measurement from participants at both baseline and follow-up.

There are several options for analyzing the data from such a trial. One option is to adjust for the baseline measurement as a covariate in a regression model that has the follow up measurement as the dependent variable. This approach is called analysis of covariance (ANCOVA). ANCOVA for independent (not clustered) observations is discussed in Section 5.4. The general topic of adjusting for baseline covariates in a parallel cluster randomized trial is discussed in Section 14.2.9.2.

In this section, we discuss another option, which is modeling the repeated measures of the outcome variable in a longitudinal model; that is, the baseline and follow up measurements together form the dependent variable vector. Confusingly, this approach is also sometimes called ANCOVA. We discuss this option for both cross-sectional and closed cohort designs. Note that adjustment for the baseline measurement as a covariate is only possible in a closed cohort design, which measures the same individuals at both timepoints. The material here is based largely on the work of Feldman and McKinlay [68] and Teerenstra et al. [215].

15.3.1 Treatment effect estimator and variance

Suppose that individuals indexed by i in a total of J clusters indexed by j are measured at times $t = 0$ for baseline and $t = 1$ for follow-up. The clusters have been assigned to two study arms indexed as $k = 0$ for control and $k = 1$ for intervention. We assume a balanced design in which there are m measurements in each cluster at baseline and at follow up. In a closed cohort design, the measurements are from m individuals measured twice. In a cross-sectional design, m individuals are measured at baseline and a different m individuals are measured at follow up.

Let μ_{kt} be the mean in arm k at time t. For this design, the cluster-period means are

	Period 0	Period 1
Arm 0 (Control)	μ_{00}	μ_{01}
Arm 1 (Intervention)	μ_{10}	μ_{11}

There are two quantities that provide unbiased estimates of the treatment effect, which we will denote γ. First, when clusters are randomized to study arms, in expectation there are no differences in means between the arms at baseline and the difference in means between study arms at follow up represents the effect of treatment. We will use $\hat{\gamma}_{fu}$ to denote this treatment effect estimator. This estimator is the difference in sample means at follow-up between intervention and control clusters,

$$\hat{\gamma}_{fu} = \hat{\mu}_{11} - \hat{\mu}_{01} = \bar{Y}_{..11} - \bar{Y}_{..01} \tag{15.16}$$

The effect of treatment can also be estimated as the mean difference in change over time between intervention and control clusters, which is

$$\hat{\gamma}_{chg} = (\hat{\mu}_{11} - \hat{\mu}_{10}) - (\hat{\mu}_{01} - \hat{\mu}_{00}) = (\bar{Y}_{..11} - \bar{Y}_{..10}) - (\bar{Y}_{..01} - \bar{Y}_{..00}). \tag{15.17}$$

Teerenstra et al. [215] show that the estimator of γ with smallest variance is the combined estimator

$$\hat{\gamma} = r\hat{\gamma}_{chg} + (1-r)\hat{\gamma}_{fu} = (\bar{Y}_{..11} - r\bar{Y}_{..10}) - (\bar{Y}_{..01} - r\bar{Y}_{..00}) \tag{15.18}$$

where r is the correlation between two cluster-periods means; see equation (15.15). This is called the ANCOVA (analysis of covariance) estimator.

Suppose that a fraction w of clusters are assigned to the control arm, so that a fraction $1-w$ are assigned to the intervention arm. For a closed cohort design, block exchangeable correlation structure as described in model (15.10) will generally be the most appropriate choice. For this model, we can find that

$$Var(\hat{\gamma}_{fu}) = \left(\frac{1}{wJ} + \frac{1}{(1-w)J}\right)\left(\sigma_c^2 + \sigma_{ct}^2 + \frac{\sigma_s^2}{m} + \frac{\sigma_{st}^2}{m}\right)$$

$$= \left(\frac{1}{w} + \frac{1}{1-w}\right)\frac{\sigma_Y^2}{mJ}[1 + (m-1)\rho_w]$$

$$Var(\hat{\gamma}_{chg}) = 2\left(\frac{1}{wJ} + \frac{1}{(1-w)J}\right)\left(\sigma_{ct}^2 + \frac{\sigma_{st}^2}{m}\right)$$

$$= 2\left(\frac{1}{w} + \frac{1}{1-w}\right)\frac{\sigma_Y^2}{mJ}(1-r)[1 + (m-1)\rho_w]$$

$$Cov(\hat{\gamma}_{fu}, \hat{\gamma}_{chg}) = \left(\sigma_{ct}^2 + \frac{\sigma_{st}^2}{m}\right)\left[\frac{1}{wJ} + \frac{1}{(1-w)J}\right].$$

The estimator can be found to have variance

$$Var(\hat{\gamma}) = \frac{\sigma_Y^2}{mJ}(1-r^2)[1 + (m-1)\rho_w]\left[\frac{1}{w} + \frac{1}{1-w}\right]. \tag{15.19}$$

For a cross-sectional design, a nested exchangeable correlation structure, as in model (15.3), is generally the most appropriate choice and the same result applies, with r defined as in equation (15.4).

15.3.2 Power

The hypothesis $H_0: \gamma = \gamma_0$ can be tested using the test statistic

$$T = \frac{\hat{\gamma} - \gamma_0}{\sqrt{\widehat{Var}(\hat{\gamma})}},$$

which has a t distribution with $J - 2$ degrees of freedom when the null hypothesis is true. When an alternative $\gamma = \gamma_A$ is true, T has a noncentral t distribution with the same degrees of freedom and noncentrality parameter

$$\lambda = \frac{\gamma_A - \gamma_0}{\sqrt{Var(\hat{\gamma})}}.$$

When using a standardized effect size $d_A = \gamma_A/\sigma_y$ and defining $d_0 = \gamma_0/\sigma_y$, we can express the noncentrality parameter as

$$\lambda = \frac{d_A - d_0}{\sqrt{\frac{(1-r^2)[1+(m-1)\rho_w]\left[\frac{1}{w}+\frac{1}{1-w}\right]}{mJ}}} \tag{15.20}$$

with r as given in (15.15). Power for a test at level α is:

$$\text{Power (lower-tail test)} = P[T \leq t_{\alpha, J-2} \mid T \sim t(J-2, \lambda)] \tag{15.21}$$
$$= \mathcal{T}_{J-2,\lambda}(t_{\alpha, J-2})$$
$$\text{Power (upper-tail test)} = P[T \geq t_{1-\alpha, J-2} \mid T \sim t(J-2, \lambda)]$$
$$= 1 - \mathcal{T}_{J-2,\lambda}(t_{1-\alpha, J-2}).$$
$$\text{Power (two-sided test)} = P[T^2 \geq f_{1-\alpha, 1, J-2} \mid T^2 \sim F(1, J-2, \Lambda)]$$
$$= 1 - \mathcal{F}_{1, J-2, \Lambda}(f_{1-\alpha, 1, J-2})$$

where $\Lambda = \lambda^2$. For a lower-tailed test, we expect λ to be negative and for an upper-tailed test, we expect λ to be positive.

What factors affect power? As shown in the expression for the noncentrality parameter (15.20), power depends on the design effect $1 + (m-1)\rho_w$ for a simple parallel cluster randomized trial, which can be considered a variance inflation factor. Power also depends on the correlation r between cluster means at baseline and follow-up. Higher values of r are expected to increase power. This makes using an ANCOVA advantageous. The value of r will be higher for higher values of CAC and SAC. In theory, r will be higher for a closed cohort design than for a cross-sectional design due to subject autocorrelation and therefore power will be higher; however, closed cohort designs may experience attrition at follow up, which can decrease power; this topic is discussed in more detail in Moerbeek [157].

15.3.3 Design effect and relative efficiency

Recall from Section 14.2.2 that the variance of the treatment effect estimator for a simple parallel cluster randomized trial with J total clusters of size m

and equal allocation is $[4\sigma_y^2/(mJ)][1+(m-1)\rho_w]$ and the design effect is $1+(m-1)\rho_w$. For an equal allocation parallel cluster randomized trial with a baseline measurement and J total clusters with m observations at both baseline and follow-up in each cluster, the variance of the treatment effect estimator is (see equation (15.19))

$$\frac{4\sigma_Y^2}{mJ}(1-r^2)[1+(m-1)\rho_w]$$

Compared to a trial without the baseline measurement, the variance is reduced by a factor of $1-r^2$. When $r=0$, the design effect is equal to that for a simple parallel cluster randomized trial.

Example 15.1. Suppose that a parallel cluster randomized trial will involve 8 clusters each in the intervention and control arms. There are 30 individuals in each cluster and they will be measured at both baseline and follow-up; this is a closed cohort design. The expected standardized effect size is 0.3, the ICC is $\rho_w = 0.05$, CAC = 0.4 and SAC = 0.5. For a two-sided test of $H_0: \gamma = 0$ at $\alpha = 0.05$, what is the power?

First, for comparison, we compute power for a trial without the baseline measurement:

```
library(powertools)
crt.parallel.cont(m = 30, J1 = 8, delta = 0.3, icc1 = 0.05, icc2 = 0.05,
    power = NULL)
[1] 0.4979796
```

Power is about 0.50. Now we compute power with the baseline measurement:crt.long.cont

```
crt.long.cont(m = 30, J1 = 8, delta = 0.3, icc = 0.05, cac = 0.4,
  sac = 0.5, power = NULL)
[1] 0.5850067
```

Power has increased to about 0.59.

If we have a cross-sectional design in which different subjects are measured in each cluster at baseline and follow-up, we would specify that SAC = 0.

```
crt.long.cont(m = 30, J1 = 8, delta = 0.3, icc = 0.05, cac = 0.4,
    power = NULL)
[1] 0.5223779
```

The power is lower, at about 0.52. In general, power will be lower for a cross-sectional design than for a closed cohort, when the sample sizes at each time point and all other parameters are equal. Note that attrition in a cohort design could reduce the sample size at the second time point.

15.3.4 Additional resources

The Shiny CRT Calculator [91] supports power calculations for parallel cluster randomized trials with baseline measurements. The calculator is implemented using a Shiny app. The app can be used via the following link: https://clusterrcts.shinyapps.io/rshinyapp. Source code and updates are located on GitHub https://github.com/karlahemming/Cluster-RCT-Sample-Size-Calculator.

15.4 Cluster randomized crossover designs

In a crossover design, participants are randomized to study arms that receive both the treatment and the control condition, but in different orders. Crossover designs in which randomization is at the individual level are discussed in Chapter 12. Here, we discuss crossover designs in which randomization is at the level of the cluster.

The most common crossover design is the 2×2 or TR/RT design, in which there are two time periods and two conditions, T and R, and participants are randomized to study arms that receive either T followed by R or R followed by T (where we are using the parlance of Chapter 12, in which we used T for treatment and R for reference). An example of a 2×2 cluster randomized crossover trial is depicted in Figure 15.1(C). In that example, three clusters are randomized to a study arm that receives the control condition and then the treatment condition and three are randomized to a study arm that receives treatment and then control. The outcomes are assessed on individuals within the clusters during each time period.

In some crossover studies, the same individuals in each cluster are measured in each period; this is a closed cohort design. In other crossover studies, different individuals in each cluster are measured in each period; this is a cross-sectional design. In a cluster randomized crossover trial, these two designs are sometimes referred to as having crossover at the cluster level (cross-sectional) or at the individual level (closed cohort) [186].

The main advantage of an individually randomized crossover trial is that the outcome of a participant under Treatment T can be contrasted with the same participant's outcome under Treatment R. This removes between-patient variation from the variance of the treatment effect estimator and makes a crossover trial potentially more efficient than a parallel group trial with the same number of outcome measurements. Cluster randomized crossover trials can potentially have greater efficiency than parallel cluster randomized trials for similar reasons. The cross-sectional subtype compares the outcomes of individuals who are in the same cluster, which removes between-cluster variation from the variance. The closed cohort subtype removes both between-cluster variation and between-individual variation from the variance [186], for potentially even greater efficiency.

In this section, we first discuss closed cohort cluster randomized crossover trials and then discuss the cross-sectional design. We restrict attention to TR/RT (that is, 2×2) crossover designs and continuous outcomes. The derivations are based largely on those of Giraudeau et al. [75] and Moerbeek [157]. Other references include [92, 186].

15.4.1 Treatment effect estimator and variance

We start with a closed cohort design and assume a total of J clusters, randomized equally to the sequences TR or RT, and m individuals measured in each time period in each cluster. Let j index cluster, i index individual within cluster and $t = 0, 1$ index time period.

The treatment effect γ can be estimated by first finding the difference between the two cluster-period means for each cluster, computed as $d_j = \bar{Y}_{\cdot j 0} - \bar{Y}_{\cdot j 1}$ for clusters allocated to the sequence TR and as $d_j = \bar{Y}_{\cdot j 1} - \bar{Y}_{\cdot j 0}$ for clusters allocated to the sequence RT, and then computing the average of these differences across all clusters,

$$\hat{\gamma} = \frac{1}{J}\sum_{j=1}^{J} d_j$$

Due to the independence of clusters, the variance of this estimate is

$$Var(\hat{\gamma}) = \frac{1}{J} Var(d_j).$$

To find $Var(d_j)$, for a closed cohort design with block exchangeable correlation structure as in model (15.10), we can find that

$$Var(\bar{Y}_{\cdot j 0}) = Var(\bar{Y}_{\cdot j 1}) = \frac{1}{m^2}[mVar(Y_{ij0}) + m(m-1)Cov(Y_{ij0}, Y_{i'j0})]$$
$$= \frac{\sigma_c^2 + \sigma_{ct}^2 + \sigma_s^2 + \sigma_{st}^2}{m} + \frac{(m-1)(\sigma_c^2 + \sigma_{ct}^2)}{m}$$
$$= \sigma_c^2 + \sigma_{ct}^2 + \frac{\sigma_s^2}{m} + \frac{\sigma_{st}^2}{m}$$

and

$$Cov(\bar{Y}_{\cdot j 0}, \bar{Y}_{\cdot j 1}) = \frac{1}{m^2}[mCov(Y_{ij0}, Y_{ij1}) + m(m-1)Cov(Y_{ij0}, Y_{i'j1})]$$
$$= \sigma_c^2 + \frac{\sigma_s^2}{m}.$$

Thus we can find that [157]

$$\begin{aligned}Var(d_j) &= Var(\bar{Y}_{\cdot j0} - \bar{Y}_{\cdot j1}) = Var(\bar{Y}_{\cdot j1} - \bar{Y}_{\cdot j0}) \\ &= 2Var(\bar{Y}_{\cdot j0}) - 2Cov(\bar{Y}_{\cdot j0}, \bar{Y}_{\cdot j1}) \\ &= \frac{2}{m}\left(\sigma_{st}^2 + m\sigma_{ct}^2\right)\end{aligned}$$

and

$$Var(\hat{\gamma}) = \frac{2\left(\sigma_{st}^2 + m\sigma_{ct}^2\right)}{mJ}. \tag{15.22}$$

We can express the variance using correlation coefficients as

$$Var(\hat{\gamma}) = \frac{2\sigma_Y^2 \left[1 - \rho_a + (m-1)(\rho_w - \rho_b)\right]}{mJ} \tag{15.23}$$

or using the CAC and SAC as

$$Var(\hat{\gamma}) = \frac{2\sigma_Y^2 \left[1 + (m-1)\rho_w - (1-\rho_w)\text{SAC} - m\rho_w\text{CAC}\right]}{mJ} \tag{15.24}$$

or using the correlation between cluster-periods means r (equation (15.15)) as

$$Var(\hat{\gamma}) = \frac{2\sigma_Y^2 \left[1 + (m-1)\rho_w\right](1-r)}{mJ} \tag{15.25}$$

To find $Var(d_j)$ for a cross-sectional design with nested exchangeable correlation structure as in model (15.3), we can find that $Var(\bar{Y}_{\cdot j0}) = Var(\bar{Y}_{\cdot j1}) = \sigma_c^2 + \sigma_{ct}^2 + \sigma_{st}^2/m$ and $Cov(\bar{Y}_{\cdot j0}, \bar{Y}_{\cdot j1}) = \sigma_c^2$. Then

$$\begin{aligned}Var(d_j) &= Var(\bar{Y}_{\cdot j0} - \bar{Y}_{\cdot j1}) = Var(\bar{Y}_{\cdot j1} - \bar{Y}_{\cdot j0}) \\ &= 2Var(\bar{Y}_{\cdot j0}) - 2Cov(\bar{Y}_{\cdot j0}, \bar{Y}_{\cdot j1}) \\ &= \frac{2}{m}\left(\sigma_{st}^2 + m\sigma_{ct}^2\right).\end{aligned}$$

Thus [75, 157]

$$Var(\hat{\gamma}) = \frac{2(\sigma_{st}^2 + m\sigma_{ct}^2)}{mJ}.$$

The variance can be expressed using correlation coefficients as

$$Var(\hat{\gamma}) = \frac{2\sigma_Y^2[1 + (m-1)\rho_w - m\rho_b]}{mJ} \tag{15.26}$$

which is equal to the expression for a closed cohort trial with ρ_a set to zero, or using the CAC as

$$Var(\hat{\gamma}) = \frac{2\sigma_Y^2 \left[1 + (m-1)\rho_w - m\rho_w\text{CAC}\right]}{mJ} \tag{15.27}$$

which is equal to the expression for a closed cohort trial with SAC set to zero. We also have

$$Var(\hat{\gamma}) = \frac{2\sigma_Y^2 \left[1 + (m-1)\rho_w\right](1-r)}{mJ}$$

for the appropriate value of r.

15.4.2 Power

To test $H_0 : \gamma = \gamma_0$, we can use the test statistic

$$T = \frac{\hat{\gamma} - \gamma_0}{\sqrt{\widehat{Var}(\hat{\gamma})}}.$$

Under the null, T has a central t distribution. The degrees of freedom of the test statistic are not straightforward to obtain and some authors present power and sample size calculations that use the normal approximation, which implies high degrees of freedom [75, 157]. It has also been suggested to calculate the degrees of freedom as the number of cluster-periods minus the number of time periods minus one [91]. Using this approach, for a two-period design with J total clusters, the degrees of freedom would be $2J - 3$.

Under an alternative $\gamma = \gamma_A$, T has a noncentral t distribution with non-centrality parameter of the form

$$\lambda = \frac{\gamma_A - \gamma_0}{\sqrt{Var(\hat{\gamma})}}$$

where any of the various expressions for the variance can be used. Power for tests at level α can be approximated as:

$$\text{Power (lower-tail test)} \approx P[T \leq t_{\alpha, 2J-3} \mid T \sim t(2J-3, \lambda)] \quad (15.28)$$
$$= \mathcal{T}_{2J-3, \lambda}(t_{\alpha, 2J-3})$$
$$\text{Power (upper-tail test)} \approx P[T \geq t_{1-\alpha, 2J-3} \mid T \sim t(2J-3, \lambda)]$$
$$= 1 - \mathcal{T}_{2J-3, \lambda}(t_{1-\alpha, 2J-3})$$
$$\text{Power (two-sided test)} \approx P[T^2 \geq f_{1-\alpha, 1, 2J-3} \mid T^2 \sim F(1, 2J-3, \Lambda)]$$
$$= 1 - \mathcal{F}_{1, 2J-3, \Lambda}(f_{1-\alpha, 1, 2J-3})$$

where $\Lambda = \lambda^2$. For a lower-tailed test, we expect $\lambda < 0$ and for an upper-tailed test, we expect $\lambda > 0$.

What factors affect power? Factors affecting power can be gleaned by inspecting the expressions for $Var(\hat{\gamma})$. Power decreases (variance increases) as ρ_w increases but power increases as ρ_b or ρ_a increases. Similarly, power increases with higher values of the CAC or SAC, and higher values of r. It is the impact of these correlations that accounts for the potential increased efficiency of the crossover design.

15.4.2.1 Design effect and relative efficiency

The variance of the treatment effect estimator for a simple parallel cluster randomized trial with J total clusters of size m and equal allocation is $[4\sigma_Y^2/(mJ)][1 + (m-1)\rho_w]$ and the design effect is $1 + (m-1)\rho_w$ (Section 14.2.2).

Comparing this to the variance of the treatment effect estimator for a cluster randomized 2×2 crossover trial (see (15.25)), the design effect is

$$[1 + (m-1)\rho_w]\left(\frac{1-r}{2}\right) \qquad (15.29)$$

where r is as given in equation (15.15). A simple parallel cluster randomized trial with a total of $2J$ clusters of size m (for a total of $2mJ$ outcome measurements) has design effect $1 + (m-1)\rho_w$. Thus for the same number of measurements, we expect a crossover trial to be more efficient than the simple parallel cluster randomized trial, with efficiency increasing as r increases. Within subtypes of crossover trials, we expect a closed cohort design to have a higher value of r and therefore to be more efficient than a cross-sectional design. However, when following both clusters and individuals within clusters longitudinally, there can be a risk of attrition at both the cluster and individual levels, which can reduce power. The impact of attrition in cluster randomized crossover trials is discussed in Moerbeek [157] and Rutterford et al. [191].

Example 15.2. We compare power for a simple parallel cluster randomized design to power for cluster randomized 2×2 crossover designs with the same total number of observations of the outcome.

Suppose that a parallel design has 8 clusters in each condition and cluster size $m = 30$, and thus a total N of 480 observations. The standardized effect size is $d = 0.3$ and the within-cluster, within-period ICC is assumed to be 0.05. Power for a two-sided test at level 0.05 can be calculated as

```
library(powertools)
crt.parallel.cont(m = 30, J1 = 8, delta = 0.3, icc1 = 0.05, icc2 = 0.05,
  power = NULL)
[1] 0.4979796
```

The power is about 0.50.

We compare this to various cluster randomized 2×2 crossover designs. To equalize the number of observations, we assume a total of 8 clusters randomized to receive TR or RT with equal allocation, and 30 observations taken in each cluster in each of the two time periods, for a total of 480 observations. For consistency, we specify the within-cluster, within-period ICC ρ_w as 0.05. We calculate power for CAC equal to 0.5 and 0.8 for a cross-sectional design; to reflect a closed cohort trial, we additionally specify a SAC of 0.6.

```
library(powertools)
crt.xo.cont(m = 30, J.arm = 4, delta = 0.3, icc = 0.05, cac = 0.5,
power = NULL)
[1] 0.6449588

crt.xo.cont(m = 30, J.arm = 4, delta = 0.3, icc = 0.05, cac = 0.8,
power = NULL)
[1] 0.775517

crt.xo.cont(m = 30, J.arm = 4, delta = 0.3, icc = 0.05, cac = 0.5,
  sac = 0.6, power = NULL)
[1] 0.815133

crt.xo.cont(m = 30, J.arm = 4, delta = 0.3, icc = 0.05, cac = 0.8,
  sac = 0.6, power = NULL)
[1] 0.9570017
```

Comparing results, we can see that power for crossover designs can be considerably higher than power of a simple parallel design and that closed cohort designs can have higher power than cross-sectional designs when the number of observations and all other parameters are equal.

This example demonstrates that a cluster randomized crossover design can have higher power than a simple parallel design with the same number of observations. However, crossover designs are not appropriate for all types of interventions. In particular, it must be possible to withdraw the intervention and restore the control condition. In addition, if the effect of a treatment would carry over to subsequent periods, a crossover design would not provide an unbiased estimate of the treatment effect [109]. Further, in cohort designs, attrition can occur and impact power.

15.4.3 Additional resources

There are two Shiny apps that perform calculations for cluster randomized crossover trials based on Moerbeek [157], with a focus on the impact of attrition. These can be found at https://utrecht-university.shinyapps.io/CRXO1/ and https://utrecht-university.shinyapps.io/CRXO2/. One app is for unanticipated attrition and the other is for anticipated attrition.

Another Shiny app is the Shiny CRT Calculator, which handles a range of cluster randomized designs, including cluster randomized crossover designs with two periods as well as a higher number of periods. The app can be found at https://clusterrcts.shinyapps.io/rshinyapp. Source code and updates are located on GitHub at https://github.com/karlahemming/Cluster-RCT-Sample-Size-Calculator. An accompanying tutorial is published in Hemming et al. [91].

Another approach to power and sample size calculations for cluster randomized crossover trials is given by Li et al. [138], who consider procedures when using a generalized estimating equation (GEE) approach. These authors consider both continuous and binary outcomes.

15.5 Stepped wedge designs

Stepped wedge trials are cluster randomized trials in which clusters are randomized to study arms that transition from the control to the treatment condition at different time points. Figure 15.1(D) displays an example of a stepped wedge design with three study arms and two clusters in each arm. All study arms begin in the control condition in Period 1, and then the study arms transition to the treatment condition at the beginning of Periods 2, 3 or 4. This is an example of a "standard" stepped wedge design, in which all clusters start in the control condition in Period 1 and then equal numbers of clusters transition to treatment at the start of each period until all clusters are exposed. Another example of a standard stepped wedge trial is depicted in Figure 15.3. This design was used by Selby et al. [200], who report on an organizational-level intervention to improve outcomes associated with acute kidney injury. In this study, five hospitals began in a usual care control condition and then the intervention was introduced sequentially at one hospital at a time at three-month intervals until all hospitals were exposed. Outcomes were measured at the patient level and included 30-day mortality and hospital length of stay.

Stepped wedge designs have several advantages over simple parallel cluster randomized trials. They include within-cluster comparisons of control and intervention conditions, which can potentially yield efficiency gains similar to that for crossover trials [234]. It may be less costly and logistically easier to roll out the intervention at staggered time points instead of simultaneously, as would occur in many parallel cluster randomized trials. Additionally, it can be viewed as more equitable to guarantee that all clusters eventually receive the intervention. A weakness of stepped wedge designs is that the treatment condition is partially confounded with time, because there are more observations in the control condition earlier in the study and more observations in the intervention condition later in the study. Stepped wedge trials also tend to take longer to complete than parallel trials, which makes they more susceptible to intercurrent events or other disruptions. **Intercurrent events** are post-randomization events that affect either the interpretation or existence of outcome data, for example, an unanticipated modification of the treatment or barrier to data collection [64, 114].

In this section, we discuss power calculation for stepped wedge trials with continuous outcomes. The designs and models that we consider cover many

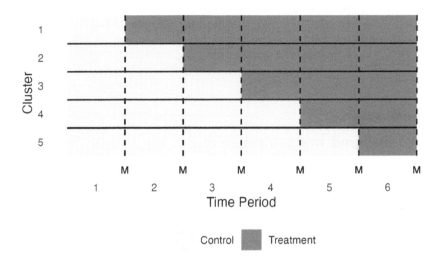

FIGURE 15.3: Schematic representation of a "standard" stepped wedge design trial with five clusters. After a baseline period in the control condition, one cluster transitions to the treatment condition at the start of each period. Measurements of outcomes (M) are taken at the end of each period.

but not all possible options. We restrict attention to complete designs, that is, designs in which observations are collected from all clusters in all periods. Considerations for the design and analysis of stepped wedge trials can get quite complex. Sections 15.5.4 and 15.5.5 provide resources and references for other outcome types and other modeling options as well as power and sample size calculation resources. The material here draws on many references [13, 49, 68, 77, 82, 88, 85, 86, 99, 100, 107, 140, 164].

15.5.1 Treatment effect estimator and variance

Stepped wedge trials usually have three or more time periods, meaning that observations are often taken over a considerable length of time. For this reason, the choice of model for the correlation structure of the data is of key importance. Models and correlation structures for longitudinal cluster randomized trials were presented in Sections 15.2.1 and 15.2.2; the reader should refer to those sections for detailed explanations of the various models and correlation structures. Here, we explain a general approach for estimating the treatment effect in a stepped wedge trial and obtaining the variance of the treatment effect estimator, and present power calculation approaches for the models presented in those sections.

Suppose that a stepped wedge trial will have J clusters indexed by j and T time periods indexed by t. Clusters are randomized to K different study

Stepped wedge designs

arms, each corresponding to a distinct sequence of conditions. Individuals within clusters are indexed by i. We assume an equal number of observations m are taken from each cluster during each period.

In their seminal paper, Hussey and Hughes [107] presented a model for a stepped wedge design with cross-sectional observations that has the form

$$Y_{ijt} = \mu + \beta_t + \gamma x_{jt} + c_j + s_{ijt} \qquad (15.30)$$

In this model, μ is the mean in the control condition during Period 1, β_t is a fixed effect for time t, modeled using $T - 1$ indicator variables, x_{jt} is an indicator of whether cluster j receives the intervention during period t, with $x_{jt} = 1$ if yes and 0 if no, and γ is the treatment effect. For example, for the design in Figure 15.1(D), the means in each arm during each period are

	Period 1	Period 2	Period 3	Period 4
Arm 1	μ	$\mu + \beta_1 + \gamma$	$\mu + \beta_2 + \gamma$	$\mu + \beta_3 + \gamma$
Arm 2	μ	$\mu + \beta_1$	$\mu + \beta_2 + \gamma$	$\mu + \beta_3 + \gamma$
Arm 3	μ	$\mu + \beta_1$	$\mu + \beta_2$	$\mu + \beta_3 + \gamma$

The random effects in the Hussey and Hughes model (15.30) correspond to those in model (15.1), which has exchangeable correlation structure.

Hussey and Hughes [107] pointed out that if the values of the variance components are known, then estimates of the fixed effects and their variances, most importantly the variance of the estimator of the treatment effect $Var(\hat{\gamma})$, can be obtained using weighted least squares (WLS). Specifically, let $\mathbf{Y}$ be a vector of all of the observations and let $\mathbf{Z}$ be the $JT \times (T+1)$ design matrix corresponding to the parameter vector $\boldsymbol{\eta} = (\mu, \beta_1, \ldots, \beta_{T-1}, \gamma)$. Then $\hat{\boldsymbol{\eta}} = (\mathbf{Z}'\mathbf{V}^{-1}\mathbf{Z})^{-1}(\mathbf{Z}'\mathbf{V}^{-1}\mathbf{Y})$ and the covariance matrix of $\hat{\boldsymbol{\eta}}$ is $(\mathbf{Z}'\mathbf{V}^{-1}\mathbf{Z})^{-1}$ where $\mathbf{V}$ is a $JT \times JT$ block diagonal matrix. Each $T \times T$ block in $\mathbf{V}$ describes the variance-covariance structure of a cluster's means across time periods. $Var(\hat{\gamma})$ is obtained as the $(T+1, T+1)$ element of $(\mathbf{Z}'\mathbf{V}^{-1}\mathbf{Z})^{-1}$.

This provides an approach for obtaining a closed-form expression for $Var(\hat{\gamma})$ that can be used in power calculations. For **exchangeable correlation** model (15.30), when we have a complete design and m observations per cluster at each period, the WLS estimator of $Var(\hat{\gamma})$ takes the form

$$Var(\hat{\gamma}) = \frac{(\sigma_Y^2/m) JT \lambda_1 \lambda_2}{(U^2 + JTU - TW - JV)\lambda_2 - (U^2 - JV)\lambda_1} \qquad (15.31)$$

where

$$\lambda_1 = 1 - \rho_w$$
$$\lambda_2 = 1 + (mT - 1)\rho_w$$

and U, W and V are design constants that depend on the assignment of clusters to sequences, with $U = \sum_j \sum_t x_{jt}$, $W = \sum_t (\sum_j x_{jt})^2$ and $V = \sum_j (\sum_t x_{jt})^2$ [107, 140].

Li et al. [140] show that expression (15.31) is a general form that applies to several other model variants. For **nested exchangeable correlation** structure, as in model (15.3), the WLS estimator of $Var(\hat{\gamma})$ takes the form of expression (15.31) with $\sigma_Y^2 = \sigma_c^2 + \sigma_{ct}^2 + \sigma_{st}^2$ and

$$\lambda_1 = 1 + (m-1)\rho_w - m\rho_b$$
$$\lambda_2 = 1 + (m-1)\rho_w + m(T-1)\rho_b.$$

The latter parameters can also be expressed using the cluster autocorrelation (CAC) rather than ρ_b by using the relationship $\rho_b = \rho_w \mathrm{CAC}$. For **exponential decay** structure [117], as in model (15.5), there is no closed-form expression for $Var(\hat{\gamma})$. However, this variance can be computed numerically given values for all of the parameters [117].

We now consider expressions for $Var(\hat{\gamma})$ for closed cohort designs. In **basic cohort** model (15.7), discussed by Baio et al. [13], $Var(\hat{\gamma})$ takes the form given in equation (15.31) when we set $\sigma_Y^2 = \sigma_c^2 + \sigma_s^2 + \sigma_{st}^2$ and

$$\lambda_1 = 1 - \rho_a$$
$$\lambda_2 = 1 + T(m-1)\rho_w + (T-1)\rho_a;$$

see [138, 140]. For the **block exchangeable correlation** model (15.3), the expression for $Var(\hat{\gamma})$ is the same as in equation (15.31) with the substitutions $\sigma_Y^2 = \sigma_c^2 + \sigma_{ct}^2 + \sigma_s^2 + \sigma_{st}^2$ and

$$\lambda_1 = 1 + (m-1)(\rho_w - \rho_b) - \rho_a$$
$$\lambda_2 = 1 + (m-1)\rho_w + (T-1)(m-1)\rho_b + (T-1)\rho_a;$$

see [140]. The latter parameters can also be expressed using the CAC and the subject autocorrelation (SAC) by using the relationships $\rho_b = \rho_w \mathrm{CAC}$ and $\rho_a = (1-\rho_w)\mathrm{SAC} + \rho_w \mathrm{CAC}$. For the **proportional decay** model, $Var(\hat{\gamma})$ has the form

$$Var(\hat{\gamma}) = \frac{(\sigma_Y^2/m) J (1-\tau^2)[1+(m-1)\rho_w]}{(JU - W)(1+\tau^2) - 2(JP - Q)\tau} \qquad (15.32)$$

where U and W are as previously defined, $P = \sum_{j=1}^{J} \sum_{t=1}^{T-1} x_{jt} x_{j,t+1}$ and $Q = \sum_{t=1}^{T-1} (\sum_{j=1}^{J} x_{jt})(\sum_{j=1}^{J} x_{j,t+1})$ [137].

15.5.2 Power

To conduct a test of $H_0: \gamma = \gamma_0$, we can use the test statistic

$$T = \frac{\hat{\gamma} - \gamma_0}{\sqrt{\widehat{Var}(\hat{\gamma})}}. \qquad (15.33)$$

Stepped wedge designs

Under the null, T has a central t distribution. The degrees of freedom of the test statistic to use for power calculations are unclear. One approach is to estimate the degrees of freedom as the number of cluster-periods minus the number of time periods minus one [91], i.e., $JT - T - 1$. Under an alternative that $\gamma = \gamma_A$, T has a noncentral t distribution with noncentrality parameter of the form

$$\lambda = \frac{\gamma_A - \gamma_0}{\sqrt{Var(\hat{\gamma})}}$$

where $Var(\hat{\gamma})$ depends on the particular design and modeling choice, as discussed in Section 15.5.1.

Power for tests at level α can be approximated as:

$$\text{Power (lower-tail test)} \approx P[T \leq t_{\alpha,df} \mid T \sim t(df, \lambda)] \quad (15.34)$$
$$= \mathcal{T}_{df,\lambda}(t_{\alpha,df})$$
$$\text{Power (upper-tail test)} \approx P[T \geq t_{1-\alpha,df} \mid T \sim t(df, \lambda)]$$
$$= 1 - \mathcal{T}_{df,\lambda}(t_{1-\alpha,df})$$
$$\text{Power (two-sided test)} \approx P[T^2 \geq f_{1-\alpha,1,df} \mid T^2 \sim F(1, df, \Lambda)]$$
$$= 1 - \mathcal{F}_{1,df,\Lambda}(f_{1-\alpha,1,df})$$

where $df = JT - T - 1$ and $\Lambda = \lambda^2$. For a lower-tailed test, we expect $\lambda < 0$ and for an upper-tailed test, we expect $\lambda > 0$. For a two-sided test, we can square the test statistic and use the F distribution:

What factors affect power? Because there are many different design and modeling options for stepped wedge trials, it is difficult to make broad statements about factors that affect power. We focus on the influence of correlation parameters on power for a standard stepped wedge design. For exchangeable or nested exchangeable correlation, higher values of ρ_w reduce power, while higher values of ρ_b or CAC increase power. In a closed cohort design, higher values of ρ_w reduce power, while higher values of ρ_b or ρ_a (or CAC and SAC) increase power [138].

For models with exponential decay, in particular, autoregressive order of 1, when values of τ are higher, there is less decay (i.e., cluster-period means are more similar over time), and power is higher. Kasza et al [117] provide more discussion and also discuss exponential decay models for a broader class of longitudinal cluster randomized trials.

Example 15.3. We compute power for the standard stepped wedge trial design in Figure 15.3. In this design, after a baseline period, one cluster switches to treatment at each time period. Suppose there are 30 subjects measured at each cluster-period. We assume a cross-sectional design with nested exchangeable correlation structure with $\rho_w = 0.05$ and CAC $= 0.5$ (and thus $\rho_b = \rho_w \text{CAC} = 0.025$). We expect a standardized effect size of $d = 0.3$.

We calculate power using the `swCRTdesign` package. This example demonstrates only some of the functionality of this package. The first step is to create a design object using the `swDsn` function. The main input to this function is a vector `clusters` that specifies the number of study arms (i.e., distinct sequences), corresponding to the length of the vector, and the number of clusters in each arm. For example, `c(6, 6, 6, 6)` specifies four study arms with 6 clusters in each arm. The default settings are for a standard design in which all study arms begin in the control condition in Period 1 and then one study arm transitions to the intervention condition at each subsequent period.

Our standard design with five study arms and one cluster per arm can be specified as follows:

```
library(swCRTdesign)
design <- swDsn(clusters = c(1, 1, 1, 1, 1))
# display a schematic of the sequence of conditions in each arm:
design$swDsn
     [,1] [,2] [,3] [,4] [,5] [,6]
[1,]   0    1    1    1    1    1
[2,]   0    0    1    1    1    1
[3,]   0    0    0    1    1    1
[4,]   0    0    0    0    1    1
[5,]   0    0    0    0    0    1
```

Power is calculated using the `swPwr` function. Inputs include `n`, the number of observations per cluster per period, `mu0`, the mean in the control condition, and `mu1`, the mean in the intervention condition.

For nested exchangeable correlation structure, we specify `icc` (ρ_w), `cac` and `sigma`, the standard deviation of observations within a cluster-period, which corresponds to σ_{st} in our notation. When using a standardized effect size, we have $\sigma_Y^2 = \sigma_c^2 + \sigma_{ct}^2 + \sigma_{st}^2 = 1$, which implies that $\sigma_c^2 + \sigma_{ct}^2 = \rho_w$ and therefore $\sigma_{st}^2 = 1 - \rho_w$; thus `sigma` is set equal to $\sqrt{1 - \rho_w}$. Power is for a two-sided test at level 0.05.

```
rho_w <- 0.05
swPwr(design = design, distn = "gaussian", n = 30, mu0 = 0, mu1 = 0.3,
    icc = rho_w, cac = 0.5, sigma = sqrt(1 - rho_w), silent = TRUE)

treatment.1
   0.557745
```

Power is about 0.56.

Suppose that we have a closed cohort design with the same parameters and SAC of 0.5, which implies that $\rho_a = (1 - \rho_w)\text{SAC} + \rho_b = 0.5$. When using a standardized effect size, we have $\sigma_Y^2 = \sigma_c^2 + \sigma_{ct}^2 + \sigma_s^2 + \sigma_{st}^2 = 1$, which implies that $\sigma_{st}^2 = 1 - \rho_w - \rho_a + \rho_b$; thus `sigma` is set equal to $\sqrt{1 - \rho_w - \rho_a + \rho_b}$. The SAC is denoted as `iac`, i.e., individual autocorrelation.

Stepped wedge designs

```
rho_w <- 0.05
rho_b <- 0.025
rho_a <- 0.5
swPwr(design = design, distn = "gaussian", n = 30, mu0 = 0, mu1 = 0.4,
   icc = rho_w, cac = 0.2, iac = 0.5, silent = TRUE,
   sigma = sqrt(1 - rho_w - rho_a + rho_b))
treatment.1
   0.8050669
```

Power is about 0.80.

15.5.3 Design effect and normal approximation sample size

Several authors present design effects for stepped wedge trials that can be useful for approximating the required sample size and examining the relative efficiency of different designs [85, 99, 100]. Hooper et al [100] present a sample size by design effect approach that applies not only to stepped wedge trials but more generally to longitudinal cluster randomized trials. Let N_{indep} be the total sample size required for a study comparing independent groups of equal size. For a cluster randomized trial with K study arms and T time periods, define $\text{DE}_{\text{longCRT}}$ as

$$\text{DE}_{\text{longCRT}} = \frac{K^2(1-r)[1+(T-1)r]}{4[KB - D + (B^2 + K(T-1)B - (T-1)D - KC)r]} \quad (15.35)$$

where r is the correlation between two cluster-periods means (see equation (15.15)), $B = \sum_k \sum_t x_{kt}$, $C = \sum_k (\sum_t x_{kt})^2$ and $D = \sum_t (\sum_k x_{kt})^2$.

When there is cross-sectional sampling of individuals, there are mT individuals per cluster. In this case, for a longitudinal cluster randomized trial to achieve the same power to detect the same effect size, the total number of individuals required is approximately

$$N \approx \text{DE}_{\text{longCRT}}[1 + (m-1)\rho_w]TN_{\text{indep}}$$

and the total number of clusters required is approximately

$$J \approx \text{DE}_{\text{longCRT}}[1 + (m-1)\rho_w]N_{\text{indep}}/m.$$

For a closed cohort, there are m individuals per cluster and the total number of individuals required is approximately

$$N \approx \text{DE}_{\text{longCRT}}[1 + (m-1)\rho_w]N_{\text{indep}}$$

with the total number of clusters required approximately equal to

$$J \approx \text{DE}_{\text{longCRT}}[1 + (m-1)\rho_w]N_{\text{indep}}/m.$$

Note that these are based on a large sample approximation and may not be very accurate for studies with small numbers of clusters.

As noted, this design effect approach can be applied broadly to various cluster randomized trial designs. For example, for a simple parallel group cluster randomized trial with no baseline measurement, we have $K = 2, T = B = C = D = 1$, and $DE_{\text{longCRT}} = 1$. For a simple parallel design with a baseline measurement, $K = T = 2, B = C = D = 1$, and $DE_{\text{longCRT}} = 1 - r^2$. For a 2×2 cluster randomized crossover trial, $K = T = B = C = D = 2$ and $DE_{\text{longCRT}} = (1-r)/2$. Multiplying each of these by $1 + (m-1)\rho_w$ gives their full design effect, as discussed in previous sections of this chapter.

For a standard stepped wedge design with K arms and $T = K+1$ periods, we have $B = K(K+1)/2$ and $C = D = K(K+1)(2K+1)/6$, and the design effect simplifies to

$$\frac{3K}{(K+1)(K-1)} \frac{(1+rK)}{(2+rK)}(1-r);$$

multiplying this by $1 + (m-1)\rho_w$ gives the full design effect. For example, for $K = 4, 5$ or 6 arms, we have

$$K = 4: \quad \left(\frac{4}{5}\right)\left(\frac{1+4r}{2+4r}\right)(1-r)$$

$$K = 5: \quad \left(\frac{5}{8}\right)\left(\frac{1+5r}{2+5r}\right)(1-r)$$

$$K = 6: \quad \left(\frac{18}{35}\right)\left(\frac{1+6r}{2+6r}\right)(1-r)$$

In general, these design effects are always lower than those for a parallel group cluster randomized trial, with or without a baseline measurement, and comparable to those for a 2×2 cluster randomized crossover trial. However, when participants are sampled cross-sectionally, the total number of measurements and thus number of participants might be larger for a stepped wedge trial due to the larger number of periods.

The statistical efficiency of a broad class of longitudinal cluster randomized trials is discussed in Girling and Hemming [77].

15.5.4 Other modeling and design options

There are various extensions and alternatives to the modeling and design options for stepped wedge trials discussed in this section, and options continue to be developed. We briefly discuss some salient issues.

Binary and count outcomes. Power for stepped wedge trials with discrete outcomes is discussed in Xia et al. [238], who propose power calculations for generalized linear models for stepped wedge designs using the Laplace approximation described in Breslow and Clayton [22] to obtain the covariance matrix of the estimated parameters. These methods are implemented in the `swCRTdesign` package using the `swGlmPwr` function. The outcome of interest can be binomial (logit link) or Poisson (log link) distributed. A cross-sectional or closed cohort sampling scheme can be specified.

Marginal models. In this chapter, we have focused on the use of mixed models, also termed conditional models, for stepped wedge trials and other longitudinal cluster randomized trial designs. Power methods that focus on the use of marginal models fit by generalized estimating equations (GEE) have been developed by several authors [138, 139, 243]. The `swdpwr` package implements marginal model as well as other methods.

Open cohort designs. In addition to closed cohort and cross-sectional designs, stepped wedge trials can have open cohort designs, which allow for individuals to enter and exit the study during its course [40]. An open cohort design generalizes the other two designs by allowing for a subject to be assessed at anywhere from one to all time points. Sample size and power calculation for longitudinal cluster randomized trials with open cohorts are discussed in Kasza et al. [118].

Incomplete designs. We have considered only stepped wedge trials with "complete" designs, in which all cluster-periods contribute data to the analysis. Some trials may use "incomplete" designs, in which data from some cluster-periods are not collected or are not used to estimate the treatment effect. For example, in staircase designs, clusters are measured only in periods immediately before and immediately after the treatment switch. Other designs allow for a transitional period during which the intervention has started implementation but has not yet become full strength, and these cluster-periods are omitted from the outcome analysis. Other designs may allow for a fractional treatment effect during transitional periods [120]. There are no closed-form expressions for power and sample size for many such incomplete designs. Power can be determined by using numerical methods to invert the variance covariance matrix to obtain the variance of the treatment effect estimator [88] or by simulation.

Varying cluster sizes. In general, cluster randomized trials with varying cluster sizes have lower power compared to trials with constant cluster sizes, as discussed in Section 14.2.6. Some investigations have found that imbalance in cluster sizes in stepped wedge trials can lead to power loss but the loss is often minimal [127, 151, 243] and is generally less than that for a parallel cluster randomized trial [76]. A conservative approach for allowing for varying cluster sizes is to replace cluster period size m with $m(1 + CV^2)$, where CV is the coefficient of variation of cluster sizes [76].

Modeling the intervention effect. The models we have discussed assume an immediate and constant treatment effect throughout the trial. Alternatives include a time-on-treatment effect model, which allows the intervention effect to depend on elapsed time since the intervention was introduced or a delayed treatment effect [105, 106, 120]. Additionally, several authors have proposed models that allow for heterogeneity of the treatment effect across clusters in a stepped wedge trial using random treatment effects [89, 90, 105, 224].

Multiple treatment conditions. Stepped wedge design variations that accommodate multiple interventions are discussed in Lyons et al. [146]. Power analysis for stepped wedge trials with two or more different treatment conditions are discussed in Sundin and Crespi [214]. R code for power calculations is available.

15.5.5 Software resources

Ouyang et al. [176] review sample size calculators for stepped wedge cluster randomized trials available on many major platforms, including R, SAS, Stata, PASS and nQuery. A companion Shiny app is available to help users select a calculator for their requirements at https://douyang.shinyapps.io/swcrt calculator/.

The swCRTdesign package, which is described in the paper by Voldal et al. [224], is a comprehensive package for computing power for stepped wedge trials. The package includes functions for both design and analysis and can handle cross-sectional or closed cohort designs as well as both continuous and discrete (binary and count) outcomes. The swDsn function creates a stepped wedge design object based on specified information on number of clusters, number of arms and time points. For normal outcomes, the swPwr function computes power for the specified design via weighted least squares, where the outcome is assumed to come from a mixed effects model with normal errors. For discrete outcomes, the swGlmPwr function does power calculations using the generalized linear mixed model framework [238]. The swSimPwr function simulates data and runs analyses using the linear mixed model or generalized linear mixed model framework. The swSim function generates individual level data consisting of response, treatment, time, time on treatment and id variables based on a specified design. Some features of the package are available as a Shiny app, available at https://swcrtdesign.shinyapps.io/stepped_wedge_power_calculation/ or to download and run locally https://github.com/swCRTdesign/Stepped-wedge-power-calculation.

The clusterPower package calculates power for cluster randomized trials including multi-arm trials, individually randomized group treatment trials, stepped wedge trials and others using closed-form analytic solutions, and estimates power using Monte Carlo methods. Only the standard stepped wedge design, with equal numbers of clusters switching from control to intervention at each step, is supported.

The swdpwr package [29] calculates power for stepped wedge cluster randomized trials with a focus on different methods for binary outcomes. The methods included in this package are based on Li et al. [138], which presents sample size procedures for continuous and binary responses in the generalized estimating equations framework, and [243], which derives the asymptotic variance of the maximum likelihood estimator for the risk difference to obtain power and sample size formulas for stepped wedge trials of binary outcomes. A Shiny app for this package can be accessed at https://jiachenchen322.shinyapps.io/swdpwr_shinyapp/. A SAS macro is also available. Other supplemental material can be found at https://ysph.yale.edu/cmips/research/software/swdpwr/.

The `SWSamp` package [13] computes power for stepped wedge trials using both closed-form formulas based on a set of specific models and simulation-based procedures that can extend the basic framework, for continuous, binary and count outcomes. It can be accessed at https://rdrr.io/github/giabaio/SWSamp/.

The `CRTpowerdist` package [175] implements simulations and approximate analytic formulae to calculate attained power. Attained power is the power conditional on the realized allocation of units to study conditions and can differ from the pre-randomization expected power. For example, a two-arm trial that is expected to allocate 20 participants to each condition will attain less than the expected power if by chance it allocates 25 and 15 participants to the conditions. The analytic formulae-based calculations are also implemented in a Shiny app.

The `SteppedPower` package has a set of tools for power and sample size calculation for longitudinal mixed model settings, with a focus on stepped wedge designs. Calculations use the WLS approach.

The National Institutes of Health Research Methods Resources website has guidance on research methods related to parallel cluster randomized trials, individually randomized group treatment trials and stepped wedge cluster randomized trials at https://researchmethodsresources.nih.gov. The website includes a sample size calculator.

Shiny CRT Calculator [91] supports power calculations for stepped wedge trials. The app can be used via https://clusterrcts.shinyapps.io/rshinyapp. Source code and updates are located on GitHub https://github.com/karlahemming/Cluster-RCT-Sample-Size-Calculator.

16

Time to event outcomes

16.1 Introduction

This chapter considers studies in which the outcome is the length of time until some event occurs. This type of data is often called survival data and the times to event are called survival times, although the event of interest could be something other than death, for example, disease progression.

A distinguishing feature of time to event studies is that the survival times for some participants may be **censored**, meaning that we do not observe the patient experience the event of interest during the study; rather, we only know that they survived longer than their last observed time. Censoring can occur when a patient is lost to follow up during the study or when the study ends; the latter situation is called administrative censoring. This feature impacts the measures that are used to compare survival between groups. For example, we typically cannot compare mean survival times because not all survival times are observed and so means cannot be computed.

Another distinguishing feature of studies with survival outcomes is that the processes of patient accrual and loss to follow up (censoring) impact power and must be modeled as part of a power or sample size calculation. As shown in Figure 16.1, such studies typically have an accrual period, during which patients are gradually enrolled into the trial and begin their observation period, then an additional period of time during which patients are followed to observe outcomes. Participants may be lost to follow up at any point after entering, causing their observations to be censored. The processes of accrual and loss to follow up affect the participants' time under observation, which affects the probability that events will be observed. This in turn affects power. For power and sample size calculations, we will typically need to make assumptions about the distribution of accrual times and loss to follow up times, in addition to the distribution of time to event in each study arm. Thus there are more aspects of the trial that need to be modeled when the outcome is a survival outcome compared to other types of outcomes.

This chapter is organized as follows. In Section 16.2, we cover key concepts such as survival and hazard functions, proportional hazards, hazard ratio, and the Kaplan-Meier (KM) estimator of a survival curve. Two different testing approaches are covered: the logrank test in Section 16.3 and various tests based on the KM estimator in Section 16.4. Given the need to specify survival,

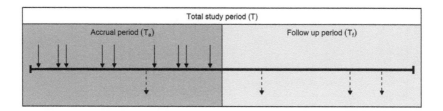

FIGURE 16.1: Depiction of accrual and loss to follow up processes. Participants enter during the accrual period (solid arrows) and may exit due to loss to follow up (dashed arrows) at any time after entry, causing their observations to be censored. The total study period length equals the length of the accrual period plus the length of the follow up period.

accrual and loss to follow up distributions in order to compute sample size and power, Section 16.5.1 discusses some commonly used distributions. Additional resources are discussed in Section 16.6.

16.2 Concepts for time to event studies

Let the random variable T be the time until an event occurs, which we expect to be a positive value $(T > 0)$. Denote its cdf as $F(t) = P(T \leq t)$ and its density function as $f(t)$. With time to event data, we often work with the survival function and/or the hazard function, which are other ways of expressing the distribution of time to event. The **survival function** $S(t)$ is defined as the probability of surviving beyond time t,

$$S(t) = P(T > t) = 1 - F(t) = \int_t^\infty f(x)dx.$$

The **hazard function** $\lambda(t)$ gives the probability that the event will occur in the next instant given that it has not yet occurred,

$$\lambda(t) = \lim_{\Delta t \to 0} \frac{P(t \leq T < t + \Delta | T \geq t)}{\Delta t} = \frac{f(t)}{S(t)} = \frac{d \log(S(t))}{dt}.$$

The survival and density functions are related to each other as $f(t) = \frac{dS(t)}{dt}$ and the survival and hazard functions are related to each other as $S(t) = \exp\left(-\int_0^x \lambda(x)dx\right)$. Because of the interrelationships among the density, survival and hazard functions, if one is specified, the other two can be derived.

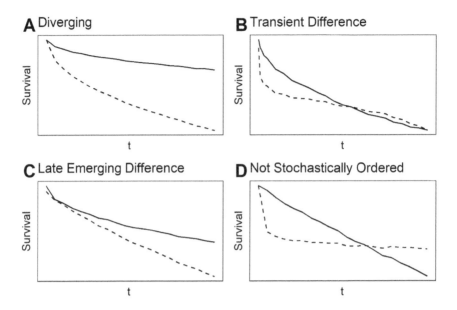

FIGURE 16.2: Examples of survival curves in two groups.

When comparing the survival times of two groups, a **proportional hazards** assumption is often made. Under the proportional hazards assumption, the ratio of the hazards in the two groups is constant, i.e., $\lambda_2(t)/\lambda_1(t) = k$; in other words, the hazards are proportional to each other and although the two hazards may change over time, their ratio does not.

The ratio $\lambda_2(t)/\lambda_1(t)$ is called the **hazard ratio**. A hazard ratio greater than one, $\lambda_2(t)/\lambda_1(t) > 1$, means that we expect a higher event rate and shorter survival times in group 2 than in group 1; $\lambda_2(t)/\lambda_1(t) < 1$ means that we expect a lower event rate and longer survival times in group 2 than in group 1.

Although it is common to assume proportional hazards, there are many ways in which the survival functions of two groups could differ. Figure 16.2 provides some examples. Panel (A) depicts survival functions that diverge early and remain divergent. In Panel (B), survival in the two groups shows a transient early difference that then disappears, while Panel (C) shows groups with a late emerging difference in survival. In Panel (D), the survival curves are not stochastically ordered; at some time point they cross such that survival probabilities are higher in one group before the curves cross and lower thereafter. In Panels (B), (C) and (D), the hazard rates are clearly not proportional. In general, one should try to anticipate the likely relationship between two survival curves and select a testing approach and corresponding power method accordingly.

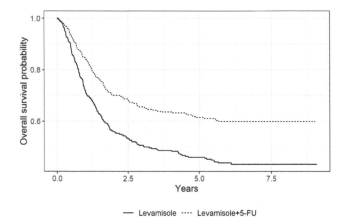

FIGURE 16.3: Example of Kaplan-Meier survival curve estimates. Time to cancer recurrence or death in patients with stage III colon cancer assigned to levamisole alone or levamisole plus fluorouracil. Data from Moertel et al. [162].

The fundamental technique for estimating and visualizing a survival function based on study data is the Kaplan-Meier (KM) estimator of the survival curve [116]. The KM estimator is built around the observed event times, denoted as t_j. Denote the distinct times of observed events as $t_1 < t_2 < \cdots < t_J$. The estimator of the survival function at time t is

$$\hat{S}(t) = \prod_{j:\, t_j \leq t} \left(1 - \frac{d_j}{Y_j}\right)$$

where d_j is the number of events that occurred at time t_j and Y_j is the number of individuals known to have survived (that is, have not yet had the event or been censored) up to time t_j. Such individuals are "at risk" of the event and are called the "risk set" at time t_j. Using this approach and assuming that the survival curve is constant between times of events, one can produce an estimate of the survival curve. An example is provided in Figure 16.3 comparing the estimated survival curves of two groups.

16.3 Logrank test

One approach to comparing survival between two groups is to compare their entire survival curves. The null hypothesis is $H_0\colon S_1(t) = S_2(t)$ for all t, that is, the survival curves coincide at all time points, while the alternative hypothesis is that they do not. This is equivalent to $H_0: \lambda_1(t) = \lambda_2(t)$ for all t because survival and hazard functions are different ways of expressing the same distribution.

The logrank test [37, 150] provides such a test. The logrank test is based on comparing the observed number of events to the expected number under the null hypothesis, with these numbers computed at the times of events. Denote the distinct times of observed events as $t_1 < t_2 < \cdots < t_J$ and index them using j. Let $i = 1, 2$ index group. For groups 1 and 2, denote the number of individuals at risk at time t_j as Y_{1j} and Y_{2j} and the observed number of events at time t_j as d_{1j} and d_{2j}, respectively. Summed across groups, at time t_j, we have $Y_j = Y_{1j} + Y_{2j}$ total individuals in the risk set and $d_j = d_{1j} + d_{2j}$ total events.

When H_0 is true, each d_{ij} has a hypergeometric distribution with parameters Y_j, Y_{ij} and d_j. Thus the expected value and variance of, say, d_{1j} under the null are

$$E_j = d_j \frac{Y_{1j}}{Y_j} \qquad (16.1)$$

$$V_j = d_j \frac{Y_{1j}}{Y_j} \left(\frac{Y_j - Y_{1j}}{Y_j} \right) \left(\frac{Y_j - d_j}{Y_j - 1} \right).$$

The next step is to compare the observed and expected number of events. Define $O_j = d_{1j}$ and further define $O = \sum_j O_j$, the total number of observed events in group 1; $E = \sum_j E_j$, the expected total number of events in group 1 under the null; and $V = \sum_j V_j$. The logrank test statistic is

$$Z_{LR} = \frac{O - E}{\sqrt{V}} = \frac{\sum_j (O_j - E_j)}{\sqrt{\sum_j V_j}}. \qquad (16.2)$$

Under H_0, $Z_{LR} \dot\sim \mathcal{N}(0, 1)$.

Logrank statistic (16.2) gives all observations the same weight, regardless of the time at which an event occurs or the size of the risk set at that time. In some studies, we may wish to emphasize certain observations more than others. This can be operationalized by using a weighted logrank test statistic,

$$Z_{WLR} = \frac{\sum_j w_j (O_j - E_j)}{\sqrt{\sum_j w_j^2 V_j}} \qquad (16.3)$$

where the weights $w_1, \ldots, w_J$ are positive constants. Setting all $w_j = 1$ yields the unweighted logrank test. Gehan-Breslow (also called Wilcoxon) weights are Y_j, the number in the risk set at time t_j; this approach gives more weight to deaths at early time points, when the risk set is larger. Tarone-Ware is similar but uses $\sqrt{Y_j}$. Many other options are available; see Collett [37] for more details.

What is the distribution of Z_{WLR} under an alternative hypothesis of a treatment benefit? To determine this, we need to make assumptions about the accrual, survival and loss to follow up distributions in the groups. Based on these distributions, we can calculate the expected number of observed events in each group at various time points and ultimately the distribution of Z_{WLR} under the alternative. Our narrative here is based on Yung and Liu [240].

Denote the proportions of patients randomized to groups 1 and 2 as p_1 and p_2, with $p_1 + p_2 = 1$. The total sample size is N. Patients are accrued into the study over a period of length T_a and then followed for an additional period T_f, for a total study duration of $T = T_a + T_f$. Let $H(t)$ represent a patient's probability of accrual into the study up to time t; this does not differ by group. For group i, $S_i(t)$ represents a patient's probability of survival to time t, $f_i(t)$ represents the survival density function at time t, $\lambda_i(t)$ represents the hazard function at time t, and $G_i(t)$ represents a patient's probability of loss to follow up before time t.

The probability that a patient in group i will still be in the risk set at time t is given by $\pi_i(t) = S_i(t)(1 - G_i(t))H(\min(T_a, T - t))$ (i.e., the patient has accrued, has not been lost to follow up, and has not experienced the event up to time t). Unconditional on group, the probability of being in the risk set at time t is $\pi(t) = p_1 \pi_1(t) + p_2 \pi_2(t)$. For group i, the expected number of observed events at time t is $v_i(t) = \int_0^t f_i(s)(1 - G_i(s))H(\min(T_a, T - s))ds$. Unconditional on group, the expected number of observed events at time t is $v(t) = p_1 v_1(t) + p_2 v_2(t)$.

Yung and Liu [240] show that $Z_{WLR} \stackrel{.}{\sim} \mathcal{N}(\sqrt{N}\Delta/\sigma, \tilde{\sigma}^2/\sigma^2)$, where Δ is a measure of treatment benefit given by

$$\Delta = \int_0^T w(s) \frac{p_1 \pi_1(s) p_2 \pi_2(s)}{\pi(s)} [\lambda_2(s) - \lambda_1(s)] ds,$$

which is interpretable as a weighted average of the difference in hazards; $\Delta = 0$ under the null hypothesis of no treatment benefit and $\Delta < 0$ under the alternative of a treatment benefit. The quantities pertaining to variance include

$$\sigma = \int_0^T w(s)^2 \frac{p_1 \pi_1(s) p_2 \pi_2(s)}{\pi(s)^2} v'(s) ds$$

where $v'(s) = H(\min(T_a, T - s)) \sum_i p_i f_i(s)(1 - G_i(s))$, the derivative of $v(\cdot)$ evaluated at s. The quantity $\tilde{\sigma}$ depends on whether simple or block randomization is used. For most practical purposes, $\tilde{\sigma}^2 \approx \sigma^2$, and we will use this simplification; see [240] for details.

Power and sample size for a two-sided test at level α can be calculated as

$$1 - \beta = 1 - \Phi\left(z_{1-\alpha/2} + \sqrt{N}\Delta/\sigma\right)$$

and

$$N = \frac{\sigma^2 (z_{1-\alpha/2} + z_{1-\beta})^2}{\Delta^2}$$

In general, the quantities Δ and σ are not trivial to calculate and calculations are performed in software based on user-specified inputs for T_a, T_f, p_1, $H(t)$, $S_1(t), S_2(t), G_1(t)$ and $G_2(t)$.

The npsurvSS package has a comprehensive set of functions for computing power and sample size for trials with survival endpoints. Yung and Liu [240] is the companion article and provides detailed derivations. We use it to illustrate a power calculation for a logrank test in the following example.

Example 16.1. Suppose that in a randomized trial with a survival endpoint, the expected median survival times in the control and treatment arms are 13 and 22 months, respectively. Accrual will occur over 6 months, followed by an additional period of observation of 12 months. If we enroll 120 patients in each arm, what is the power for an unweighted logrank test at two-sided $\alpha = 0.05$?

In the npsurvSS package, the first step is to create objects that specify the assumptions about sample size, accrual and follow up period durations, and the accrual, survival and loss to follow-up distributions for each study arm. Suppose that we are willing to assume that survival times follow an exponential distribution. Then we can solve for the exponential rate parameters as $\lambda \approx \log(2)/\text{median}$, yielding (see Section 16.5.1 for explanation)

```
lambda1 <- log(2) / 13 ; lambda1
[1] 0.05331901
lambda2 <- log(2) / 22 ; lambda2
[1] 0.03150669
```

Note that the assumption of exponential distributions for survival times entails a proportional hazards assumption, since the hazard ratio is λ_2/λ_1, which is constant over time.

We assume loss to follow up is exponential with rate parameter $\eta = 0.005$, which translates to a probability of loss of $1 - \exp(-12\eta)$ after 12 months, which calculates to about 5.8% (see Section 16.5.1 for explanation):

```
1 - exp(-12 * 0.005)
[1] 0.05823547
```

Now we create objects with the assumptions for each arm:

```
library(npsurvSS)
arm1 <- create_arm(size = 120, accr_time = 6, follow_time = 12,
   surv_scale = lambda1, loss_scale = 0.005)
arm2 <- create_arm(size = 120, accr_time = 6, follow_time = 12,
   surv_scale = lambda2, loss_scale = 0.005)
```

Here, surv_scale and loss_scale are scale parameters for the Weibull distribution. One can also define shape parameters; the default for shape parameters is 1, which yields the exponential distribution.

The default test is the logrank test with default weight of 1:

```
power_two_arm(arm1, arm2)
[1] 0.7714754
```

Power is about 0.77.

The npsurvSS package has various options for specifying distributions, different weights and different large-sample approximations, as well as options for block or simple randomization.

16.3.1 Proportional hazards

The most commonly used regression model for survival analysis is the Cox proportional hazards model [37, 41]. Sample size for Cox regression with a single covariate indicating treatment group can be viewed as a special case of the unweighted logrank test assuming proportional hazards [33]. Suppose that the hazard ratio $\lambda_2(t)/\lambda_1(t)$ is constant at all t, meaning that we have proportional hazards. Let θ represent the log of the hazard ratio, $\log(\lambda_2(t)/\lambda_1(t))$. If there are N total subjects and p_E is the probability that a patient in either group will have an event during the study, then $d_E = Np_E$ is the expected number of observed events. In this case, the logrank test statistic is approximately normal with mean $\theta\sqrt{Np_E p_1 p_2}$ and unit variance; see Schoenfeld [197]. For a two-sided test at level α, for power of $1-\beta$, we have

$$d_E = Np_E = \frac{(z_{1-\alpha/2} + z_{1-\beta})^2}{p_1 p_2 \theta^2}. \tag{16.4}$$

A common approach to sample size calculation is to calculate d_E using this formula and then determine the enrolled sample size N based on the accrual, survival and loss to follow up distributions and the study duration [37].

Sample size formula (16.4) has the property that as long as θ is correctly specified, the power remains the same even if the accrual, survival and/or loss to follow-up distributions are misspecified [240]. However, the formula is only valid under the assumption of proportional hazards and when the unweighted log-rank test is used to test the null hypothesis.

A useful relationship is that when the proportional hazard assumption is met, when Z is the logrank statistic and D is the number of events observed, the log of the hazard ratio can be estimate as $\hat{\theta} \approx Z/\sqrt{p_1 p_2 D}$, with $\hat{\theta} \approx 2Z/\sqrt{D}$ for equal allocation. This relationship allows one to approximate the underlying hazard ratio when Z and D are given (e.g., in a published article).

Example 16.2. An article on the results of a two-arm randomized trial reports that 44 participants had an observed time of death and gives the value of the logrank test statistic as 2.11. The trial used equal allocation. Then under the assumption of proportional hazards, the log of the hazard ratio can be approximated as $\theta \approx 2Z/\sqrt{D} = 2 \times 2.11/\sqrt{44} = 0.636$.

16.4 Tests based on the Kaplan-Meier estimator

The logrank test has a number of limitations [240]. If the proportional hazards assumption is violated, it may be less efficient [94]. It is not a directional (one-sided) test, which makes it unsuitable for tests of noninferiority or superiority by a margin. It may be misleading under various patterns of nonproportional hazards (see Figure 16.2 for examples). In addition, it does not correspond to a readily interpretable measure of treatment benefit.

Some authors have advocated for the use of nonparametric tests that have clearly interpretable measures of treatment efficacy [217]. These include the difference in survival probability, the difference in p^{th} percentile survival, and the difference in restricted mean survival time (RMST) at a milestone time t^*. One can also consider the ratios of these quantities in the two groups. These measures are based on the Kaplan-Meier estimate of the survival function (see Section 16.2). We briefly discuss the comparison of milestone survival probability and RMST.

To compare survival probabilities between two groups at some prespecified time t^*, the null hypothesis is $H_0\colon S_1(t^*) - S_2(t^*) = 0$ and can be tested using the Wald statistic

$$Z_S = \frac{\hat{S}_1(t^*) - \hat{S}_2(t^*)}{\sqrt{\widehat{Var}(\hat{S}_1(t^*)) + \widehat{Var}(\hat{S}_2(t^*))}}.$$

The prespecified time t^* could be selected as a fixed clinically meaningful duration (for example, $t^* = 2$ years), or minimax (minimum of the two arms' maximum) event time [240]. The test can be one-sided, which allows for tests of noninferiority and superiority by a margin.

The restricted mean survival time $RMST(t^*)$ is the mean survival time in patients followed to a prespecified time t^*. This is equivalent to the area under the survival curve up to time t^*. The null hypothesis $H_0\colon RMST_1(t^*) - RMST_2(t^*) = 0$ can be tested using the Wald statistic

$$Z_{\text{RMST}} = \frac{\widehat{RMST}_1(t^*) - \widehat{RMST}_2(t^*)}{\sqrt{\widehat{Var}(\widehat{RMST}_1(t^*)) + \widehat{Var}(\widehat{RMST}_2(t^*))}}.$$

Tests based on the Kaplan-Meier estimator

Power and sample size calculations for such tests can be implemented in the npsurvSS package. Options for tests in this package include survival difference, survival ratio, RMST difference, RMST ratio, and percentile difference and ratio. Yung and Liu [240] is the companion article and provides detailed derivations.

Example 16.3. We provide an illustration of computing power for a test of the difference in survival probabilities or the restricted mean survival time at a milestone time point. We specify the survival curves using the piecewise exponential approach, which is an approach for modeling nonproportional hazards. We expect that the survival curves will be similar early in the trial and then diverge more rapidly starting at around 6 months, when the control group has a higher hazard rate. Figure 16.4 displays the survival curves. Other specifications are as in Example 16.1.

```
library(npsurvSS)
library(ggplot2)
arm1 <- create_arm(size = 120, accr_time = 6, follow_time = 12,
    surv_interval = c(0, 6, 12, Inf), surv_scale = c(0.04, 0.06, 0.06),
    loss_scale = 0.005)
arm2 <- create_arm(size = 120, accr_time = 6, follow_time = 12,
    surv_interval = c(0, 6, 12, Inf), surv_scale = c(0.03, 0.03, 0.03),
    loss_scale = 0.005)
t <- seq(from = 1, to = 20, by = 1)
s1 <- psurv(q = t, arm = arm1, lower.tail = F)
s2 <- psurv(q = t, arm = arm2, lower.tail = F)
p = ggplot() +
    geom_line(aes(x = t, y = s1), linetype = "dashed") +
    geom_line(aes(x = t, y = s2), linetype = "solid") +
    xlab("Month") + ylim(0, 1) + ylab("Survival")
print(p)
```

We compute power for comparing the difference in survival probabilities and RMST at 15 months:

```
power_two_arm(arm1, arm2, list(test = "survival difference",
    milestone = 15))
[1] 0.7494031
power_two_arm(arm1, arm2, list(test = "rmst difference",
    milestone = 15))
[1] 0.5288692
```

Power for survival probability difference at 15 months is about 75%, whereas power for RMST difference at 15 months is about 53%.

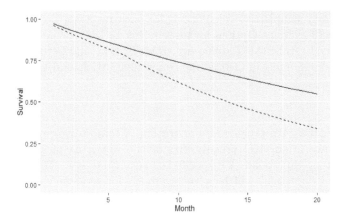

FIGURE 16.4: Survival curves from Example 16.3.

16.5 Distributions for survival, accrual and loss to follow up

As discussed, to conduct power or sample size calculations for time to event studies, one needs to make assumptions about the survival, accrual and loss to follow up (censoring) distributions. In this section, we discuss some commonly used distributions.

16.5.1 Survival distributions

A common assumption is that time to event has an **exponential distribution**. When T has an exponential distribution with rate parameter λ, denoted $T \sim \text{Exp}(\lambda)$, the density, survival and hazard functions are $f(t) = \lambda e^{-\lambda t}, S(t) = e^{-\lambda t}$ and $\lambda(t) = \lambda$. Figure 16.5 displays exponential survival and hazard functions for $\lambda = 0.2$.

The defining property of the exponential distribution is that the hazard function is constant; the probability of the event occurring at any time t does not depend on t, i.e., it does not depend on how much time has elapsed. This is referred to as the "lack of memory" or "no-aging" property of the exponential distribution. This property can seem unrealistic for modeling survival times, since we often expect the probability of the event to change with time (e.g., for older adults, the probability of death increases with age). However, it can be reasonable to assume a constant hazard rate when modeling survival over relatively short time intervals.

The survival times of a sample are often summarized as the **median survival time**, that is, the time to which 50% of the sample survived. When

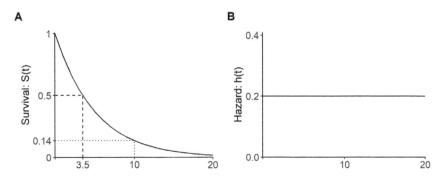

FIGURE 16.5: Exponential distribution $Y \sim \text{Exp}(0.2)$, for which the median survival time is $\log(2)/0.2 = 3.5$. (A) Survival function $S(t)$, showing $S(3.5) = 0.5$ and $S(10) = 0.14$. (B) Hazard function $h(t) = 0.2$ for all t.

survival times have an exponential distribution, median survival time can be used to solve for the hazard rate as $\lambda = \log(2)/\text{median}$.

Example 16.4. Suppose the median survival time in a population is 6 months. If survival times are exponentially distributed, the hazard rate is $\lambda = \log(2)/6 = 0.1155$ months^{-1}, that is, events occur at the rate of 0.1155 per month.

If the survival times in two groups are exponentially distributed, then they both have constant hazard rates and the hazard ratio is also constant. This implies proportional hazards, which may not hold in practice. Distributions that allow for nonproportional hazards include piecewise exponential, which partitions follow up into intervals and assumes a separate exponential within each interval, and the Weibull distribution. The Weibull distribution has two parameters, which we denote as $\lambda > 0$, a scale parameter, and $k > 0$, a shape parameter. The density function is

$$f(t) = \lambda k (\lambda t)^{k-1} \exp(-(\lambda t)^k)$$

When $k = 1$, the Weibull reduces to the exponential distribution. The hazard ratio will not be constant over time (i.e., nonproportional hazards) if the shape parameter k is set to different values for different groups. Another option that allows for proportional or nonproportional hazards is the mixture cure model [19], which models survival as a mixture of a cure fraction and survival function of uncured patients,

$$S(t) = c + (1-c)S^*(t)$$

where c denotes the fraction of the population that is cured and will not experience the event and $S^*(t)$ is the cumulative distribution of time to event for uncured patients.

16.5.2 Accrual distributions

A commonly used distribution for accrual is the **uniform distribution**. Uniform patient entry over an interval $[0, T_a]$ is represented by the cumulative distribution function $H(t) = t/T_a$. However, it is quite common to have nonuniform accrual. In multisite trials, the accrual rate is often low early in the trial and increases as more recruitment sites become fully operational. Or, if the pool of eligible patients is limited, accrual may be highest at the beginning and then diminish over time as the pool becomes exhausted. An option for these situations is the **truncated exponential distribution**, which is an exponential distribution that is defined only over a certain region, e.g., $[0, T_a]$. The density function for a truncated exponential distribution with rate parameter γ is

$$h(t) = \frac{\gamma e^{-\gamma t}}{1 - e^{-\gamma T_a}}, \ 0 \leq t \leq T_a.$$

For $\gamma > 0$, this distribution is convex and the accrual rate decreases over time. For $\gamma < 0$, the distribution is concave and the accrual rate increases over time. Another option is a piecewise uniform distribution, which partitions the accrual period into intervals and allows a different uniform accrual rate within each interval.

16.5.3 Loss to follow up distributions

Loss to follow up (censoring) times are typically given less consideration than the survival and accrual distributions. They are often assumed to have an exponential distribution, or a Weibull distribution might be used if censoring is expected to happen at different rates early versus late during follow up. If assumed to be exponential, a handy relationship is that the probability of a patient being lost within t months of follow-up, independent of event and administrative censoring, can be equated to $1 - \exp(-\eta t)$. This allows one to solve for the rate of loss parameter η given a probability of loss to follow up by time t.

Example 16.5. Suppose that 10% of patients are expected to be lost to follow up after 12 months in the study. If loss to follow up times are $\text{Exp}(\eta)$, the hazard rate parameter for loss can be found by solving $0.1 = 1 - \exp(-12\eta)$, which gives $\eta = -\log(0.9)/12 = 0.008780043$ months^{-1}.

16.6 Additional resources

The trial designs that we have discussed are "time-driven" trials, in which the final analysis for the trial is triggered at time $T = T_a + T_f$ after the first patient is enrolled. An alternative is an "event-driven" trial, in which the final analysis is triggered when a predetermined number of events is reached. See [240] for more discussion.

We have focused on the use of the npsurvSS package, which is currently one of the most comprehensive. A list of sample size programs for survival trials is available as Web Table 1 of a supplemental material file to Yung and Liu [240] at https://onlinelibrary.wiley.com/doi/10.1111/biom.13196. Other packages include Hmisc (the cpower function), PWEALL and SSRMST. Some simple approaches are also available in the designsize and powerSurvEpi packages. The package gsDesign derives group sequential designs for continuous, binary and time to event outcomes.

17

Multiple primary endpoints

17.1 Introduction

Often, a study has one primary outcome or endpoint, and the sample size requirement is based on ensuring adequate power for that single endpoint. However, in some studies, there may be two or more outcomes or endpoints that are considered important in terms of concluding whether the intervention is beneficial or not. Having more than one primary endpoint affects power and sample size requirements, as we discuss in this chapter.

We use the term "endpoint" in this chapter because it helps provide clarity in some situations. Consider a study that measures the same outcome variable at several different time points; for example, a study might measure depressive symptoms at baseline, 3-month, 6-month and 12-month assessments. If we deem that the 6- and 12-month assessments are both of key importance, we might designate these two assessments as primary endpoints. Note that these assessments involve measuring the same outcome variable, but they are distinct endpoints because the measurements are at different times.

We can classify multiple primary endpoints as co-primary endpoints or alternative primary endpoints. With **co-primary endpoints**, we seek to reject the null hypothesis and conclude that the alternative hypothesis is true for *all* of the primary endpoints. For example, we may want to demonstrate that a new treatment is both safe AND effective; there is a safety endpoint and an efficacy endpoint, and both are important for concluding that the study is a "success". In other trials, there may be no single variable that is deemed sufficient to capture the range of clinically relevant treatment benefits, and so the trial is designed with more than one co-primary efficacy endpoint.

Studies with co-primary endpoints use "all-or-none" testing procedures and only declare the trial to be a "success" if all endpoints are affirmed. In this setting, there is no danger that the type I error rate will be inflated and no adjustment is needed to control the type I error rate for multiple tests. However, the type II error rate, that is, the probability of failing to reject the null hypothesis when it is false, will increase as the number of endpoints increases, which will impact power and sample size requirements.

In other studies, we may seek to reject the null hypothesis for *at least one* of the primary endpoints. This is called **multiple** or **alternative primary endpoints**. We will use the term "alternative". The associated testing

Model

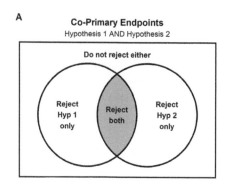 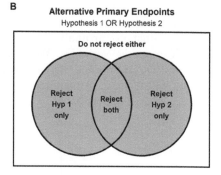

FIGURE 17.1: Venn diagram representing co-primary versus alternative primary endpoints. (A) Two co-primary endpoints: both null hypotheses must be rejected in order to conclude "success". (B) Two alternative primary endpoints: rejecting either null hypothesis is sufficient to conclude "success".

procedure is sometimes called an "at-least-one" procedure. With alternative endpoints, inflation of the type I error rate is a concern and procedures are needed to control it. The Bonferroni procedure is an example of one such procedure. Such procedures will impact power and sample size requirements.

The distinction between co-primary and alternative primary endpoints is illustrated in Figure 17.1 for the case of two endpoints. When there are two co-primary endpoints, both null hypotheses must be rejected in order to conclude "success"; that is, success requires the intersection of two events. When there are two alternative primary endpoints, rejecting either null hypothesis is sufficient to conclude "success"; success corresponds to the union of two events.

Sample size and power determination in the setting of multiple endpoints is discussed in Sozu et al. [209] and much of this chapter is based on that reference. The R functions are also based on R code provided by this reference. We discuss only continuous endpoints.

17.2 Model

The following model for the data will apply to both the co-primary endpoint and alternative primary endpoint situation. Continuous outcome variables are assumed.

Suppose we are planning a trial that will compare a treatment condition to a control condition on the means of $K \geq 2$ outcome variables. In this setting, each participant provides a vector of responses of length K. Denote these vectors as $\mathbf{Y}_{iT} = (Y_{iT1}, ..., Y_{iTK})'$ for participant i in the treatment condition and $\mathbf{Y}_{iC} = (Y_{iC1}, ..., Y_{iCK})'$ for participant i in the control condition.

To conduct power analysis, we need to consider the joint distribution of these K outcome variables. We will assume that the K outcome variables have multivariate normal distributions with mean vectors $(\mu_{T1}, ..., \mu_{TK})'$ and $(\mu_{C1}, ..., \mu_{CK})'$ for treatment and control participants, respectively, and a common covariance matrix $\boldsymbol{\Sigma}$,

$$\boldsymbol{\Sigma} = \begin{bmatrix} \sigma_1^2 & \cdots & \rho_{1K}\sigma_1\sigma_K \\ \vdots & \ddots & \\ \rho_{1K}\sigma_1\sigma_K & \cdots & \sigma_K^2 \end{bmatrix}$$

where $Var(Y_{iTk}) = Var(Y_{iCk}) = \sigma_k^2$. This reflects an assumption that each outcome variable has a variance that is equal across treatment and control groups, and $Corr(Y_{iTk}, Y_{iTk'}) = Corr(Y_{iCk}, Y_{iCk'}) = \rho_{kk'}$, i.e., each pair of outcome variables is correlated, with the degree of correlation allowed to differ for different pairs.

17.3 Co-primary endpoints

Studies with co-primary endpoints use "all-or-none" testing procedures and only declare the trial to be a "success" if all endpoints are affirmed. Suppose we are planning a trial that will compare a treatment condition to a control condition on the means of $K \geq 2$ outcome variables. Assuming that higher values correspond to better outcomes, for co-primary endpoints, we hope to conclude that $\mu_{Tk} - \mu_{Ck} > 0$ for all k. The hypotheses are

$$H_0: \mu_{Tk} - \mu_{Ck} \leq 0 \text{ for at least one } k \quad (17.1)$$
$$H_A: \mu_{Tk} - \mu_{Ck} > 0 \text{ for all } k.$$

We reject H_0 and conclude that H_A is true if and only if we reject $\mu_{Tk} - \mu_{Ck} \leq 0$ and conclude $\mu_{Tk} - \mu_{Ck} > 0$ for all K endpoints. The event of rejecting H_0 is the intersection of K events, $H_0 = \cap_{k=1}^{K} H_{0k} : \{\mu_{Tk} - \mu_{Ck} \leq 0\}$, as depicted in Figure 17.1(A).

17.3.1 Covariance matrix known

First, we derive power assuming the covariance matrix is known, in particular, that the variances of the outcome variables are known and do not need to be estimated, which leads to z test statistics. The next section considers the more realistic situation that the covariance matrix is not known and the variances must be estimated, which leads to t test statistics.

Co-primary endpoints

Suppose there are n_T participants in the treatment group and n_C in the control group. If the variances σ_k^2 were known, we could test each hypothesis using the test statistic for a two-sample z test,

$$Z_k = \frac{\bar{Y}_{Tk} - \bar{Y}_{Ck}}{\sigma_k \sqrt{\frac{1}{n_T} + \frac{1}{n_C}}} \qquad (17.2)$$

where $\bar{Y}_{Tk}$ and $\bar{Y}_{Ck}$ are the sample means, $\bar{Y}_{Tk} = \frac{1}{n_T} \sum_{i=1}^{n_T} Y_{iTk}$ and $\bar{Y}_{Ck} = \frac{1}{n_C} \sum_{i=1}^{n_C} Y_{iCk}$. For one-sided tests at level α, we reject H_{0k} if $Z_k > z_{1-\alpha}$. The power to reject H_{0k} for all K co-primary endpoints, when each is tested with a one-sided test at level α, is the probability of the intersection,

$$1 - \beta = P\left[\cap_{k=1}^{K} \{Z_k > z_{1-\alpha}\}\right]. \qquad (17.3)$$

To compute power, we need to compute this probability when some alternative is true. Denote the true standardized difference in means for endpoint k as $d_k = \frac{\mu_{Tk} - \mu_{Ck}}{\sigma_k}$. If we subtract $d_k/\sqrt{1/n_T + 1/n_C}$ from both sides of the inequality in (17.3), we arrive at

$$1 - \beta = P\left[\cap_{k=1}^{K} \{Z_k^* > c_k\}\right]$$

where $Z_k^* = Z_k - d_k/\sqrt{1/n_T + 1/n_C}$ and $c_k = z_{1-\alpha} - d_k/\sqrt{1/n_T + 1/n_C}$. The vector $(Z_1^*, ..., Z_K^*)'$ has a K-variate normal distribution with a zero mean vector and covariance matrix equal to the correlation matrix of the K outcome variables,

$$\begin{bmatrix} Z_1^* \\ Z_2^* \\ \vdots \\ Z_K^* \end{bmatrix} \sim \mathcal{N}_K \left(\begin{bmatrix} 0 \\ 0 \\ \vdots \\ 0 \end{bmatrix}, \begin{bmatrix} 1 & \rho_{12} & \cdots & \rho_{1K} \\ \rho_{21} & 1 & \cdots & \vdots \\ \vdots & \vdots & \ddots & \vdots \\ \rho_{K1} & \cdots & \cdots & 1 \end{bmatrix} \right). \qquad (17.4)$$

We denote this distribution as $\mathcal{N}_K(\mathbf{0}, \boldsymbol{\rho}_K)$. Power can be calculated as $\Phi_K(-c_1, \ldots, -c_K)$, where Φ_K is the cumulative distribution function of $\mathcal{N}_K(\mathbf{0}, \boldsymbol{\rho}_K)$. Note that $\mathcal{N}_K(\mathbf{0}, \boldsymbol{\rho}_K)$ reduces to a univariate standard normal distribution, $\mathcal{N}(0, 1)$, when $K = 1$.

Example 17.1. Consider a study with 2 co-primary endpoints with 100 participants in each group, standardized mean differences $d_1 = 0.4$ and $d_2 = 0.5$, and correlation $\rho_{12} = \rho_{21} = 0.3$ between endpoints. For $\alpha = 0.025$ for each one-sided test, what is the power to reject the null for each endpoint separately and the power to reject both? First, we compute power for each test singly:

```
library(powertools)
ztest.2samp(n1 = 100, delta = 0.4, sd1 = 1, alpha = 0.025,
   power = NULL, sides = 1)
[1] 0.8074296

ztest.2samp(n1 = 100, delta = 0.5, sd1 = 1, alpha = 0.025,
   power = NULL, sides = 1)
[1] 0.9424375
```

Now we compute the power to reject both null hypotheses:

```
library(powertools)
# This function assumes one-sided tests
coprimary.z(K = 2, n1 = 100, delta = c(0.4, 0.5), sd = c(1, 1),
   rho = 0.3, alpha = 0.025, power = NULL)
[1] 0.772327
```

Note that the power to reject both components of the null hypothesis is lower than the power to reject either one singly.

The smallest sample size that will achieve overall power of $1 - \beta$ with significance level α for each test can be found as the smallest integer n satisfying

$$1 - \beta \geq \Phi_K(-c_1, \ldots, -c_K).$$

There is no closed-form solution to this equation. The sample size can be found in software that uses numerical methods, such as the coprimary.z function in the following example.

Example 17.2. Continuing with Example 17.1, suppose we want to find the sample size that will achieve 80% power.

```
library(powertools)
coprimary.z(K = 2, n1 = NULL, delta = c(0.4, 0.5), sd = c(1, 1),
   rho = 0.3, alpha = 0.025, power = 0.8)
[1] 105.9794
```

The smallest sample size that attains the desired level of power is 106 per group.

17.3.2 Covariance matrix unknown

Usually the covariance matrix of the outcome variables is not known and variances need to be estimated in order to perform hypothesis tests. To test for a difference in means for each endpoint k, we use a test statistic equivalent to that for a two-sample t test with equal variance,

$$T_k = \frac{\bar{Y}_{Tk} - \bar{Y}_{Ck}}{s_k \sqrt{\frac{1}{n_T} + \frac{1}{n_C}}} \quad (17.5)$$

where $s_k^2 = \frac{\sum_{i=1}^{n_T}(Y_{iTk}-\bar{Y}_{Tk})^2 + \sum_{i=1}^{n_C}(Y_{iCk}-\bar{Y}_{Ck})^2}{n_T+n_C-2}$ is the pooled estimate of the variance for endpoint k. Power to reject the null (17.1) is

$$1 - \beta = P\left[\cap_{k=1}^{K}\{T_k > t_{1-\alpha,n_T+n_C-2}\}\right]. \quad (17.6)$$

When there is a single endpoint, the test statistic has a noncentral t distribution, as discussed in previous chapters. The joint distribution of the K test statistics $(T_1, ..., T_K)$ has a type of multivariate t distribution [130] for which there is no closed form expression. However, the distribution can be approximated using simulation. A key step involves simulating values of the covariance matrix using the Wishart distribution. For additional details, see Sozu et al. [208]. The coprimary.t function performs the simulations.

Example 17.3. We continue Example 17.1 but use coprimary.t, which assumes that the covariance matrix is not known. The input M is the number of simulations. In the function, values of the covariance matrix are simulated, power is calculated for each value, and the M values of power are averaged.

```
library(powertools)
coprimary.t(K = 2, n1 = 100, delta = c(0.4, 0.5), sd = c(1, 1),
    rho = 0.3, alpha = 0.025, power = NULL, M = 10000)
[1] 0.7675367
```

The power is slightly lower compared to the power computed assuming the covariance matrix is known. Because of the use of simulation, there is Monte Carlo error and the result will vary. Increasing the number of simulations increases the precision of the result but is more computationally intensive.

To find the sample size needed to attain a desired level of power, power needs to be computed iteratively until finding the smallest n that meets the desired power level. Software can do this for us.

Example 17.4. Continuing the previous example, suppose we want to find sample size that will achieve 80% power. The function coprimary.t performs a search from min.n to max.n. Since coprimary.z indicated that we would need 106 in each group when the covariance matrix was known, we specify min.n and max.n to search through somewhat higher values:

```
library(powertools)
coprimary.t(K = 2, n1 = NULL, n.ratio = 1, delta = c(0.4, 0.5),
    sd = c(1, 1), rho = 0.3, alpha = 0.025, power = 0.8, M = 10000,
    min.n = 105, max.n = 110)
[1] 106.9586
```

The results indicate that we need about 107 per group. Due to the use of simulation, there is Monte Carlo error and the result will vary. The function needs to compute power for various values of sample size and so a number of iterations are performed.

The computations can be intensive, especially for $K > 2$. As a practical matter, the sample size required when the covariance matrix is unknown is generally about 1 participant per group larger than that assuming known covariance [209]. Hence for a good approximation, one can use the formula for known covariance and add one per group.

Example 17.5. In Example 17.2, assuming the covariance matrix was known, we calculated that we needed 106 per group. To account for unknown covariance, we can approximate the required sample size as 107 per group. This matches the required sample size that we obtained using the more computationally intensive method.

What factors affect power? When we have co-primary endpoints, in addition to the factors that affect power and sample size for each endpoint singly, we need to consider the correlation between the endpoints and their relative effect sizes. The impacts of these factors are illustrated in Table 17.1. The table provides the sample sizes per group needed for 80% power for two co-primary endpoints with standardized mean differences d_1 and d_2, assuming equal allocation, for correlation between endpoints ranging from 0.0 to 1.0, assuming known covariance. E_1 and E_2 are the sample sizes per group calculated separately for each endpoint, that is, assuming single primary endpoints. For any given combination of effect sizes, as the correlation between endpoints increases, the required sample size per group decreases. Thus higher correlation can lead to lower sample sizes. The table also shows that when effect sizes are unequal, the required sample size is driven by the smaller effect size, and the correlation between endpoints no longer has much impact.

The impact of correlation between co-primary endpoints on power is illustrated schematically in Figure 17.2. In Panel (B), the two endpoints are more

Co-primary endpoints

TABLE 17.1: Sample sizes needed for 80% power for two co-primary endpoints with one-sided tests, $\alpha = 0.025$, equal allocation, for correlation between endpoints ranging from 0.0 to 1.0, assuming known covariance. d_1 and d_2 are standardized mean differences. E_1 and E_2 are the sample sizes per group needed when an endpoint is the single primary endpoint. Adapted from Table 2.1 of Sozu et al. [209].

d_1	d_2	\multicolumn{5}{c}{ρ}	E_1	E_2
		0.0	0.3	0.5	0.8	1.0		
0.20	0.20	516	503	490	458	393	393	393
0.20	0.30	402	399	397	393	393	393	175
0.20	0.40	393	393	393	393	393	393	99
0.30	0.30	230	224	218	204	175	175	175
0.30	0.40	186	183	181	176	175	175	99
0.40	0.40	129	126	123	115	99	99	99

highly correlated than in Panel (A). When two endpoints are more highly correlated, the intersection of the two events of rejecting the two null hypotheses is larger and it is more likely that both nulls will be rejected. This leads to higher levels of power and less of an increase in required sample size.

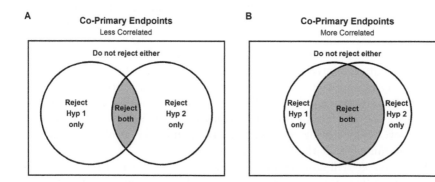

FIGURE 17.2: Venn diagram showing the impact of correlation on power for two co-primary endpoints, for which both null hypotheses must be rejected in order to conclude "success". In Panel (B), the two endpoints are more highly correlated than in Panel (A). This leads to a greater probability of rejecting both null hypotheses in (B) compared to (A).

17.4 Alternative primary endpoints

In studies with alternative or at-least-one primary endpoints, hypothesis tests are conducted for several outcomes and the trial is declared a "success" if at least one of the null hypotheses is rejected. This is a version of the "multiple comparisons" problem that was discussed in Section 5.2.4 with regard to multiple comparisons in ANOVA; see that section for more background on this topic. In this section, we focus more specifically on the case of multiple continuous alternative endpoints.

Suppose that a randomized trial will compare a treatment and a control condition on $K \geq 2$ alternative primary endpoints. Assuming a higher mean is better, the hypotheses are

$$H_0: \mu_{Tk} - \mu_{Ck} \leq 0 \text{ for all } k$$
$$H_A: \mu_{Tk} - \mu_{Ck} > 0 \text{ for at least one } k.$$

We reject H_0 and conclude H_A if we reject $\mu_{Tk} - \mu_{Ck} \leq 0$ and conclude $\mu_{Tk} - \mu_{Ck} > 0$ for any of the K endpoints. The event of rejecting H_0 is the union of K events, $H_0 = \cup_{k=1}^{K} H_{0k}: \{\mu_{Tk} - \mu_{Ck} \leq 0\}$, as depicted in Figure 17.1(B).

In such studies, we are often concerned about controlling the probability of making type I errors. In general, if we conduct several tests, each at a type I error rate of α, then the overall probability of making one or more type I errors will exceed α. A common approach to avoid an inflated type I error rate is to specify a familywise error rate (FWER), which is the probability of rejecting H_0 for at least one endpoint when H_0 is true, and use a testing procedure that guarantees that the FWER will not exceed the specified value.

A variety of approaches have been developed to control the FWER in the context of alternative endpoints. We will consider the widely used Bonferroni procedure. The Bonferroni procedure controls the FWER for K hypothesis tests at level α by testing each outcome at significance level α/K. This approach guarantees that the FWER will not exceed α.

As before, we will assume a higher outcome is better and the use of one-sided tests. When the covariance matrix is known, the test statistics are $Z_1, \ldots, Z_K$ as in equation (17.2), and the null hypothesis for any endpoint k is rejected if Z_k exceeds the multiplicity adjusted critical value $z_{1-\alpha/K}$. The rejection region is a union, $\cup_{k=1}^{K} \{Z_k > z_{1-\alpha/K}\}$, meaning that we reject the null if any $Z_k > z_{1-\alpha/K}$. Power under the Bonferroni procedure can be calculated as

$$1 - \beta = P\left[\cup_{k=1}^{K} \{Z_k > z_{1-\alpha/K}\}\right]$$
$$= 1 - P\left[\cap_{k=1}^{K} \{Z_k \leq z_{1-\alpha/K}\}\right].$$

Alternative primary endpoints

Using the same approach as in Section 17.3.1, we subtract $d_k/\sqrt{1/n_T + 1/n_C}$ from both sides of the inequality and arrive at

$$1 - \beta = 1 - P\left[\cap_{k=1}^{K}\{Z_k^* \leq c_k\}\right]$$

where $Z_k^* = Z_k - d_k/\sqrt{1/n_T + 1/n_C}$ and $c_k = z_{1-\alpha/K} - d_k/\sqrt{1/n_T + 1/n_C}$. The vector $(Z_1^*, ..., Z_K^*)'$ has a K-variate normal distribution with a zero mean vector and covariance matrix equal to the correlation matrix of the K outcome variables, ρ_K. Thus power can be calculated as $1 - \Phi(c_1, ..., c_K)$, where $\Phi(\cdot)$ is cumulative distribution function of $N_K(\mathbf{0}, \rho_K)$.

When the covariance matrix is not known, the test statistics are $T_1, ..., T_K$ as in equation (17.5), and power under the Bonferroni procedure is equal to

$$1 - \beta = 1 - P\left[\cap_{k=1}^{K}\{T_k \leq t_{1-\alpha/K, n_T+n_C-2}\}\right]$$

The joint distribution of the K test statistics $(T_1, ..., T_K)$ has a type of multivariate t distribution [130] that can be approximated using simulation. For additional details, see Sozu et al. [208].

Example 17.6. We use the same parameter values as in Example 17.1 but suppose that the two endpoints are alternative endpoints; we will reject the null and conclude the alternative if we reject the null for either endpoint. Using the Bonferroni procedure with a one-sided FWER of 0.025, what is the power to reject the null for one or both endpoints? We assume a known covariance matrix. To use a Bonferroni correction for K endpoints, alpha should be specified as FWER/K.

```
library(powertools)
altprimary(K = 2, n1 = 100, delta = c(0.4, 0.5), sd = c(1, 1),
    rho = 0.3, alpha = 0.025 / 2, power = NULL)
[1] 0.9534408
```

Power is over 0.95. This is considerably higher than when we handled these endpoints as co-primary.

What factors affect power? Table 17.2 shows sample sizes per group needed for 80% power when using a Bonferroni adjustment for two alternative endpoints for a range of standardized mean effect sizes and correlation values. For each set of effect sizes, the sample size requirement increases as the correlation between the two endpoints increases. Thus higher correlation between endpoints is associated with reduced power and a larger required sample. Figure 17.3 provides more insights on the impact of correlation on alternative endpoints. When there is higher correlation, the union (rejecting the null for one or both endpoints) becomes smaller and its complement (failing to reject the null for either endpoint) becomes proportionally larger.

TABLE 17.2: Sample sizes needed for 80% power for two alternative ("at least one") primary endpoints using Bonferroni adjustment, equal allocation, for correlation between endpoints ranging from 0.0 to 1.0, assuming known covariance. d_1 and d_2 are standardized mean differences. E_1 and E_2 are the sample sizes per group calculated separately for each endpoint at $\alpha/2$. Adapted from Table 5.1 of Sozu et al. [209].

		ρ						
d_1	d_2	0.0	0.3	0.5	0.8	1.0	E_1	E_2
0.20	0.20	282	316	342	394	476	476	476
0.20	0.30	169	185	195	209	212	476	212
0.20	0.40	106	112	116	119	119	476	119
0.30	0.30	126	141	152	175	212	212	212
0.30	0.40	89	99	105	116	119	212	119
0.40	0.40	71	79	86	99	119	119	119

▶ For alternative (at-least-one) primary endpoints, higher correlation between endpoints leads to lower power. This stands in contrast to co-primary endpoints, for which higher correlation increases power.

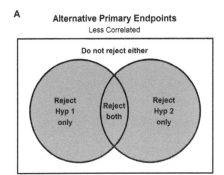
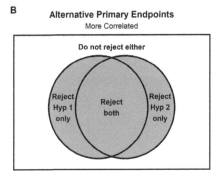

FIGURE 17.3: Venn diagram showing the impact of correlation on power for two alternative primary endpoints, for which "success" is concluded if either null hypotheses is rejected. In Panel (B), the two endpoints are more highly correlated than in Panel (A). The intersection of the two events is larger but overall, the union is smaller. This leads to a lower probability of rejecting one or both null hypotheses in (B).

17.5 Additional resources

There is a vast literature on control of type I error probability under multiple testing (see, for example, [54]), which we have referred to as alternative or at-least-one endpoints, although less literature on sample size and power methods. Table 1.1 of Sozu et al. [209] has a summary of references discussing sample size methods for clinical trials with multiple endpoints for endpoint scales including continuous, binary, time-to-event, and mixed. Some helpful references include Vickerstaff et al. [222] and Wilson et al. [231].

R packages implementing sample size calculations that control the familywise error rate for multiple testing include the rPowerSampleSize package, which is discussed in Lafaye de Micheaux et al. [130]. The FDRsampsize and pwrFDR packages have functions that can be used to compute average power and sample size for studies that use the false discovery rate as the measure of statistical significance. Computing power using simulation is also a good option for many studies that involve multiple alternative endpoints.

Bibliography

[1] Adams G, Gulliford MC, Ukoumunne OC, Eldridge S, Chinn S, Campbell MJ. Patterns of intra-cluster correlation from primary care research to inform study design and analysis. Journal of Clinical Epidemiology, 57(8):785–794, 2004.

[2] Agresti A. On logit confidence intervals for the odds ratio with small samples. Biometrics, 55(2):597–602, 1999.

[3] Agresti A, Caffo B. Simple and effective confidence intervals for proportions and differences of proportions result from adding two successes and two failures. The American Statistician, 54(4):280–288, 2000.

[4] Agresti A, Coull BA. Approximate is better than "exact" for interval estimation of binomial proportions. The American Statistician, 52(2): 119–126, 1998.

[5] Ahn C, Hu F, Skinner CS. Effect of imbalance and intracluster correlation coefficient in cluster randomized trials with binary outcomes. Computational Statistics & Data Analysis, 53(3):596–602, 2009.

[6] Ahn C, Heo M, Zhang S. Sample Size Calculations for Clustered and Longitudinal Outcomes in Clinical Research. CRC Press/Taylor and Francis Group, Boca Raton, FL, 2015.

[7] Albers C, Lakens D. When power analyses based on pilot data are biased: Inaccurate effect size estimators and follow-up bias. Journal of Experimental Social Psychology, 74:187–195, 2018.

[8] Anderson TW. An Introduction to Multivariate Statistical Analysis. New York: John Wiley & Sons, 2nd edition, 1984.

[9] Ankenman BE, Aviles AI, Pinheiro JC. Optimal designs for mixed-effects models with two random nested factors. Statistica Sinica, 13: 385–401, 2003.

[10] Anscombe FJ. The transformation of Poisson, binomial and negative-binomial data. Biometrika, 35(3/4):246–254, 1948.

[11] Armitage P, Berry G, Matthews JNS. Statistical Methods in Medical Research. John Wiley & Sons, 2008.

[12] Ataneka A, Kelcey B, Dong N, Bulus M, Bai F. PowerUp R Shiny App (Version 0.9) Manual, 2023. Available at https://www.causalevaluation.org/power-analysis.html.

[13] Baio G, Copas A, Ambler G, Hargreaves J, Beard E, Omar RZ. Sample size calculation for a stepped wedge trial. Trials, 16(1):1–15, 2015.

[14] Beal SL. Sample size determination for confidence intervals on the population means and on the difference between two population means. Biometrics, 45(3):969–977, 1989.

[15] Benjamini Y, Hochberg Y. Controlling the false discovery rate: a practical and powerful approach to multiple testing. Journal of the Royal Statistical Society: Series B (Methodological), 57(1):289–300, 1995.

[16] Benjamini Y, Yekutieli D. The control of the false discovery rate in multiple testing under dependency. Annals of Statistics, 29(4):1165–1188, 2001.

[17] Berger RL. Multiparameter hypothesis testing and acceptance sampling. Technometrics, 24:295–300, 1982.

[18] Berger RL, Hsu JC. Bioequivalence trials, intersection-union tests and equivalence confidence sets. Statistical Science, 11(4):283–319, 1996.

[19] Berkson J, Gage RP. Survival curve for cancer patients following treatment. Journal of the American Statistical Association, 47(259):501–515, 1952.

[20] Blackwelder WC. Sample size and power for prospective analysis of relative risk. Statistics in Medicine, 12(7):691–698, 1993.

[21] Bloom HS, Richburg-Hayes L, Black AR. Using covariates to improve precision for studies that randomized schools to evaluate educational interventions. Evaluation and Policy Analysis, 29:30–59, 2007.

[22] Breslow NE, Clayton DG. Approximate inference in generalized linear mixed models. Journal of the American Statistical Association, 88(421):9–25, 1993.

[23] Bretz F, Hothorn T, Westfall P. Multiple Comparisons Using R. CRC Press, 2016.

[24] Brown LD, Cai TT, DasGupta A. Interval estimation for a binomial proportion. Statistical Science, 16(2):101–133, 2001.

[25] Campbell MJ, Walters SJ. How to Design, Analyse and Report Cluster Randomised Trials in Medicine and Health-Related Research. John Wiley & Sons Ltd, Chichester, UK, 2014.

[26] Candel MJ, Van Breukelen GJ. Varying cluster sizes in trials with clusters in one treatment arm: Sample size adjustments when testing treatment effects with linear mixed models. Statistics in Medicine, 28(18):2307–2324, 2009.

[27] Candel MJ, Van Breukelen GJ. Sample size adjustments for varying cluster sizes in cluster randomized trials with binary outcomes analyzed with second-order PQL mixed logistic regression. Statistics in Medicine, 29(14):1488–1501, 2010.

[28] Casagrande JT, Pike MC, Smith PG. An improved approximate formula for calculating sample sizes for comparing two binomial distributions. Biometrics, 34:483–486, 1978.

[29] Chen J, Zhou X, Li F, Spiegelman D. swdpwr: A SAS macro and an R package for power calculations in stepped wedge cluster randomized trials. Computer Methods and Programs in Biomedicine, 213:106522, 2022.

[30] Cho SH, Han S, Ghim JL, Nam MS, Yu S, Park T, Kim S, Bae J, Shin JG. A randomized, double-blind trial comparing the pharmacokinetics of CT-P16, a candidate bevacizumab biosimilar, with its reference product in healthy adult males. BioDrugs, 33:173–181, 2019.

[31] Chou YM. A bivariate noncentral t-distribution with applications. Communications in Statistics: Theory and Methods, 21(12):3427–3462, 1992.

[32] Chow SC, Liu JP. Design and Analysis of Bioavailability and Bioequivalence Studies. Chapman & Hall/CRC Taylor & Francis Group, Boca Raton, FL, 2009.

[33] Chow SC, Shao J, Wang H, Lokhnygina Y. Sample Size Calculations in Clinical Research. Chapman & Hall/CRC Taylor & Francis Group, Boca Raton, FL, 3rd edition, 2018.

[34] Clarkson JE, Ramsay CR, Averley P, Bonetti D, Boyers D, Campbell L, Chadwick GR, Duncan A, Elders A, Gouick J, et al. IQuaD dental trial; improving the quality of dentistry: a multicentre randomised controlled trial comparing oral hygiene advice and periodontal instrumentation for the prevention and management of periodontal disease in dentate adults attending dental primary care. BMC Oral Health, 13:1–12, 2013.

[35] Cochran WG. The comparison of percentages in matched samples. Biometrika, 37(3/4):256–266, 1950.

[36] Cohen J. Statistical Power Analysis for the Behavioral Sciences. Lawrence Erlbaum Associates, Hillsdale, New Jersey, 2nd edition, 1988.

[37] Collett D. Modeling Survival Data in Medical Research. Chapman & Hall, Boca Raton, FL, 2015.

[38] Commenges D, Jacqmin H. The intraclass correlation coefficient: distribution-free definition and test. Biometrics, 50(2):517–526, 1994.

[39] Connor RJ. Sample size for testing differences in proportions for the paired-sample design. Biometrics, 43:207–211, 1987.

[40] Copas AJ, Lewis JJ, Thompson JA, Davey C, Baio G, Hargreaves JR. Designing a stepped wedge trial: three main designs, carry-over effects and randomisation approaches. Trials, 16:1–12, 2015.

[41] Cox DR, Oakes D. Analysis of Survival Data. Chapman & Hall, New York, NY, 1984.

[42] Crespi CM. Cluster randomized trials. In Halabi S, Michiels S, editors, Textbook of Clinical Trials in Oncology: A Statistical Perspective. CRC Press/Taylor and Francis Group, 2019.

[43] Crespi CM, Ziehl K. Cluster-randomized trials of cancer screening interventions: Has use of appropriate statistical methods increased over time? Contemporary Clinical Trials, 123:106974, 2022.

[44] Crespi CM, Maxwell AE, Wu S. Cluster randomized trials of cancer screening interventions: are appropriate statistical methods being used? Contemporary Clinical Trials, 32(4):477–484, 2011.

[45] Cui X, Dickhaus T, Ding Y, Hsu JC. Handbook of Multiple Comparisons. Chapman & Hall, New York, NY, 2022.

[46] Cumming G. Understanding the New Statistics: Effect Sizes, Confidence Intervals, and Meta-analysis. Routledge, 2012.

[47] Cundill B, Alexander ND. Sample size calculations for skewed distributions. BMC Medical Research Methodology, 15:1–9, 2015.

[48] Davenport Jr EC, El-Sanhurry NA. Phi/phimax: review and synthesis. Educational and Psychological Measurement, 51(4):821–828, 1991.

[49] de Hoop E. Efficient designs for cluster randomized trials with small numbers of clusters: Stepped wedge and other repeated measurements designs. Available at http://hdl.handle.net/2066/134179. PhD thesis, Radboud University, 2015.

[50] Dean A, Voss D, Draguljic D. Design and Analysis of Experiments. Springer International Publishing AG, 2nd edition, 2017.

[51] Demidenko E. Sample size determination for logistic regression revisited. Statistics in Medicine, 26:3385–3397, 2007.

[52] Demidenko E. Sample size and optimal design for logistic regression with binary interaction. Statistics in Medicine, 27:36–46, 2008.

[53] DiSantostefano RL, Muller KE. A comparison of power approximations for Satterthwaite's test. Communications in Statistics-Simulation and Computation, 24(3):583–593, 1995.

[54] Dmitrienko A, Tamhane A, Bretz F, editors. Multiple Testing Problems in Pharmaceutical Statistics. Oxford University Press, 2010.

[55] Donald A, Donner A. Adjustments to the Mantel–Haenszel chi-square statistic and odds ratio variance estimator when the data are clustered. Statistics in Medicine, 6(4):491–499, 1987.

[56] Dong N, Maynard R. Powerup!: A tool for calculating minimum detectable effect sizes and minimum required sample sizes for experimental and quasi-experimental design studies. Journal of Research on Educational Effectiveness, 6(1):24–67, 2013.

[57] Donner A. An empirical study of cluster randomization. International Journal of Epidemiology, 11(3):283–286, 1982.

[58] Donner A, Klar N. Design and Analysis of Cluster Randomization Trials in Health Research. Oxford University Press, New York, New York, USA, 2000.

[59] Duffy SW. Asymptotic and exact power for the McNemar test and its analogue with R controls per case. Biometrics, 40(4):1005–1015, 1984.

[60] Dumville J, Hahn S, Miles J, Torgerson D. The use of unequal randomisation ratios in clinical trials: a review. Contemporary Clinical Trials, 27(1):1–12, 2006.

[61] Eldridge SM, Ashby D, Feder GS, Rudnicka AR, Ukoumunne OC. Lessons for cluster randomized trials in the twenty-first century: a systematic review of trials in primary care. Clinical Trials, 1(1):80–90, 2004.

[62] Eldridge SM, Ashby D, Kerry S. Sample size for cluster randomized trials: effect of coefficient of variation of cluster size and analysis method. International Journal of Epidemiology, 35(5):1292–1300, 2006.

[63] Eldridge SM, Ukoumunne OC, Carlin JB. The intra-cluster correlation coefficient in cluster randomized trials: a review of definitions. International Statistical Review, 77:378–394, 2009.

[64] European Medicines Agency. ICH E9 (R1) Addendum on Estimands and Sensitivity Analysis in Clinical Trials to the Guideline on Statistical Principles for Clinical Trials. Available at https://www.ema.europa.eu/en/documents/scientific-guideline/ich-e9-r1-addendum-estimands-sensitivity-analysis-clinical-trials-guideline-statistical-principles/en.pdf, 2021.

[65] Fagerland MW, Sandvik L, Mowinckel P. Parametric methods outperformed non-parametric methods in comparisons of discrete numerical variables. BMC Medical Research Methodology, 11:1–8, 2011.

[66] Fagerland MW, Lydersen S, Laake P. Recommended confidence intervals for two independent binomial proportions. Statistical Methods in Medical Research, 24(2):224–254, 2015.

[67] Farrington CP, Manning G. Test statistics and sample size formulae for comparative binomial trials with null hypothesis of non-zero risk difference or non-unity relative risk. Statistics in Medicine, 9(12):1447–1454, 1990.

[68] Feldman H, McKinlay S. Cohort versus cross-sectional design in large field trials: precision, sample size, and a unifying model. Statistics in Medicine, 13:61–78, 1994.

[69] Ferguson GA. The factorial interpretation of test difficulty. Psychometrika, 6(5):323–329, 1941.

[70] Fisher RA. The logic of inductive inference. Journal of the Royal Statistical Society, 98(1):39–82, 1935.

[71] Freidlin B, Korn EL. Two-by-two factorial cancer treatment trials: is sufficient attention being paid to possible interactions? Journal of the National Cancer Institute, 109(9):djx146, 2017.

[72] Gart JJ. Alternative analyses of contingency tables. Journal of the Royal Statistical Society Series B: Statistical Methodology, 28(1):164–179, 1966.

[73] Gart JJ, Nam JM. Approximate interval estimation of the ratio of binomial parameters: a review and corrections for skewness. Biometrics, 44(2):323–338, 1988.

[74] Gatsonis C, Sampson AR. Multiple correlation: exact power and sample size calculations. Psychological Bulletin, 106:516–524, 1989.

[75] Giraudeau B, Ravaud P, Donner A. Sample size calculation for cluster randomized cross-over trials. Statistics in Medicine, 27(27):5578–5585, 2008.

[76] Girling AJ. Relative efficiency of unequal cluster sizes in stepped wedge and other trial designs under longitudinal or cross-sectional sampling. Statistics in Medicine, 37(30):4652–4664, 2018.

[77] Girling AJ, Hemming K. Statistical efficiency and optimal design for stepped cluster studies under linear mixed effects models. Statistics in Medicine, 35(13):2149–2166, 2016.

[78] Goulão B, MacLennan G, Ramsay C. The split-plot design was useful for evaluating complex, multilevel interventions, but there is need for improvement in its design and report. Journal of Clinical Epidemiology, 96:120–125, 2018.

[79] Grieve A, Beal SL. Confidence intervals and sample sizes. Biometrics, 47(4):1597–1603, 1991.

[80] Guenther WC. Sample size formulas for normal theory t tests. The American Statistician, 35(4):243–244, 1981.

[81] Gupta S, Jain S, Yeh J, Guddati AK. Unequal allotment of patients in phase III oncology clinical trials. American Journal of Cancer Research, 11(7):3735, 2021.

[82] Hargreaves JR, Copas AJ, Beard E, Osrin D, Lewis JJ, Davey C, Thompson JA, Baio G, Fielding KL, Prost A. Five questions to consider before conducting a stepped wedge trial. Trials, 16(1):1–4, 2015.

[83] Hayes RJ, Moulton LH. Cluster Randomised Trials. Taylor & Francis Group, LLC, Boca Raton, FL, USA, 2nd edition, 2017.

[84] Hedges LV, Olkin I. Statistical Methods for Meta-Analysis. Academic Press, 2014.

[85] Hemming K, Taljaard M. Sample size calculations for stepped wedge and cluster randomised trials: a unified approach. Journal of Clinical Epidemiology, 69:137–146, 2016.

[86] Hemming K, Taljaard M. Reflection on modern methods: when is a stepped-wedge cluster randomized trial a good study design choice? International Journal of Epidemiology, 49(3):1043–1052, 2020.

[87] Hemming K, Girling AJ, Sitch AJ, Marsh J, Lilford RJ. Sample size calculations for cluster randomised controlled trials with a fixed number of clusters. BMC Medical Research Methodology, 11(1):1–11, 2011.

[88] Hemming K, Lilford R, Girling AJ. Stepped-wedge cluster randomised controlled trials: a generic framework including parallel and multiple-level designs. Statistics in Medicine, 34(2):181–196, 2015.

[89] Hemming K, Taljaard M, Forbes A. Analysis of cluster randomised stepped wedge trials with repeated cross-sectional samples. Trials, 18:1–11, 2017.

[90] Hemming K, Taljaard M, Forbes A. Modeling clustering and treatment effect heterogeneity in parallel and stepped-wedge cluster randomized trials. Statistics in Medicine, 37(6):883–898, 2018.

[91] Hemming K, Kasza J, Hooper R, Forbes A, Taljaard M. A tutorial on sample size calculation for multiple-period cluster randomized parallel, cross-over and stepped-wedge trials using the Shiny CRT Calculator. International Journal of Epidemiology, 49(3):979–995, 2020.

[92] Hemming K, Taljaard M, Weijer C, Forbes AB. Use of multiple period, cluster randomised, crossover trial designs for comparative effectiveness research. BMJ, 371:m3800, 2020.

[93] Hettmansperger TP. Statistical Inference Based on Ranks. Wiley, New York, 1984.

[94] Hill C. Asymptotic relative efficiency of survival tests with covariates. Biometrika, 68(3):699–702, 1981.

[95] Hochberg Y. A sharper Bonferroni procedure for multiple tests of significance. Biometrika, 75(4):800–802, 1988.

[96] Hoenig JM, Heisey DM. The abuse of power: the pervasive fallacy of power calculations for data analysis. The American Statistician, 55(1): 19–24, 2001.

[97] Holm S. A simple sequentially rejective multiple test procedure. Scandinavian Journal of Statistics, 6(2):65–70, 1979.

[98] Hommel G. A stagewise rejective multiple test procedure based on a modified Bonferroni test. Biometrika, 75(2):383–386, 1988.

[99] Hooper R, Bourke L. Cluster randomised trials with repeated cross sections: alternatives to parallel group designs. BMJ, 350:h2925, 2015.

[100] Hooper R, Teerenstra S, deHoop E, Eldridge S. Sample size calculation for stepped wedge and other longitudinal cluster randomised trials. Statistics in Medicine, 35(26):4718–4728, 2016.

[101] Hoover DR. Clinical trials of behavioural interventions with heterogeneous teaching subgroup effects. Statistics in Medicine, 21(10):1351–1364, 2002.

[102] Hsieh FY, Bloch DA, Larsen MD. A simple method of sample size calculation for linear and logistic regression. Statistics in Medicine, 17: 1623–1634, 1998.

[103] Hu FB, Goldberg J, Hedeker D, Flay BR, Pentz MA. Comparison of population-averaged and subject-specific approaches for analyzing repeated binary outcomes. American Journal of Epidemiology, 147(7): 694–703, 1998.

[104] Huang S, Fiero MH, Bell ML. Generalized estimating equations in cluster randomized trials with a small number of clusters: review of practice and simulation study. Clinical Trials, 13(4):445–449, 2016.

[105] Hughes JP, Granston TS, Heagerty PJ. Current issues in the design and analysis of stepped wedge trials. Contemporary Clinical Trials, 45: 55–60, 2015.

[106] Hughes JP, Lee WY, Troxel AB, Heagerty PJ. Sample size calculations for stepped wedge designs with treatment effects that may change with the duration of time under intervention. Prevention Science, 2023. URL https://doi.org/10.1007/s11121-023-01587-1.

[107] Hussey MA, Hughes JP. Design and analysis of stepped wedge cluster randomized trials. Contemporary Clinical Trials, 28(2):182–191, 2007.

[108] Johnson NL, Kotz S, Balakrishnan N. Continuous Univariate Distributions, volume 2. John Wiley and Sons, 1995.

[109] Jones B, Kenward MG. Design and Analysis of Cross-over Trials. Chapman and Hall/CRC, 3rd edition, 2014.

[110] Jones B, Jarvis P, Lewis JA, Ebbutt AF. Trials to assess equivalence: the importance of rigorous methods. British Medical Journal, 313:36–39, 1996.

[111] Julious SA. Sample Sizes for Clinical Trials. Taylor and Francis Group, 2010.

[112] Jung SH. Randomized Phase II Cancer Clinical Trials. Chapman & Hall/CRC, Boca Raton, FL, 2013.

[113] Jung SH, Lee TY, Kim KM, George S. Admissible two-stage designs for phase II cancer clinical trials. Statistics in Medicine, 23:561–569, 2004.

[114] Kahan BC, Hindley J, Edwards M, Cro S, Morris TP. The estimands framework: a primer on the ICH E9 (R1) addendum. BMJ, 384:e076316, 2024.

[115] Kang SH, Ahn CW, Jung SH. Sample size calculation for dichotomous outcomes in cluster randomization trials with varying cluster size. Drug Information Journal, 37(1):109–114, 2003.

[116] Kaplan E, Meier P. Nonparametric estimation from incomplete observations. Journal of the American Statistical Association, 53(282):457–481, 1958.

[117] Kasza J, Hemming K, Hooper R, Matthews J, Forbes A. Impact of non-uniform correlation structure on sample size and power in multiple-period cluster randomised trials. Statistical Methods in Medical Research, 28(3):703–716, 2019.

[118] Kasza J, Hooper R, Copas A, Forbes AB. Sample size and power calculations for open cohort longitudinal cluster randomized trials. Statistics in Medicine, 39(13):1871–1883, 2020.

[119] Katz D, Baptista J, Azen S, Pike M. Obtaining confidence intervals for the risk ratio in cohort studies. Biometrics, 34(3):469–474, 1978.

[120] Kenny A, Voldal EC, Xia F, Heagerty PJ, Hughes JP. Analysis of stepped wedge cluster randomized trials in the presence of a time-varying treatment effect. Statistics in Medicine, 41(22):4311–4339, 2022.

[121] Keppel G, Wickens TD. Design and Analysis: A Researcher's Handbook. Pearson Prentice-Hall, Upper Saddle River, NJ, 4th edition, 2004.

[122] Kerby DS. The simple difference formula: An approach to teaching nonparametric correlation. Comprehensive Psychology, 3:1, 2014.

[123] Kerry SM, Bland JM. Unequal cluster sizes for trials in English and Welsh general practices: implications for sample size calculations. Statistics in Medicine, 20:377–390, 2001.

[124] Khatri C. A note on a large sample distribution of a transformed multiple correlation coefficient. Annals of the Institute of Statistical Mathematics, 18(1):375–380, 1966.

[125] Koopman P. Confidence intervals for the ratio of two binomial proportions. Biometrics, 40(2):513–517, 1984.

[126] Korn EL, Freidlin B. Non-factorial analyses of two-by-two factorial trial designs. Clinical Trials, 13(6):651–659, 2016.

[127] Kristunas CA, Smith KL, Gray LJ. An imbalance in cluster sizes does not lead to notable loss of power in cross-sectional, stepped-wedge cluster randomised trials with a continuous outcome. Trials, 18:1–11, 2017.

[128] Kugler KC, Dziak JJ, Trail J. Coding and interpretation of effects in analysis of data from a factorial experiment. In Collins LM, Kugler KC, editors, Optimization of Behavioral, Biobehavioral, and Biomedical Interventions, pages 175–205. Springer, 2018.

[129] Lachin JM. Power and sample size evaluation for the McNemar test with application to matched case-control studies. Statistics in Medicine, 11(9):1239–1251, 1992.

[130] Lafaye deMicheaux P, Liquet B, Marque S, Riou J. Power and sample size determination in clinical trials with multiple primary continuous correlated endpoints. Journal of Biopharmaceutical Statistics, 24(2):378–397, 2014.

[131] Lake S, Kammann E, Klar N, Betensky R. Sample size re-estimation in cluster randomization trials. Statistics in Medicine, 21(10):1337–1350, 2002.

[132] Lakens D. Calculating and reporting effect sizes to facilitate cumulative science: a practical primer for t-tests and ANOVAs. Frontiers in Psychology, 4:863, 2013.

[133] Lakens D, Caldwell AR. Simulation-based power analysis for factorial analysis of variance designs. Advances in Methods and Practices in Psychological Science, 4(1):69–70, 2021.

[134] Landau S, Stahl D. Sample size and power calculations for medical studies by simulation when closed form expressions are not available. Statistical Methods in Medical Research, 22(3):324–345, 2013.

[135] Lee EW, Dubin N. Estimation and sample size considerations for clustered binary responses. Statistics in Medicine, 13(12):1241–1252, 1994.

[136] Lehmann EL. Nonparametrics: Statistical Methods Based on Ranks. Prentice Hall, Upper Saddle River, New Jersey, 1998.

[137] Li F. Design and analysis considerations for cohort stepped wedge cluster randomized trials with a decay correlation structure. Statistics in Medicine, 39(4):438–455, 2020.

[138] Li F, Turner EL, Preisser JS. Sample size determination for GEE analyses of stepped wedge cluster randomized trials. Biometrics, 74(4):1450–1458, 2018.

[139] Li F, Forbes AB, Turner EL, Preisser JS. Power and sample size requirements for GEE analyses of cluster randomized crossover trials. Statistics in Medicine, 38(4, SI):636–649, 2019.

[140] Li F, Hughes JP, Hemming K, Taljaard M, Melnick ER, Heagerty PJ. Mixed-effects models for the design and analysis of stepped wedge cluster randomized trials: an overview. Statistical Methods in Medical Research, 30(2):612–639, 2021.

[141] Liang KY, Zeger SL. Longitudinal data analysis using generalized linear models. Biometrika, 73(1):13–22, 1986.

[142] Liu XS. Statistical Power Analysis for the Social and Behavioral Sciences. Routledge, New York, New York, 2013.

[143] Lohr S, Schochet PZ, Sanders E. Partially Nested Randomized Controlled Trials in Education Research: A Guide to Design and Analysis. NCER 2014-2000. National Center for Education Research, 2014.

[144] Lu B, Preisser JS, Qaqish BF, Suchindran C, Bangdiwala SI, Wolfson M. A comparison of two bias-corrected covariance estimators for generalized estimating equations. Biometrics, 63(3):935–941, 2007.

[145] Lumley T, Diehr P, Emerson S, Chen L. The importance of the normality assumption in large public health data sets. Annual Review of Public Health, 23(1):151–169, 2002.

[146] Lyons VH, Li L, Hughes JP, Rowhani-Rahbar A. Proposed variations of the stepped-wedge design can be used to accommodate multiple interventions. Journal of Clinical Epidemiology, 86:160–167, 2017.

[147] Manatunga AK, Hudgens MG, Chen S. Sample size estimation in cluster randomized studies with varying cluster size. Biometrical Journal, 43: 75–86, 2001.

[148] Mancl LA, DeRouen TA. A covariance estimator for GEE with improved small-sample properties. Biometrics, 57(1):126–134, 2001.

[149] Mann HB, Whitney DR. On a test of whether one of two random variables is stochastically larger than the other. The Annals of Mathematical Statistics, 18:50–60, 1947.

[150] Mantel N. Evaluation of survival data and two new rank order statistics arising in its consideration. Cancer Chemotherapy Reports, 50(3):163–170, 1966.

[151] Martin JT, Hemming K, Girling A. The impact of varying cluster size in cross-sectional stepped-wedge cluster randomised trials. BMC Medical Research Methodology, 19:1–11, 2019.

[152] Maxwell SE. Sample Size and Multiple Regression Analysis. Psychological Methods, 5:434–458, 2000.

[153] McCullagh P. Regression models for ordinal data. Journal of the Royal Statistical Society: Series B (Methodological), 42(2):109–127, 1980.

[154] McNemar Q. Note on the sampling error of the difference between correlated proportions or percentages. Psychometrika, 12:153–157, 1947.

[155] Miettinen O, Nurminen M. Comparative analysis of two rates. Statistics in Medicine, 4(2):213–226, 1985.

[156] Moerbeek M. Power and money in cluster randomized trials: When is it worth measuring a covariate? Statistics in Medicine, 25:2607–2617, 2006.

[157] Moerbeek M. The cluster randomized crossover trial: The effects of attrition in the AB/BA design and how to account for it in sample size calculations. Clinical Trials, 17(4):420–429, 2020.

[158] Moerbeek M, Teerenstra S. Power Analysis of Trials with Multilevel Data. CRC Press/Taylor & Francis Group, Boca Raton, Florida, 2016.

[159] Moerbeek M, Wong WK. Sample size formulae for trials comparing group and individual treatments in a multilevel model. Statistics in Medicine, 27(15):2850–2864, 2008.

[160] Moerbeek M, van Breukelen GJP, Berger MPF. Design issues for experiments in multilevel populations. Journal of Educational and Behavioral Statistics, 25(3):271–284, 2000.

[161] Moerbeek M, van Breukelen GJP, Berger MPF. Optimal experimental designs for multilevel logistic models. Journal of the Royal Statistical Society: Series D (The Statistician), 50(1):17–30, 2001.

[162] Moertel CG, Fleming TR, Macdonald JS, Haller DG, Laurie JA, Tangen CM, Ungerleider JS, Emerson WA, Tormey DC, Glick JH, et al. Fluorouracil plus levamisole as effective adjuvant therapy after resection of stage iii colon carcinoma: a final report. Annals of Internal Medicine, 122(5):321–326, 1995.

[163] Morikawa T, Yoshida M. A useful testing strategy in Phase III trials: combined test of superiority and test of equivalence. Journal of Pharmaceutical Statistics, 5(3):297–306, 1995.

[164] Murray DM. Design and Analysis of Group-Randomized Trials. Oxford University Press, New York, NY, USA, 1998.

[165] Murray DM, Blitstein JL. Methods to reduce the impact of intraclass correlation in group-randomized trials. Evaluation Review, 27(1):79–103, 2003.

[166] Nas J, Thannhauser J, Vart P, Robert-Jan vanGeuns P, Muijsers HEC, Mol JQ, Aarts GWA, Konijnenberg LSF, Gommans DHF, Ahoud-Schoenmakers SGAM, Vos JL, vanRoyen N, Bonnes JL, Brouwer MC. Effect of face-to-face vs virtual reality training on cardiopulmonary resuscitation quality: A randomized clinical trial. JAMA Cardiology, 5(3):328–335, 2020.

[167] Neuhaus JM, Kalbfleisch JD. Between-and within-cluster covariate effects in the analysis of clustered data. Biometrics, 54(2):638–645, 1998.

[168] Newcombe RG. Interval estimation for the difference between independent proportions: comparison of eleven methods. Statistics in Medicine, 17(8):873–890, 1998.

[169] Neyman J, Iwaszkiewicz K. Statistical problems in agricultural experimentation. Supplement to the Journal of the Royal Statistical Society, 2(2):107–180, 1935.

[170] Neyman J, Tokarska B. Errors of the second kind in testing "Student's" hypothesis. Journal of the American Statistical Association, 31(194):318–326, 1936.

[171] Noether GE. Two confidence intervals for the ratio of two probabilities and some measures of effectiveness. Journal of the American Statistical Association, 52(277):36–45, 1957.

[172] Noether GE. Sample size determination for some common nonparametric tests. Journal of the American Statistical Association, 82(398): 645–647, 1987.

[173] O'Brien TE, Funk GM. A gentle introduction to optimal design for regression models. The American Statistician, 57(4):265–267, 2003.

[174] Okada K. Is omega squared less biased? A comparison of three major effect size indices in one-way ANOVA. Behaviormetrika, 40(2):129–147, 2013.

[175] Ouyang Y, Xu L, Karim ME, Gustafson P, Wong H. CRTpowerdist: An R package to calculate attained power and construct the power distribution for cross-sectional stepped-wedge and parallel cluster randomized trials. Computer Methods and Programs in Biomedicine, 208:106255, 2021.

[176] Ouyang Y, Li F, Preisser JS, Taljaard M. Sample size calculators for planning stepped-wedge cluster randomized trials: a review and comparison. International Journal of Epidemiology, 51(6):2000–2013, 2022.

[177] Ouyang Y, Hemming K, Li F, Taljaard M. Estimating intra-cluster correlation coefficients for planning longitudinal cluster randomized trials: a tutorial. International Journal of Epidemiology, 52(5):1634–1647, 2023.

[178] Owen DB. A special case of a bivariate non-central t-distribution. Biometrika, 52(3/4):437–446, 1965.

[179] Pals SL, Murray DM, Alfano CM, Shadish WR, Hannan PJ, Baker WL. Individually randomized group treatment trials: a critical appraisal of frequently used design and analytic approaches. American Journal of Public Health, 98(8):1418–1424, 2008.

[180] Phillips KF. Power of the two one-sided tests procedure in bioequivalence. Journal of Pharmacokinetics and Biopharmaceutics, 18(2):137–144, 1990.

[181] Proschan MA. Sample size re-estimation in clinical trials. Biometrical Journal, 51(2):348–357, 2009.

[182] Proschan MA, Brittain EH. A primer on strong vs weak control of familywise error rate. Statistics in Medicine, 39(9):1407–1413, 2020.

[183] Raudenbush SW. Statistical analysis and optimal design for cluster randomized trials. Psychological Methods, 2:173–185, 1997.

Bibliography

[184] Raudenbush SW, Liu X. Statistical power and optimal design for multisite randomized trials. Psychological Methods, 5(2):199–213, 2000.

[185] Richardson JTE. Eta squared and partial eta squared as measures of effect size in educational research. Educational Research Review, 6: 135–147, 2011.

[186] Rietbergen C, Moerbeek M. The design of cluster randomized crossover trials. Journal of Educational and Behavioral Statistics, 36(4):472–490, 2011.

[187] Roberts C, Roberts S. Design and analysis of clinical trials with clustering effects due to treatment. Clinical Trials, 2(2):152–162, 2005.

[188] Rosner B. Fundamentals of Biostatistics. Duxbury, 6th edition, 2006.

[189] Ross S. A First Course in Probability. Prentice Hall, 1997.

[190] Rothman KJ, Greenland S. Planning study size based on precision rather than power. Epidemiology, 29(5):599–603, 2018.

[191] Rutterford C, Copes A, Eldridge S. Methods for sample size determination in cluster randomized trials. International Journal of Epidemiology, 44(3):1051–1067, 2015.

[192] Ruvuna F. Unequal center sizes, sample size, and power in multicenter clinical trials. Drug Information Journal, 38(4):387–394, 2004.

[193] Salminen P, Helmio M, Ovaska J, Juuti A, Leivonen M, Peromaa-Haavisto P, Hurme S, Soinio M, Nuutila P, Victorzon M. Effect of laparoscopic sleeve gastrectomy vs laparoscopic Roux-en-Y gastric bypass on weight loss at 5 years among patients with morbid obesity: The SLEEVEPASS randomized clinical trial. JAMA, 319(3):241–254, 2018.

[194] Satterthwaite FE. An approximate distribution of estimates of variance components. Biometrics Bulletin, 2:110–114, 1946.

[195] Schlesselman JJ. Sample size requirements in cohort and case-control studies of disease. American Journal of Epidemiology, 99(6):381–384, 1974.

[196] Schochet PZ. Statistical power for random assignment evaluations of education programs. Journal of Educational and Behavioral Statistics, 33:62–87, 2008.

[197] Schoenfeld D. The asymptotic properties of nonparametric tests for comparing survival distributions. Biometrika, 68(1):316–319, 1981.

[198] Schork MA, Williams GW. Number of observations required for the comparison of two correlated proportions: Number of observations required for the comparison. Communications in Statistics-Simulation and Computation, 9(4):349–357, 1980.

[199] Schuirmann DJ. A comparison of the two one-sided tests procedure and the power approach for assessing the equivalence of average bioavailability. Journal of Pharmacokinetics and Biopharmaceutics, 15:657–680, 1987.

[200] Selby NM, Casula A, Lamming L, Stoves J, Samarasinghe Y, Lewington AJ, Roberts R, Shah N, Johnson M, Jackson N, et al. An organizational-level program of intervention for AKI: a pragmatic stepped wedge cluster randomized trial. Journal of the American Society of Nephrology, 30(3): 505–515, 2019.

[201] Senn SS. Cross-over Trials in Clinical Research. John Wiley & Sons, 2002.

[202] Shieh G, Jan SL, Randles RH. On power and sample size determinations for the Wilcoxon–Mann–Whitney test. Journal of Nonparametric Statistics, 18(1):33–43, 2006.

[203] Shih WJ. Sample size and power calculations for periodontal and other studies with clustered samples using the method of generalized estimating equations. Biometrical Journal, 39(8):899–908, 1997.

[204] Simon R. Optimal two-stage designs for phase II clinical trials. Controlled Clinical Trials, 10(1):1–10, 1989.

[205] Skovlund E, Fenstad GU. Should we always choose a nonparametric test when comparing two apparently nonnormal distributions? Journal of Clinical Epidemiology, 54(1):86–92, 2001.

[206] Snijders T, Bosker R. Modeled variance in two-level models. Sociological Methods and Research, 22(3):342–363, 1994.

[207] Snijders TAB, Bosker RJ. Multilevel Analysis. SAGE Publications, 2nd edition, 2012.

[208] Sozu T, Kanou T, Hamada C, Yoshimura I. Power and sample size calculations in clinical trials with multiple primary variables. Japan Journal of Biometrics, 27:83–96, 2006.

[209] Sozu T, Sugimoto T, Hamasaki T, Evans SR. Sample Size Determination in Clinical Trials with Multiple Endpoints. Springer International Publishing, Switzerland, 2015.

[210] Spybrook J, Bloom H, Congdon R, Hill C, Martinez A, Raudenbush S. Optimal Design Plus Empirical Evidence: Documentation for the "Optimal Design" Software. Technical report, http://hlmsoft.net/od/od-manual-20111016-v300.pdf, Oct. 2011.

[211] Stuart A, Ord JK. Distribution Theory. Vol. 1 of Kendall's Advanced Theory of Statistics. Edward Arnold, Baltimore, 6th edition, 1994.

[212] Suissa S, Shuster JJ. The 2 x 2 matched-pairs trial: exact unconditional design and analysis. Biometrics, 47(2):361–372, 1991.

[213] Sullivan S, Swain JM, Woodman G, Antonetti M, De La Cruz-Munoz N, Jonnalagadda SS, Ujiki M, Ikramuddin S, Ponce J, Ryou M, Reynoso J, Chhabra R, Sorenson GB, Clarkson WK, Edmundowicz SA, Eagon JC, Mullady DK, Leslie D, Lavin TE, Thompson CC. Randomized sham-controlled trial evaluating efficacy and safety of endoscopic gastric plication for primary obesity: The ESSENTIAL trial. Obesity, 25(2): 294–301, 2017.

[214] Sundin P, Crespi CM. Power analysis for stepped wedge trials with multiple interventions. Statistics in Medicine, 41(8):1498–1512, 2022.

[215] Teerenstra S, Eldridge S, Graff M, deHoop E, Borm GF. A simple sample size formula for analysis of covariance in cluster randomized trials. Statistics in Medicine, 31(20):2169–2178, 2012.

[216] Tian Z, Esserman D, Tong G, Blaha O, Dziura J, Peduzzi P, Li F. Sample size calculation in hierarchical 2×2 factorial trials with unequal cluster sizes. Statistics in Medicine, 41(4):645–664, 2022.

[217] Uno H, Claggett B, Tian L, Inoue E, Gallo P, Miyata T, Schrag D, Takeuchi M, Uyama Y, Zhao L, et al. Moving beyond the hazard ratio in quantifying the between-group difference in survival analysis. Journal of Clinical Oncology, 32(22):2380, 2014.

[218] U.S. Department of Health and Human Services, Food and Drug Administration. Guidance for Industry: Statistical Approaches to Establishing Bioequivalence, January 2001.

[219] van Belle G. Statistical Rules of Thumb. John Wiley and Sons, 2nd edition, New York, New York. 2008.

[220] van Breukelen GJ, Candel MJ, Berger MP. Relative efficiency of unequal versus equal cluster sizes in cluster randomized and multicentre trials. Statistics in Medicine, 26(13):2589–2603, 2007.

[221] van Breukelen GJ, Candel MJ, Berger MP. Relative efficiency of unequal cluster sizes for variance component estimation in cluster randomized and multicentre trials. Statistical Methods in Medical Research, 17(4): 439–458, 2008.

[222] Vickerstaff V, Omar RZ, Ambler G. Methods to adjust for multiple comparisons in the analysis and sample size calculation of randomised controlled trials with multiple primary outcomes. BMC Medical Research Methodology, 19:1–13, 2019.

[223] Vierron E, Giraudeau B. Sample size calculation for multicenter randomized trial: Taking the center effect into account. Contemporary Clinical Trials, 28(4):451–458, 2007.

[224] Voldal EC, Hakhu NR, Xia F, Heagerty PJ, Hughes JP. swCRTdesign: an R package for stepped wedge trial design and analysis. Computer Methods and Programs in Biomedicine, 196:105514, 2020.

[225] Wasserstein RL, Lazar NA. The ASA's statement on p-values: context, process, and purpose. The American Statistician, 70(2):129–133, 2016.

[226] Welch BL. The generalization of 'Student's' problem when several different population variances are involved. Biometrika, 34:28–35, 1947.

[227] Westlake WJ. Response to T.B.L. Kirkwood: Bioequivalence testing–a need to rethink. Biometrics, 37:589–594, 1981.

[228] Whitehead J. Sample size calculations for ordered categorical data. Statistics in Medicine, 12(24):2257–2271, 1993.

[229] Whittemore AS. Sample size for logistic regression with small response probability. Journal of the American Statistical Association, 76(373): 27–32, 1981.

[230] Wilcoxon F. Individual comparisons by ranking methods. Biometrics Bulletin, 1(6):80–83, 1945.

[231] Wilson DT, Hooper R, Brown J, Farrin AJ, Walwyn RE. Efficient and flexible simulation-based sample size determination for clinical trials with multiple design parameters. Statistical Methods in Medical Research, 30(3):799–815, 2021.

[232] Wilson EB. Probable inference, the law of succession, and statistical inference. Journal of the American Statistical Association, 22(158):209–212, 1927.

[233] Winer BJ, Brown DR, Michels KM. Statistical Principles in Experimental Design. McGraw-Hill, 3rd edition, New York, New York, 1991.

[234] Woertman W, de Hoop E, Moerbeek M, Zuidemac S, Gerritsen D, Teerenstra S. Stepped wedge designs could reduce the required sample size in cluster randomized trials. Journal of Clinical Epidemiology, 66:752–758, 2013.

[235] Woodward M. Epidemiology: Study Design and Data Analysis. CRC Press/Taylor & Francis Group, Boca Raton, Florida, 2014.

[236] Woolf B. On estimating the relation between blood group and disease. Annals of Human Genetics, 19(4):251–253, 1955.

[237] Wu S, Crespi CM, Wong WK. Comparison of methods for estimating the intraclass correlation coefficient for binary responses in cancer prevention cluster randomized trials. Contemporary Clinical Trials, 33(5): 869–880, 2012.

[238] Xia F, Hughes JP, Voldal EC, Heagerty PJ. Power and sample size calculation for stepped-wedge designs with discrete outcomes. Trials, 22:1–10, 2021.

[239] Yates F. Contingency tables involving small numbers and the χ^2 test. Supplement to the Journal of the Royal Statistical Society, 1(2):217–235, 1934.

[240] Yung G, Liu Y. Sample size and power for the weighted log-rank test and Kaplan-Meier based tests with allowance for nonproportional hazards. Biometrics, 76(3):939–950, 2020.

[241] Zeger SL, Liang KY. Longitudinal data analysis for discrete and continuous outcomes. Biometrics, 42(1):121–130, 1986.

[242] Zhang Z, Yuan KH. Practical Statistical Power Analysis. ISDSA Press, Granger, Indiana, 2018.

[243] Zhou X, Liao X, Kunz LM, Normand SLT, Wang M, Spiegelman D. A maximum likelihood approach to power calculations for stepped wedge designs of binary outcomes. Biostatistics, 21(1):102–121, 2020.

[244] Zhu H, Lakkis H. Sample size calculation for comparing two negative binomial rates. Statistics in Medicine, 33(3):376–387, 2014.

Index

ANOVA_design (in Superpower), 99
BSDA package, 30
CRTpowerdist package, 261, 301
FDRsampsize package, 327
H2x2Factorial package, 268
MESS package, 61, 126, 139, 146
MKpower package, 64, 68
NBDesign package, 202
PWEALL package, 315
PowerTOST package, 81, 162, 215
PowerUpR package, 236, 261, 267
SSRMST package, 315
SWSamp package, 301
SimEngine package, 31
SteppedPower package, 301
Superpower package, 31, 99, 114, 117
TrialSize package, 61, 132, 156
WebPower package, 196, 201, 236, 260, 261
afex package, 99
altprimary, 325
anova1way.F.bal, 91
anova1way.F.unbal, 92
anova1way.c.bal, 96
anova2way.F.bal, 104
anova2way.c.bal, 112
anova2way.se.bal, 113
aov_car (in afex), 99
chisq.gof, 149
chisq.indep, 152
ci.meandiff, 165, 166
ci.mean, 161, 162
clinfun package, 140, 142, 144

clusterPower package, 261, 266, 300
coprimary.t, 321
coprimary.z, 320
corr.1samp, 177
corr.2samp, 178
cpower (in Hmisc), 315
create_arm (in npsurvSS), 308
crsize (in designsize), 208, 212
crt.parallel.bin, 255
crt.parallel.cont, 243, 245, 246, 248, 249, 251, 252, 284, 289
crt.varexplore, 255
crt.xo.cont, 289
dchisq, 4
designsize package, 208, 212, 215, 315
df, 4
dnorm, 2
dt, 4
es.anova.f, 94
es.h, 127
es.q, 178
fe.power (in clinfun), 145
fe.ssize (in clinfun), 145
gsDesign package, 129, 315
irgtt.bin, 266
irgtt.cont, 264
md_prec (in pwr2ppl), 165
mlrF.overall, 184, 185, 188
mlrF.partial, 190, 191
ms.varexplore, 234
multisite.bin, 235
multisite.cont, 224, 229, 230
multisite.hte, 232

nBinomial (in gsDesign), 129
n_risk_ratio (in precisely), 172
npsurvSS package, 308, 315
pchisq, 4
pf, 4
ph2simon (in clinfun), 142
ph2single (in clinfun), 140
pnorm, 2
power.fisher.test (in statmod), 144
powerSurvEpi package, 315
power_binom_test (in MESS), 63, 139
power_mcnemar_test (in MESS), 146
power_prop_test (in MESS), 126
power_two_arm (in npsurvSS), 308
prec_cor (in presize), 177
prec_meandiff (in presize), 165
prec_mean (in presize), 161
prec_or (in presize), 174
prec_prop (in presize), 167, 168
prec_riskdiff (in presize), 169, 170
prec_riskratio (in presize), 171
prec_sens (in presize), 169
prec_spec (in presize), 169
precisely package, 172, 174
presize package, 161, 165, 167–171, 174, 177
prop.1samp, 120
prop.2samp, 125, 129, 258
prop.paired, 135
prop.test.equiv, 130
propodds, 156
pt, 4
pwr.2way (in pwr2), 106
pwr.anova.test (in pwr), 94
pwr2ppl package, 165
pwr2 package, 94, 106
pwrAB package, 61
pwrFDR package, 327
pwrss.z.2corrs (in pwrss), 179
pwrss.z.corr (in pwrss), 177

pwrss.z.logistic (in pwrss), 202
pwrss.z.poisreg (in pwrss), 202
pwrss package, 117, 156, 177, 179, 202
pwr package, 94, 127
qchisq, 4
qf, 4
qnorm, 2
qt, 4
rPowerSampleSize package, 327
ranksum, 67
re.clustsize.cont, 248
relrisk, 132
round_any (in plyr), 227
sampleN.TOST (in PowerTOST), 83
samplesize package, 68
signedrank, 65
signtest, 63
sim.ssize.wilcox.test (in MKpower), 65
simglm package, 202
skewsamp package, 202
slr, 180
statmod package, 144
swCRTdesign package, 295, 296, 299, 300
swDsn (in swCRTdesign), 296
swPwr (in swCRTdesign), 296
swdpwr package, 299, 300
ttest.1samp, 36
ttest.2samp, 48, 76, 246
ttest.paired, 61
wmwpowd (in wmwpow), 67
wmwpow package, 67
wp.logistic (in WebPower), 196, 260
wp.poisson (in WebPower), 201
z.test (in BSDA), 30
ztest.1samp, 26
ztest.2samp, 27, 319
ztest.paired, 27

acceptance region, 10
additive equivalence, 79, 84

Index

allocation ratio, 47, 52
alternative endpoints, 316, 324
analysis of covariance, 114
ANCOVA, 114
ANOVA effect size, 93
attrition adjustment, 27

balanced design, 89
Bernoulli random variable, 118
binomial distribution, 118
bioequivalence, 79
block exchangeable correlation structure, 278
blocking, 218
Bonferroni procedure, 324

carryover effect, 203
case-control study, 172
categorical methods, 148
censoring, 302
chi-square test of independence, 150
closed cohort design, cluster randomized, 271
cluster autocorrelation, 274, 278
cluster randomized crossover trial, 269, 285
cluster randomized trial, parallel design, 238
cluster randomized trial, sample size, 243
cluster randomized trials, 237, 269
cluster randomized trials, longitudinal, 269
cluster sampling, 217
cluster-level proportions model, 256
co-primary endpoints, 79, 316, 318
coefficient of multiple determination, 183
coefficient of variation, 56, 228, 247
comparisonwise error rate, 97
compound symmetry, 240, 272
confidence interval width, 157

contamination, 218
contingency coefficient, 152
contrast, 95, 111
contrast coefficients, 95
correlation coefficient, 175–177, 179, 186
count data, 200
Cox proportional hazards regression, 309
critical value, 10
cross-sectional design, cluster randomized, 271
crossover design, 203
crossover design, cluster randomized, 285
cumulative distribution function, 2
cumulative logit model, 155

design effect, cluster randomized crossover trial, 289
design effect, cluster randomized trial, 243
design effect, multisite trial, 226
discordant proportion ratio, 134
distribution of sample proportion, 118
dropout adjustment, 27

effect coding, 218
effect size, 23
effect size, η^2, 93
effect size, d, 23
effect size, f, 93
effect size, h, 126
effect size, ANOVA, 93
effect size, chi-square test, 151
effect size, linear regression, partial F test, 192
effect size, one correlation, 177
effect size, overall F test, multiple linear regression, 184
effect size, standardized mean, 23
effect size, two correlations, 178
effect size, two proportions, 126

endpoint, 316
equality test, 71
equivalence test, 79, 130, 207
eta effect size, 93
eta-squared, 93, 95
exact binomial test, 137
exchangeable correlation, 240, 259, 272, 293
exponential decay structure, 275
exponential distribution, 312

false discovery rate, 98, 327
familywise error rate, 98, 324
Fisher z transformation, 175
Fisher exact test, 143

generalized estimating equations, 259, 299
generalized linear regression, 193
goodness-of-fit test, 148
grand mean, 89, 219

halfwidth of confidence interval, 158
hazard function, 303
hazard ratio, 304
Hedge's g effect size, 55
heterogeneity of the treatment effect, 218, 230
hypergeometric distribution, 144
hypothesis testing, 9

individually randomized group treatment trial, 237, 261
inequality test, 71, 72
intention to treat analysis, 87
interaction in ANOVA, 108
intercurrent events, 291
intraclass correlation coefficient, 221, 240

linear contrast, 95
linear regression, 175
logistic regression, 195
lognormal data, 56
lognormal distribution, 56

logrank test, 305
lower-tailed test, 10

main effects in ANOVA, 103
Mann-Whitney U test, 66
Mann-Whitney-Wilcoxon test, 156
margin of error, 158
margin of noninferiority, 74
margin of superiority, 77
marginal models, 299
McNemar test, 132, 145
median survival time, 312
minimum detectable effect size, 24
multilevel data, 216
multilevel trials, 266
multiple comparisons, 97, 324
multiple correlation coefficient, 183
multiple endpoints, 324
multiple linear regression, 182
multiple primary endpoints, 316
multiplicative equivalence, 84
multisite trials, 216
multistage sampling design, 217, 237

negative binomial regression, 202
nested compound symmetry correlation structure, 274
nested exchangeable correlation structure, 274
noncentral χ^2 distribution, 42
noncentral F distribution, 42
noncentral t distribution, 34
noncentrality parameter, 3
nonequality test, 71
noninferiority test, 73, 127
nonparametric tests, 62
normal distribution R functions, 1
notation, 3
null distribution, 9

odds ratio, 132, 172, 195
omega-squared, 95
omnibus F test, one-way ANOVA, 90

Index

one sample t test, 33
one-sample z test, 12
one-sided test, 10
one-way ANOVA, 88
ordinal variables, 154
overall F test, 183
Owen's Q function, 162, 166

paired t tests, 59
parallel cluster randomized trials, 237
parallel group designs, 203
parametric test, 62
partial F test, 189
partial correlation coefficient, 191
partially clustered design, 237
per protocol analysis, 87
period effect, 203
phi coefficient, 135, 152
Poisson distribution, 200
Poisson regression, 200
post hoc power, 31
power, 12
power of a confidence interval, 160, 164
power, attained, 261
precision analysis, 157
precision analysis, difference between two means, 163
precision analysis, difference between two proportions, 169
precision analysis, odds ratio, 172
precision analysis, one mean, 158
precision analysis, one proportion, 167
precision analysis, relative risk, 171
precision analysis, risk ratio, 171
precision analysis, sensitivity, 169
precision analysis, specificity, 169
probability density function, 1
probability of early termination, 142
proportional decay model, 279

proportional hazards assumption, 304
proportional odds, 155
proportions, correlated, 132
proportions, exact methods, 137
proportions, independent, 124, 153
proportions, noninferiority, 127
proportions, superiority by a margin, 127
proportions, test for nonequality, 124, 153

quantile, 3
quantile function, 2

range rule, 181, 229, 248, 257
rank-sum test, 66
rejection region, 10
relative efficiency, 54, 212, 228, 247
relative efficiency, unequal cluster sizes, 228, 247
relative risk, 131, 171
restricted mean survival time, 310
retrospective power, 31
risk ratio, 122, 131, 171

sample size, 7
sample size re-estimation, 247
sensitivity, 135, 169
sequence effect, 204
sign test, 62
signed-rank test, 64
significance level, 12
simple effects, 113
simple linear regression, 179
simulation, 29
single arm study design, 137
specificity, 169
split-plot design, 267
standard deviation of the effects in ANOVA, 93
standard deviations of the effects, ANOVA, 105

standardization of a normal random variable, 6
standardized effect sizes, ANOVA, 91
standardized halfwidth of a confidence interval, 159
standardized mean effect size, 23, 47
stepped wedge design, 269, 291
subject autocorrelation, 276, 278
super-superiority, 77
superiority by a margin test, 77, 127
superiority test, 71
survival function, 303
survival outcomes, 302

target number of events, 123
test for location, 62
test statistic, 9
time to event outcomes, 302
truncated exponential distribution, 314
two sample t test, 46
two-sided test, 10
two-stage designs, 141
two-way ANOVA, 100
type I error, 11
type II error, 11

unbalanced design, 89
unequal allocation, 47
unequal allocation, cluster randomized trials, 249
unequal allocation, multisite trials, 225
uniform distribution, 314
upper-tailed test, 10

vaccine efficacy, 122, 131
variance inflation factor, 199, 243
variance ratio, 223
variance stabilizing transformation, 126

Weibull distribution, 313
Welch-Satterthwaite degrees of freedom, 49, 263
Wilcoxon signed-rank test, 64
Wilcoxon-Mann-Whitney rank-sum test, 66